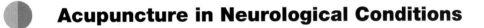

Acupuncture in Neurological Conditions

Commissioning Editor: Karen Morley
Development Editors: Alison McMurdo, Barbara Simmons
Project Manager: Sruthi Viswam
Designer: Stewart Larking
Illustration Manager: Bruce Hogarth

Acupuncture in Neurological Conditions

Val Hopwood PhD FCSP Dip Ac Nanjing
Course Director, MSc Acupuncture,
Coventry University, Coventry, UK

Clare Donnellan MSc MCSP Dip Shiatsu MRSS
Clinical Specialist Physiotherapist in Neuro-rehabilitation,
Nottingham University Hospitals NHS Trust,
Nottingham, UK

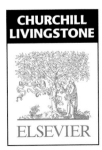

CHURCHILL LIVINGSTONE

ELSEVIER

Edinburgh London New York Oxford Philadelphia St Louis Sydney Toronto 2010

CHURCHILL
LIVINGSTONE
ELSEVIER

ISBN 9780 7020 3020 8

British Library Cataloguing in Publication Data
A catalogue record for this book is available from the British Library

Library of Congress Cataloging in Publication Data
A catalog record for this book is available from the Library of Congress

 your source for books, journals and multimedia in the health sciences
www.elsevierhealth.com

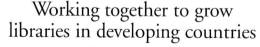
Working together to grow libraries in developing countries

www.elsevier.com | www.bookaid.org | www.sabre.org

ELSEVIER   BOOK AID International   Sabre Foundation

The Publisher's policy is to use paper manufactured from sustainable forests

Printed in China

Contents

Section 1 Backgrounds – Chinese and Western

Section 2 Clinical conditions

Section 3 Marrying East and West

Acknowledgements

Thanks to Alison Attenborough, Penny Bulley, Jeanne Burnett, Victoria Butterell, Isabel Carey, Claire Herlihy, Sarah Lindsey, Sally Lyons, Emma Martin, Sharon Meldrum, Marie Roberts, Gillian Robinson, Lal Russell, Louise Selwood and Rachel Tomasevic for providing patient cases.

Thanks to Lynn Pearce for Figures 12.4 and 12.5. Thanks also to Lal Russell and Ann Childs for helpful comments on Chapters 3 and 4.

This book is intended as a bridge between the evidence-based medicine practised by health professionals in the UK in the 21st century and the more intuitive form of medicine inherited from the Chinese traditions. More specifically it is an attempt to explore the application of these forms of medicine in a range of neurological diseases, identifying common strands and ideas. It is our hope that patient care will be improved by the combination of the two paradigms. Although there is still uncertainty, we hope to encourage the wider use of acupuncture in this field, whilst remembering the maxim 'first do no harm'.

Most physiotherapists with an advanced training in acupuncture attempt to combine traditional Chinese medicine (TCM) ideas with clinical reasoning emerging from Western medicine research. This has not always been an easy task.

We have three problems: one is that the Western acupuncture research is not looking at the conditions neurophysiotherapists deal with; the second is that the Chinese research is simply not rigorous enough, although it is improving. Finally, the TCM texts are often useful but it is hard to describe them as an 'evidence base'.

Over the years since acupuncture for pain relief was introduced into physiotherapy practice, many physiotherapists were nervous of using it in other situations, particularly conditions like stroke or multiple sclerosis. This has always seemed to be a great loss, to both potential patients and to the profession.

There is a strong impetus now to gain further knowledge and physiotherapists working in neurology are becoming very enthusiastic, so this seems to be a good time to set out the facts and options. Professional acupuncturists are less reluctant to use this modality with neurological patients but are unlikely to have the handling expertise that physiotherapists have. Clinical, anecdotal evidence appears to indicate that acupuncture could be useful. Scientific research in the west has so far not given such a favourable verdict but is very mixed in quality.

The traditional Chinese acupuncture books have not been very helpful, because the general medical theories and how neurological problems are considered do not take the nervous system, as such, into consideration and the way the text is written tends to alienate a neurological specialist. It is often just a question of language and we will endeavour to explain some of the Chinese thinking in order to make the basic theories more accessible to westerners. We will also highlight some of the more important links.

We have spent several years working in acupuncture research generally and more specifically in the neurological field and have discovered some useful information which is worth taking to a larger audience. Our aim is to inform the clinical reasoning process and assist therapists of all kinds in making treatment choices.

This book is intended primarily for physiotherapists already using acupuncture, or interested in gaining an acupuncture qualification, particularly those working in neurological units or outpatient physiotherapy departments. It may also be useful to other medical staff working in these fields. It should also be of interest to professional acupuncturists seeking insights into possible applications of scientific research in neurological problems, as well as those needing a little more confidence when working with this client group. Our aim is to see the two professions better able to work together with this important group of patients.

Val Hopwood
Clare Donnellan

Coventry, Nottingham 2010

Note on case histories

Case histories are included to clarify the application of acupuncture. We have divided these case studies into three categories:

Level 1

A simple intervention, either Western medical acupuncture or TCM, aimed at changing a single symptom, i.e. pain, numbness, nausea. This will be written in a relatively brief format.

Level 2

Describing a more complex or chronic situation where it has been necessary to look at the underlying problems, again either Western medicine or TCM. This is likely to involve a relatively short treatment period, and may be suitable for additional courses of treatment. These cases will provide more detail of the patient's condition.

Level 3

These will be written in more detail, describing long-term treatment of a complex situation requiring the mix of Western medicine and TCM clinical reasoning for success.

Section 1

Backgrounds – Chinese and Western

History and background of traditional Chinese medicine in neurological conditions

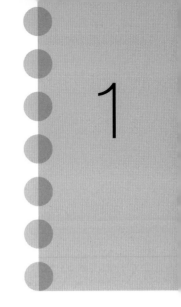

1

KEY POINTS

- The concept of 'neurology' is a relatively modern one, with no real place in traditional Chinese medicine (TCM). This is only partly because there is no historical concept of the 'brain' in TCM physiology.
- There have been many schools of Chinese medicine: some included ideas that we would recognize as 'neurology', whereas others did not.
- The ideas informing the Zang Fu consider different emotions, understanding that they may have a pathogenic influence, and consequently attribute them to appropriate organs.
- There are three syndrome groups that are particularly concerned with neurological symptoms: Bi, Wei and Feng.
- The Bi subgroups are usually defined by the type of Pathogenic invasion but also by the tissue most affected.
- Wei or atrophy syndromes are characterized by limb weakness.
- Feng syndromes are associated with muscle tremor or spasm.
- Acupuncture can often be effective in treating Wei syndromes in their early and middle stages.

Historical development

The combination of the ancient art of acupuncture, part of the equally venerable tradition of Chinese medicine, and what is perceived by Western medicine at least as the most modern of sciences, neurology, seems at first to be quite a challenge. On the one hand we have a tradition of consensus medicine where ideas and theories were handed down from father to son or from master to apprentice and, while there was a great deal of documented debate, no reductionist analysis has been recorded.

On the other hand, the type of evidence required for general acceptance of any medical intervention in our current society, the controlled clinical trial, is relatively new in the world of acupuncture and, while there is an explosion of work in the field of acupuncture for pain control, neurological problems have, thus far, been mostly ignored.

One reason for this lies within the relatively alien ideology and structure of Chinese medicine, but equal blame lies within the fundamental ideologies of Western medicine. Neurology is a complex branch of medicine but tends to be described in two dimensions, being either 'on' or 'off', like an electrical circuit.

Another very good reason for the relative lack of research into acupuncture and neurological conditions is the complexity of the symptomatology and sheer difficulty of isolating a homogeneous patient group of sufficient numbers to be accepted as a definitive randomized controlled clinical trial.

The history of acupuncture is a long and complex one. It is not necessary, perhaps, to understand every detail but it is very useful to understand how the thoughts of the ancient sages can inform the modern practice of acupuncture. There is an inherent difficulty even in the preceding statement in that actually knowing what is meant by some of the terms is very difficult. Terms gain their meaning through context and the historical contextual background is further complicated by influential modern schools of thought. For instance, the teachings of Worsley, an originator of much of the modern Five-Element theory, lay great emphasis on the 'Spirit' of the acupuncture point, even though there is little agreement among Chinese scholars as to what is meant by the term 'Spirit' or even what exactly was meant by the names of the points. The possibility for confusion is built in from the start of recorded ideas.

While many Chinese characters can have more than one English equivalent, a majority are well suited by one term. Most sources translate Shen as Spirit, so the question is, what do we really mean by this term? The Chinese context of Spirit is an integral part of the paradigm and, as difficult as it may be to understand, we must make the effort. Otherwise, we only superimpose our own cultural attitudes and beliefs on Chinese medicine.

The seminal written accounts of Chinese medicine theories are over 1000 years old and even in our own culture we are aware of the subtle changes in meaning of seemingly simple words and concepts. The word 'gay' would be a good example; it raises no eyebrows when it occurs in the writings of Jane Austen, for example, but when included in today's prose it would be interpreted rather differently.

Chinese medicine has been used over many hundreds of years. It has a long recorded history: the first written records, the *Huang Di Nei Jing*, date from about 200 BC. It has evolved as part of the traditional Chinese medical paradigm, together with Chinese herbal medicine. The origins of traditional Chinese medicine (TCM) are closely associated with demonology and ancestor worship, this being usefully defined as a ritualized propitiation and, possibly, invocation of dead relatives. Ancestor worship is firmly based on the belief that the spirits of the dead continue to dwell in the natural world, and have the power to influence the fortune and fate of the living.

Although mysterious forces such as gods, demons or ancestors were originally called on to provide explanations for the phenomena of the perceptible world, a great deal of the original Chinese philosophy underpinning TCM was the attempt to explain these phenomena as natural occurrences. Medicine and religion were closely linked in the early history of the area now known as China and cultural changes were reflected in the accounts we have of medical practices.

In the sense that what you think and believe about what is happening to you will affect how you respond psychologically to any illness, the original shamanistic ideas must have had a huge effect on the recovery of patients treated in the Shang and early Zhou dynasties. Nowadays this might well be defined as merely a placebo response but nobody will deny that a placebo response can nonetheless be powerful. A white-coated doctor in an NHS surgery with a stethoscope is still a powerful placebo!

The history of acupuncture cannot be divorced from the history of Chinese culture. The Middle and Late Zhou dynasties were particularly important and much of the theory accepted today was first recorded then. Various theories were widely discussed and some gained temporary dominance.

It would be fair to say that the origins of Chinese medicine are obscure. Some of the great heroes, Fu Xi, Shen Nong and Huang Di, were said to have lived in the Shang dynasty but were not actually written about until much later.

The recorded history of acupuncture starts from about 1520 BC and comes nearly to an end in 1911. It is useful to remind ourselves of this long history and vast wealth of empirical evidence. It is also interesting to see where theories relating to what we now understand as neurological problems fit in to the overall picture of Zang Fu physiology.

Zang Fu, the origins of physiology

The Zang Fu organs are perhaps the most fascinating aspect of TCM theory. The ancient Chinese medical practitioners did not have the advantage of meticulous dissection and careful histological studies to help them understand the body. Gross functions could be understood but the complexity and subtlety of human physiology could only be guessed at by observation and trial and error when administering herbs or acupuncture. Nonetheless, when used to define treatment protocols the observations made in the past still appear quite valid.

Many of these ideas originated in a martial society and the metaphors for function and control tend to sound like elements of military campaign. It will be useful to describe each organ in turn and discuss the links to the others. Disease patterns generally involve more than one organ at a time, and sometimes these indicate where there may be relevance to neurological conditions. The primary focus may be identifiable from the associated symptoms, but unless the practitioner has a good working knowledge of all the Zang Fu characteristics and connections, the secondary foci and possibly the origins of the problem may be hard to decide. Chinese medicine defines disease as disorders within these Zang Fu relationships rather than as a single failing organ. It is difficult to separate Western ideas of organ function from the Chinese concepts but it is important

to do so before it is possible to see the patterns. Many of the functions seem arbitrary to a Western eye but the fundamental theories informing them are often very logical.

Firstly we will give a quick explanation of the major functions of the Zang Fu organs. These functions are seen as inextricably linked and interdependent and lead to TCM diagnoses of some complexity. We are indebted to Worsley, an influential Western teacher and practitioner (and also originally a physiotherapist) for some useful ideas about the Zang Fu organs in general [1]. Most texts offer two lists of six pairs of organs, some functions of which correspond to those understood by Western medicine and some which plainly do not (Table 1.1).

However, Worsley suggested that the Zang Fu should be considered as 10 organs and two functions. That is very helpful to those of us working with neurological conditions. The two he selects as functions, the Sanjiao and the Pericardium, have extended influence throughout the body physiology. The Sanjiao, or, as it is often known, the Triple Heater, has a wide-ranging function particularly concerned with the circulation of fluid throughout the body and described as being responsible for the opening-up of passages and general irrigation. The fluid thus regulated is associated with both the interstitial spaces and the major organs.

The Pericardium is clearly defined in orthodox modern Chinese texts as the Heart Protector and little more. However, since it is so intimately connected to the Heart it takes on some of the characteristics of that organ.

Table 1.1 Zang Fu organs

Zang organs (Yin)	Fu organs (Yang)
Heart (Xin)	Small Intestine (Xiao Chang)
Lungs (Fei)	Large Intestine (Da Chang)
Liver (Gan)	Gall Bladder (Dan)
Spleen (Pi)	Stomach (Wei)
Kidney (Shen)	Urinary Bladder (Pang Guan)
Pericardium (Xin Bao)	**Sanjiao**
(Extra Uterus)	(Extra Brain)

Heart (Xin)

The Heart is the 'emperor' within the body and as such has control over everything. It is said to govern all the other organs and is pictured as a benevolent and enlightened ruler. It regulates the flow of Blood and Qi and governs the Blood in two ways. TCM sources see it as a pump which is responsible for the circulation of blood in the vessels, as understood in Western medicine. This makes it responsible for the innate health of the vessels too. The Heart propels the Blood through the tissues, communicating with every part and suffusing the body with consciousness and feeling.

The relationship between the Heart and the Blood is important and determines the strength of the constitution of an individual. Tongue diagnosis can give an indication of the relative strength of the constitution. The presence of a clear crack down the centre of the tongue would alert a TCM practitioner to the possibility of a deficiency of Heart Qi or energy. The state of the blood vessels and general circulation reflects the strength of the Heart Qi, as does the condition of the Heart pulse. Since the Heart controls the blood vessels and circulation, deficient Heart energy leads to a very noticeable bright, white complexion, often seen in Parkinson's disease patients.

Since Blood and Body Fluids are thought to have a common origin, sweat is considered to be controlled by the Heart and to be found in the spaces just under the skin. If there is a lack of fluid within the circulation it can be replenished from this source. If there is too much heat within the body it is 'steamed off' and discharged through the pores. Whatever the true physiology, Heart points appear to have a clinical influence on otherwise unexplained hyperhydrosis problems.

In addition to the clear links with the mechanism of circulation, the Heart also houses the Mind or Shen. This is where the psychological influences become apparent, affecting five functions, all of which are involved in our response to any neurological illness:

1. mental activity
2. consciousness
3. memory
4. thinking
5. sleep.

The term 'Shen' is also sometimes used to indicate vitality. The involvement of the Heart with all of the above means that it must be considered when treating mental illness and, indeed, Heart 7, Shenmen, is a useful point to calm and relax a patient, or to treat insomnia or depression. 'Shenmen' translates as 'Gateway to the Spirit'. The Heart has a strong influence over sleep patterns. If the Heart is deficient in energy the mind is said to have no residence and it will float at night, causing disturbed sleep or excessive dreaming, should sleep come at all.

The connection between the Heart and the emotions is well understood in folk legend in most countries but there is little scientific proof that this could have any foundation. However there are some interesting ideas in a paper by Rosen [2], where the internal memory of the heart cells with regard to physiological process is recognized and discussed. It is suggested that the heart does remember, 'making use of mechanisms similar to those in other systems that manifest memory, the brain, the gastrointestinal tract and the immune system'.

The emotion of joy is most closely associated with the Heart. Joy is said to slow down the Qi and affects the Heart in this way. Since the Heart controls the Mind or Spirit and hence the emotions, it follows that an excess, i.e. over-joy or extreme anxiety, will damage the balance of Qi in this Zang Fu organ. Excess joy is said to disturb the Xin Qi so much that the Shen becomes confused and scattered. Over-joy is quite a violent emotion and in TCM a sudden laughing fit is thought to be able to trigger a heart attack. The effect of emotional lability, often found in multiple sclerosis (MS), mimics this imbalance.

The concept of a 'broken heart' is far from alien to TCM. When the Heart is overwhelmed by strong emotion, usually in this case shock or sorrow, the Shen will be able to break free, thinking becomes disordered and confused and the resulting anxiety will be evident in the abnormal circulation. The impaired circulation will lead to stagnation of the Blood, blood pressure decreases and the patient will show signs of heart disease, angina or chest pain. Shock and fright have an opposite effect on the Heart and are said to cause the Shen to contract.

The most extreme disharmonies of the emotions arise from imbalances within Xin (Heart) and Gan (Liver) and it is sometimes difficult to differentiate between a lack of joie de vivre caused by Xin deficiency and the sorrow and melancholy caused by depression of Gan Qi.

A further disharmony that will give rise to confusing symptoms is that between the Heart and the Kidney. This is often considered in terms of Yin and Yang or Fire and Water. The water aspect of the Kidneys must control the Fire aspect of the Heart, but if the Yin aspect of the Kidney energy is deficient then it will not control and cool the Heart Fire, which then flares up, causing symptoms like insomnia and irritability.

The Heart is said to be the most important Zang Fu organ but, although it is intimately concerned with feelings and emotions, it has little or no influence on the movements and physical activities that we understand to be controlled by the brain. The Governing Vessel, or Du meridian, in its anterior pathway passes through the Heart and is said to penetrate the brain posteriorly at GV 16 Fengfu.

Since the Du meridian is also closely associated with the Kidneys at Du 4 or Mingmen, both these points can be used to influence Heart function (Figure 1.1).

A useful comparison with the TCM function of the Heart is with that of the cerebral cortex, an integrative function, giving rise to the capacity for individual thought and memory. This is further expressed through speech, the voice and facial expression. The intimate link with the Pericardium means that some of the Heart functions can be influenced by treating points on the Pericardium meridian. It is commonly held that this is a 'gentler' form of treatment.

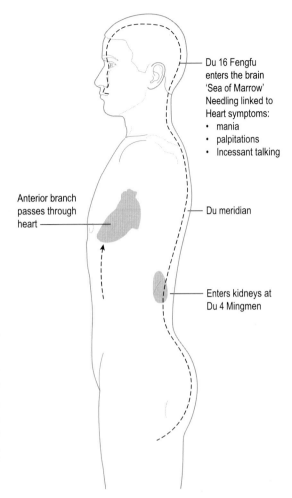

Figure 1.1 • Du meridian: Marrow and Heart linked.

Du 16 Fengfu enters the brain 'Sea of Marrow' Needling linked to Heart symptoms:
• mania
• palpitations
• Incessant talking

Anterior branch passes through heart

Du meridian

Enters kidneys at Du 4 Mingmen

Lungs (Fei)

The Lung is characterized as a diplomatic foreign minister, conducting affairs of state and determining foreign boundaries, thus effectively governing the relationship between the inside and outside of the body. The Lungs are the most external of all the organs, having direct contact with the outer air. Because the Lung is so susceptible to Pathogenic invasion it is sometimes referred to as the 'tender organ'.

The Lungs control respiration and are responsible for the intake of clean air, which they convert into 'Clear Qi'. Together with the Qi produced from substances that are eaten and drunk, this goes to make up the Post Heaven or renewable Qi within the body. The rhythm of the Lungs sets the rate for all other body functions, starting with the first breath taken by the newborn baby. The clean air or Qi from the Lungs condenses into fluid and passes down through the Sanjiao to the Kidneys, where it is heated, vaporizes and ascends to the Lungs again, forming a sort of energy cycle effectively controlling water circulation within the body (Figure 1.2).

The emptying of the Lungs, expiration, slows the movement of Qi whereas the act of filling them, inspiration, speeds it up.

Some teachers compare the activity of the lungs to that of the parasympathetic system, an inhibitory action, but it could be argued that they are just as likely to be involved in a sympathetic mode. Either way, they may be peripherally affected when central nervous system control is damaged in any neurological condition.

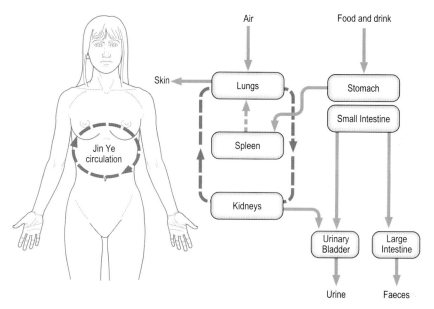

Figure 1.2 • Jin Ye circulation. (Reproduced with permission from Hopwood V. Acupuncture in Physiotherapy. Oxford: Butterworth Heinemann: 2004.)

The Lung controls the condition of the hair and also the state of the pores. The skin is sometimes referred to as the 'third lung'. If the skin is in poor condition the pores may remain more open than usual, allowing the invasion of exogenous pathogens. The Lung is also said to produce and control the Wei Qi, or Defensive Qi. This is the first line of defence against Pathogenic invasion of the body and circulates in the spaces just underneath the skin. The link with the Kidneys and water circulation coupled with the control of the pore size means that it also has an effect on sweating, along with the Heart.

The Lung opens into the nose, and is vulnerable to the External Pathogens Wind and Cold. The common cold is said to be an invasion of a combination of Wind and Cold. The sense of smell and the loudness of the voice are dependent on Lung health. A husky voice and a runny or blocked nose are therefore not surprising as common cold symptoms.

The Lung houses the Corporeal Soul or Hun. It is particularly sensitive to grief or sadness, and often affected by bereavement. It is associated with the pain of loss, of letting go, sorrow, loneliness, anxiety and melancholy. The effect of sorrow on the Lung can result in a lack of desire to face the world. Sadness of this kind tends to produce stagnation of Qi in the chest and this in turns inhibits the function of both the Lungs and the Heart. This could result

in the subsequent stagnation of Blood throughout the body.

Treatment of LU 7 or Lieque can have a powerful release effect in constrained emotional conditions. The link between sorrow and the function of the Lung has been suggested as the reason for many recently bereaved elderly patients contracting fatal chest infections while still grieving.

Liver (Gan)

The Liver is often characterized as a General, directing his troops; this is a useful analogy because it allows us to think of this organ as concerned in the balance of energies. The Liver has a controlling action on the circulation of blood but this activity depends on whether the body is at rest or active. The Liver sends blood through the vessels when the body is in movement but gathers it back into itself and stores it when at rest.

Some authorities describe this as a rhythm, similar to that of the Lungs, but differing in that it is a voluntary rhythm depending on the circumstances [3]. Ideas of fight and flight, as understood in Western neurology, are clearly appropriate here.

The Liver is responsible for the smooth movement of Qi and body fluids throughout the body. The Liver is involved in the process of digestion, providing energy for the transportation of the Gu Qi produced by the Stomach and Spleen. The Qi from each organ has a characteristic direction of flow, actually controlled by the Liver, ensuring the TCM physiological pathways. The Liver is the source of endurance in times of mental stress or physical exertion. If the Liver Qi is weak, one is easily exhausted, finding it difficult to get out of bed in the morning. Diseases such as MS are thought to attack and weaken Liver Qi.

Liver Qi should flow freely in all directions. If it is constrained it is said to invade the Stomach, Spleen or Lung. 'Liver invading Spleen' is fast becoming a common modern syndrome, perhaps because of the combined effect of unsuitable diet and stress on the liver triggering a chain reaction throughout the Zang Fu [4]. The Liver functions as a gentle regulator of the Spleen and Stomach and is thus a regulator of digestion. In addition, bile, under the control of the Liver, aids in the digestive process.

Storage of Blood is seen as integral to Liver function. The Liver releases blood for the start of menstruation and continues to do this regularly, in appropriate quantity, throughout the fertile life of the female. Menstrual problems, such as amenorrhoea and dysmenorrhoea, are primarily treated by restoring Liver function. The Liver has an influence on the even movement of Blood around the body in both sexes. Stagnation is often seen as a result of poor Liver function since Blood and Qi flow together and Qi is said to clear and smooth the channels to allow the accompanying Blood flow.

The Liver controls normal muscle tone in the body. Disturbance of this function leads to muscle tremor, twitching, spasm or even convulsions. This would be said to be the result of an 'insufficiency of the Yin and Blood in the Liver', resulting in malnutrition of the tissues. Many of the muscle impairments present in neurological disorders, such as tremor in Parkinson's disease and progressive paralysis in MS, are associated with Liver Qi imbalance. The Liver is also said to influence the muscle tendons. The fingernails are considered by TCM to be extensions of the tendons; thus, dry, flaky and ridged nails are indicative of an energy deficiency in the Liver.

A link with the eye means that the condition of the Liver can also be detected through examination of the 'white of the eye'. Conversely, it also means that Liver points can be used to treat eye problems, particularly LR 2 for problems of an inflammatory nature. The fluids most closely associated with the Liver, apart from Blood, are the tears. The syndrome 'stirring of the inner Wind of the Liver' can cause poor vision, night blindness and abnormal movements of the eye.

Failure of the free-flowing function of the Liver may be associated with both frustration and depression and outbursts of uncontrolled anger. The Liver requires a calm internal environment, with an even disposition. It is very sensitive to being obstructed in any way. It is interesting that the English language equates being 'liverish' with being irritable. The Hun or ethereal soul is housed in the Liver; it is injury to the Hun which causes insomnia, so Liver Qi stagnation in neurological diseases such as MS needs to be addressed to relieve insomnia.

Blazing Gan Fire is linked with severe and violent outbursts of rage. Feelings of irritation and moderate anger are also associated with Liver imbalance and often ascribed to deficient Liver Yin or hyperactive Liver Yang, both of which cause the even tenor of life to become a little more bumpy. Stagnation of the Liver Qi, often produced by anger, can also have a profound effect on the Stomach and Spleen Qi and disturb digestion.

Spleen (Pi)

The Spleen is an interesting organ from a TCM point of view but has never excited much enthusiasm in Western medicine. It occupies the very last pages in *Gray's Anatomy* and has always been regarded as generally superfluous to requirements. Splenectomy is not regarded as a life-threatening situation, although antibiotics are required to maintain health afterwards.

The spleen is said to store blood and to have some blood-manufacturing properties but the important part played in the digestive process is not recognized in the West. Interestingly, it has been observed to increase in size during digestion, although no conclusions appear to have been drawn from this.

In TCM the Spleen is regarded as the minister of agriculture, able to control and regulate the production and distribution of essential nourishment. The Spleen is said to govern transformation and transportation. It is the main digestive organ in TCM and responsible, along with the Stomach, for the breaking down or transformation of ingested food and drink and its subsequent transportation to the other sites in the body where it will be utilized. The Spleen is said to incorporate and then distribute Nutritive Essence in order to diminish or augment body mass [5]. It is responsible for forming and reconstituting the internal milieu, gathering and holding together the substance of the body.

Overeating can damage the Spleen; being continually full slows metabolism and assimilation of nutrients. Food will sit undigested in the stomach, uncomfortably inflating the abdomen with stagnant fluid and gases. Lacking sufficient energy from the food ingested, the possible gain from this new food decreases steadily. This leads to a form of weight increase that could be described as more mass than energy. Retarded digestion engenders an urge for a quick fix of sugar and starch. Hence a frequent symptom of Spleen imbalance is a craving for sweet foods or chocolate. Since this obviously applies to patients losing normal mobility, for whatever reason, nutritional advice with the TCM Spleen in mind can be helpful.

The Spleen has a direct influence on muscle bulk since the transformation and transport of food substances help to maintain this. It adjusts the quantity of pure fluid or Essence produced by the digestive process and released into circulation, a function rather like providing additional fuel when the tank is emptying. Stomach and Spleen can be compared to storehouse and granary: the food substances are refined, stored and subsequently transported for use. The whole process is vital to nutrition. Hence Spleen points are recommended where there is evidence of muscle wasting. In addition, the control exerted over the water content of the tissues affects muscle bulk. In Wei syndrome (or 'withering'), when a decrease in muscle bulk is marked, a combination of Spleen and Stomach points is useful.

This organ is also closely involved with the control of the fluid balance throughout the body, so the Spleen channel is frequently used when there is an excess of fluid, oedema, particularly in the lower limbs. The Spleen itself is said to prefer dryness; this means that it is adversely affected by the Western habit of excessive consumption of icy, sweet drinks and forced to use too much energy in the breakdown of uncooked foods like salads.

The Spleen controls or supervises the Blood, keeping it in the blood vessels and preventing bleeding. If the Blood seeps from the vessels, causing superficial bruising with no perceived cause, then this is thought to be a weakness of Spleen Qi failing to keep it within the vessels. If the Spleen fails in this role the walls of the blood vessels may become fragile and even collapse and marked extravasation occurs, with unexplained bruising appearing on the body surface. Blood may also appear in the stools, which are characteristically loose in any Spleen syndrome. Deficient Yang Qi in the spleen will also adversely affect the formation of Blood.

The Spleen has a centralizing and uplifting effect, holding all organs in their proper places in the body. In practical terms this is said to explain why Spleen points are used to control prolapsed, particularly of the uterus or rectum. Spleen points are very useful when treating haemorrhoids.

The Spleen opens into the mouth and the lips indicate the general state of the Spleen, which should be a healthy red colour. Spleen Qi deficiencies are indicated by pale, thin lips. The associated body fluid is saliva.

The Spleen houses thought and is associated with the act of thinking. If the balance is wrong then excessive or obsessive worrying will be the sign, with general lack of energy and lassitude as the result. There is an obvious link here with the Heart. The Spleen influences our capacity for thinking, studying, concentrating, focusing and memorizing, whereas in TCM the Heart actually does it. The Spleen is damaged by long periods of intensive study or chronic anxiety and several Spleen syndromes are made worse by comfort eating, overdependence on chocolate, which of course is brought about in the first place by low-grade stress. Some scholars have also suggested that it has a connection with compassion and the emotion of caring, but this link may be perceived because, at a time when the Spleen is overwhelmed, the capacity for these emotions is lost.

Symptoms of Spleen Qi deficiency include a disinclination to talk, a low indistinct voice, sallow or pale complexion and general lassitude. Another important symptom associated with imbalance in the Spleen is loss of the sense of smell and, associated with this, the sense of taste. There may also be chronic diarrhoea due to excessive dampness. Swelling or oedema in the lower part of the body, particularly the legs and ankles, is common. Strengthening the Spleen always accompanies a similar treatment for the Stomach and is frequently used to invigorate Blood and the circulation and expel the Pathogen Damp.

Kidney (Shen)

The Kidney is characterized as a Minister of the Interior who conserves natural resources, storing them for use in times of need, growth, crisis or transition. It is of fundamental importance in TCM and said to be the root of life. The Shen Kidney stores Jing or Essence, which is derived from each of the parents and established at conception. This in turn controls the Yang aspects of sexual potency. The Yin and Yang of the Kidneys serve as the foundation for that of the rest of the body. Kidney Yin is the fundamental substance for birth, growth and reproduction while Kidney Yang is the motive force for all physiological processes. Although, according to the Five-Element theory, the Kidneys belong to Water, they are also said to be the source of Fire in the body. This is called Fire of the Gate of Vitality.

The Pre-heaven Essence determines constitutional strength and vitality. It is also associated with individual creativity, and is the basis of sexual life. Impotence and infertility can be linked with it. The Kidneys store Post-heaven Qi or Essence, the refined energy extracted from food through the transforming power of the internal organs. Kidney Essence is the original material substance that forms the basis of all other tissues. It is compared to the genetic information encoded in DNA. Essence is finite and the length of life is dependent upon the quantity and quality. After birth, through childhood and youth, through maturity and old age, all the normal development and ageing processes are associated with the Kidney Essence. When it is abundant the body has the facility to develop and grow. The changes associated with old age are all symptomatic of Kidney deficiency: loss of hair, blurring of vision, low-back pain, tinnitus and loose teeth.

Since it is the origin of both vitality and endurance the Kidney is important in many ways. It represents our own personal link in the continuous chain of existence. The Kidney energy of the fetus and newborn is manifesting the Pre-heaven Qi. The Post-heaven Qi is still potential; consider a small mulberry bush. We see the little thing beginning to grow: the berries that contain the seed haven't formed yet, and won't for years, but they are still there deep within the being.

It is ultimately responsible for the instinct to procreate and thus survive. If Kidney Qi is abundant, a long and vigorous sex life is expected since it supports the reproductive organs, material and activity.

When stress – the negative kind – occurs in a normal person, tension occurs, the circulation contracts, breathing is less natural or optimum, and the lack of perceived freedom or even joy creates the internal stagnations that subsequently become bad choices, low expectations and a self-fulfilling self-originating skewed world view. Growth decline and disease follows.

Since the Kidneys belong to Water and they govern the transformation and transportation of Body Fluids in many ways, they act like a gate which opens and closes to control the flow of fluids in the Lower Jiao or lower third of the body cavity. This flow is regulated by the Kidney Yang which in turn controls Kidney Yin. All forms of body fluid are derived from the synthesis of acquired and inherited body essence. This includes tears, saliva, mucus, urine, sweat, cerebrospinal fluid, synovial fluid, plasma and semen.

If too much fluid accumulates in the lower Jiao (Figure 1.2), it stagnates, giving rise to swelling at the knees and ankles, gravitational oedema, abdominal bloating and, occasionally, puffiness beneath the eyes. The build-up of fluid will have a direct effect on the lungs and eventually the heart, leading to further swelling in the upper part of the body.

Because of this involvement in the circulation of water, the Kidneys have a more direct effect on the functions of the Lung. They are said to control and promote respiration. If the Kidney energy is low, the energy necessary to 'steam' the pure fluids and send them back up to the Lung will be lacking. The connected descent of the heavier fluid down to the Kidney will not occur, with a build-up of fluid in the lung tissues for a different reason. This type of accumulated fluid causes wheezing and is identified as late-onset asthma.

The Kidneys are said to open into the ear, making Kidney points useful for the treatment of deafness and tinnitus. TCM associates deafness with the idea of extra-thick bone being laid down in the ear, and therefore being under the control of the Kidney. Hair growth is dependent on Essence and Blood and its loss is a result of poor supply. The whitening of the hair in the elderly is connected to the state of the Kidney Essence. There is a saying: 'the function of the kidney reflects in the glossiness of the hair'. This is interesting because the Lung is also credited with playing a part in the condition of the hair. Perhaps it just serves to emphasize the connection between these two Zang organs.

Fear is the emotion most strongly associated with the Kidneys. It is closely linked to the desire for self-preservation and consequently encompasses true terror. The basic physiological responses, fight or flight, are involved and the other Zang Fu organs are brought into play. The type of fear that immobilizes or paralyses involves weakness of Dan (Gall Bladder) and, when linked to anger, involves Gan

(Liver). If caused by worry, then the Spleen may be involved; if a result of anxiety, then the Lung also shows symptoms.

The failure of the Kidney energy to support the body-healing process is implicit in many of the neurological conditions discussed in this book. Use of points to stimulate both Kidney Yin and Kidney Yang energy is usually recommended; the best, all-round point is KI 3, Taixi.

Pericardium (Xin Bao)

The Pericardium is closely related to the Heart; traditionally it is thought to shield the Heart from the invasion of External Pathogenic factors. It is also known as the Heart Protector. The ancient manuscripts, most particularly the *Spiritual Pivot* [6], do not grant the Pericardium true Zang Fu status, describing the Heart as the master of the five Zang and the six Fu. The Heart is considered to be the dwelling of the Shen and no Pathogen can be allowed past the barrier of the Pericardium in case the Heart is damaged and the Shen departs and death occurs. The Pericardium displays some of the characteristics of Xin Heart but is far less important, in that it only assists with the government of Blood and housing the Mind.

However, as stated earlier, Worsley considered the Pericardium more of a function than an entity and the points on the channel are often used to treat emotional problems, having a perceived cheering effect [1]. They are also frequently used for their sedative effect. The meridian is also used in treatment of the Heart but is considered to be a less intense form of therapy than the use of Heart points.

In effect the Pericardium is considered as the active mechanism of the Heart, the physical pumping activity, whereas the Heart itself is more involved with containing the Spirit and maintaining full consciousness.

In spite of this lesser importance in Zang Fu terms, the meridian is a very useful one with many internal connections and wide-ranging physiological effects.

Fu organs

Small Intestine (Xiao Chang)

The Small Intestine does not differ greatly in function from what is understood in the West but the description of its connections is rather different. The Small Intestine receives food and drink from the stomach and separates the clean or reusable fraction from that which is dirty. The clean part is then transported by the Spleen to all parts of the body. The dirty or turbid part is transmitted to the Large Intestine for excretion as stools and to the Bladder to form the urine. This means that the Small Intestine has a direct functional relationship with the Bladder and influences urinary function. The Small Intestine thus plays a minor part in the Jin Ye or body water circulation.

The Small Intestine is paired with the Heart and is said to have an effect on dreams, although it is not so strong as the Heart itself. The Small Intestine is linked with the Heart through the purification of the substances that enter the Blood, thus protecting the Shen or Spirit. The traditional pairing with the Heart is rather tenuous and only really evident when heat from Fire in the Xin Heart shifts downwards into the Small Intestine and disturbs the Lower Jiao. This relationship is only relevant in the psychological sense. The Small Intestine is said to have an influence on judgement, and on making the best choices.

Large Intestine (Da Chang)

The digestive function of the Large Intestine, as described in TCM, is very similar to that understood in Western medicine. In some Chinese texts it is described as 'passing and changing', referring to what happens to the faecal matter. However, many of the normal functions of the Large Intestine are also ascribed to the Spleen. The most important action is the reception of food and drink from the Small Intestine, and the reabsorption of a proportion of the fluid. The remainder goes to make up the faeces and is excreted.

The Large Intestine is the final part of the digestive system and will reflect any imbalances occurring in the other organs of digestion in terms of quantity or quality.

Deficient Yang energy in the Spleen is also called Deficient Energy in the Large Intestine because both tend to result in the same symptoms. This means that the Large Intestine is part of the fluid balance mechanism of the body. The Large Intestine is linked to the Lung both interiorly and exteriorly via the meridians and can therefore have an influence on the Lung/Kidney water cycle. The Lung is said to disperse water while the Large Intestine absorbs it. Equally the Lung takes in air while the Large Intestine discharges gas. If there is Heat in the Lung the faeces will be dry and if the function of the Lung is weak the faeces tend to be loose. Simple stagnation of food in the Large Intestine or constipation can give rise to a degree of breathlessness.

If the Large Intestine is functioning poorly the mind becomes unclear and muddled. It is as though the failure to eliminate the waste leaves feelings of staleness and lifelessness. Many neurological patients suffering from constipation will describe the effect of it in just this way, as will those suffering from a drug-induced constipation. Optimum functioning of the body requires elimination of that which is no longer of use, both physically and psychologically.

Gall Bladder (Dan)

The main function of the Gall Bladder is perceived to be that of assisting the Spleen and Stomach in the process of digestion. The bile from the Gall Bladder is discharged into the Small Intestine under the control of the Liver. If this flow is impaired the digestion process is affected and there will be loss of appetite, abdominal pain and distension with diarrhoea.

This Fu organ is closely connected to the Liver. In TCM terms it is thought that Gan, the Liver, produces the bile and Dan, the Gall Bladder, stores it. The Gall Bladder is not always included in the list of Fu organs and is sometimes termed a 'Curious Organ' because it is hollow and secretes a pure fluid (making it more Zang than Fu). It has much in common with the pancreas, and, since the pancreas is not mentioned in the Zang Fu, is sometimes regarded as serving in that capacity too.

The Gall Bladder is said to be responsible for making decisions while the Liver is responsible for smooth planning. Both are affected by the emotional Pathogens Anger and Irritability. A deficiency in Gall Bladder energy leads to timidity, indecision or procrastination. The Gall Bladder is said to give an individual courage and increase drive and vitality. A man with a serene character and firmness of resolve could be referred to as 'having a large Gall Bladder' or a 'thick Liver' and regarded as most valuable in a military sense by Eastern philosophers.

The Liver and Gall Bladder are so closely linked that it is difficult to regard their disharmonies

individually. The balance of energy within the Liver will have a bearing on the storage and release of bile and the subsequent symptoms of poor digestion may result in jaundice, hepatitis or cholecystitis.

A graphic illustration of the interconnectedness of the Zang Fu organs comes from Dey's translation of Zhang Cong Zheng in his book on treating schizophrenia:

> when the Liver constantly plans, and the Gall Bladder is constantly indecisive, by being bent over without stretching, and holding anger that is not discharged, the Heart blood grows dryer by the day. Spleen humor does not move and phlegm then confounds the orifices of the Heart, forming Heart Wind [7].

Stomach (Wei)

The Stomach is the most important of the Fu organs and has a vital role in digestion. Together with the Spleen it is known as the root of Post-heaven Qi. Digestion was understood by the ancient Chinese to be a rotting or fermenting process, in which the stomach was described graphically as the 'Chamber of Maceration'. This process prepares for the action of the Spleen, which then separates and extracts the refined Essence from the food and drink. It has also been compared to a bubbling cauldron.

After the transformation process, which takes place in the Stomach, the food passes into the Small Intestine for further breakdown and absorption. The Stomach is always considered as the true origin of acquired Qi or Gu Qi and is vital for a healthy constitution. For this reason it is often necessary to tonify Stomach Qi when there is any disease process present. The most commonly used acupuncture point is Zusanli Stomach 36, often described as a boost to the system or Qi metabolism. The Stomach has a similar role to that of the Spleen in transporting the food Qi to all the tissues, most particularly the limbs. Weak muscles and general fatigue may indicate a lack of Stomach Qi.

The Stomach sends transformed food down to the Small Intestine and is described as having a descending function. If this is absent or impaired the food stagnates, leading to fullness, distension, sour regurgitation, belching, hiccups, nausea and vomiting. Vomiting is often described as 'rebellious Stomach Qi'. Under normal conditions the Liver Qi has a hand in this smooth downward flow, so it often needs to be treated alongside the Stomach in digestive disorders.

In order to perform the ripening and rotting task assigned to it, the Stomach requires large quantities of fluid to dissolve the valuable parts of the food. It is, of course, itself a source of fluid but it works best when damp and is damaged by dryness and the Pathogen Heat. Eating large meals late at night depletes the fluids of the Stomach and sets up disharmonies right through the system.

Since it is easily damaged by Heat the Stomach is susceptible to Excess patterns, such as Fire or Phlegm Fire, and can eventually produce mental states similar to mania. Mild cases are likely to suffer from confusion and severe anxiety.

The state of the Stomach may be seen quite clearly in the tongue coating, which is formed as a byproduct of the rotting process. A thin white coating is normal. Absence of a coating implies impaired function and a yellow coating indicates Heat in the Stomach.

The Stomach and the Spleen are so closely interlinked in physiology and function that they are always treated together. While the Stomach controls the downward movement of the less pure elements in the food, the Spleen governs the upward movement of the clear fraction, linking with the Lung. Any type of illness pattern that involves the malabsorption of food and subsequent diminishing Qi production requires both Stomach and Spleen points to be stimulated. This is often apparent in any type of wasting disease where muscle bulk diminishes visibly.

The link between digestion and the mental state has often been considered in the West and common sense tells us that one affects the other. It is rare to see it considered from the Chinese perspective, however, and an article by McMillin et al. [8] throws some light on the sympathetic and parasympathetic nerve connections, which serve to reinforce the Zang Fu attributes.

Urinary Bladder (Pang Guan)

The Urinary Bladder holds few surprises. It secretes and stores urine, using energy from the Kidney, and releases it when appropriate. It is closely involved in the circulation of fluid around the body, receiving fluids separated by the Small Intestine and transforming them into urine. Energy in the Lower Jiao, particularly that of the Kidney, ensures the maintenance of clear water passages.

The Urinary Bladder tends to be susceptible to the Pathogen Heat, producing the painful symptoms of cystitis if this occurs. Incontinence of urine is directly attributable to the Bladder but is usually caused by deficient Kidney Qi. The Urinary Bladder is also said to have control of the urethral, anal and cervical sphincters, regulating the discharge of all body fluids in this area.

The Bladder is thought to be linked to negative emotions such as jealousy and the holding of long-standing grudges. Another saying associated with the Urinary Bladder is: 'when the Bladder is deficient one dreams of voyages'.

Sanjiao

The Sanjiao or Triple Energizer is a fascinating concept peculiar to Chinese medicine, demonstrating the fundamental holistic concept of the physiological body. It is an explanation of the predominant functions in distinct areas of the trunk and the TCM theory demonstrates the interconnectedness of everything. It is a uniquely Chinese concept and is the subject of much speculation. The word Sanjiao means 'three chambers' or 'three spaces'.

To understand the Sanjiao one needs to reconsider the circulation of Qi, Blood and Body Fluids. The Upper Jiao is said to contain the Lungs and Heart and is known as the 'chamber of mist'. It is clearly defined as being the portion of the trunk above the diaphragm. The Middle Jiao is just below, between the diaphragm and the navel, and contains the Spleen and Stomach. This region is particularly concerned with the digestion and absorption of food. It is known as the Chamber of Ripening and Rotting or sometimes the Chamber of Maceration.

Since the predominant direction of Stomach Qi is downwards and that of the Spleen is upwards it is clear that the Middle Jiao acts as a kind of junction. The Lower Jiao contains all the other organs, even the Liver and Gall Bladder, although true anatomical location is somewhat inaccurate here. Of major importance physiologically, however, are the Kidneys and Bladder, giving the region the general name of 'Drainage Ditch' and controlling the storage and excretion of water.

The Sanjiao is really the summary of the physiology of the Zang Fu organs and points on that meridian (designated Triple Energizer, or TE, by the World Health Organization) can be utilized in coordination of function, particularly fluid circulation. Figure 1.2 shows the contents of the three Jiaos with the predominant direction of Qi flow. In fact all the Zang Fu organs are interlinked in some way, either by fluid circulation or Qi production, so any diagram can become very complex once every factor is taken into account.

The Sanjiao has a very close link with the Kidneys, both Yin and Yang aspects. Since it controls water metabolism it relies on Kidney energy to accomplish this.

Zang Fu in neurology

The link between Chinese medicine and the brain is tenuous at best. As defined within the Zang Fu system the brain is one of the Curious Organs, so called because they are hollow, resembling the Fu organs and also functioning as stores rather than excreting. The other recognizable organs in this group are the Uterus and the Gall Bladder. Also considered under this heading, however, are the bones, the circulation system of blood and bone marrow. As Ross notes: 'These tissues, in their aspect as the Curious Organs, have relatively little theoretical or practical importance and are generally treated via other systems' [9].

The extraordinary organs are those about which there has been some doubt: either they were not really identified in the ancient writings or they did not fully qualify in their assigned classification. Also, as in the case of the Uterus, not everybody had them!

The Brain (Nao)

The brain is referred to as the 'sea of Marrow'. Zang Fu theory dictates that the pathology and physiology of the brain belong to the Heart, which is described as 'the monarch of all the organs who is in charge of spiritual activities', so in reality the Brain has little function in TCM terms, although the connection with the Du meridian is considered important.

In more modern texts it is designated a true Zang Fu (although one of the Curious Organs) and allotted functions that correlate closely with what we understand from our modern studies [10].

So the brain controls memory, concentration, motor activity and mental activity. It also controls the senses – sight, hearing, taste, smell and touch.

Some texts also claim that Kidney Essence produces the Marrow which gathers to fill the brain and spinal cord, but this is rather a lazy way of thinking. If the brain can really be classified in the Zang Fu system then borrowing function from Western medicine is disingenuous at best. Nonetheless, one of the recent textbooks [10] has a wonderful list, owing its content to a cheerful mix of paradigms. Claiming that there are three parts to the brain, it characterizes function and offers selected acupoints, as shown in Table 1.2, giving somewhere to start in the general complexity.

Introducing the important syndromes

When considering the problem of diagnosing and identifying the many neurological conditions it is necessary to understand the TCM-defined syndromes. There is a case for proposing one all-purpose 'neuro-syndrome', making it slightly easier to define. The traditional syndrome format does not require the patient to be suffering from every symptom listed, just a majority, as opposed to any other syndrome. In any case more than one syndrome can be present at any one time, adding further confusion. Perhaps surprisingly, some of the TCM ideas have their echoes in modern medical thinking; for instance, the cause of Wei syndrome is held to be a febrile disease and this may link with some ideas about the causes of MS.

'Stagnation' is a TCM term generally used to describe the inhibition of movement, often the most obvious symptom in neurological diseases. The word refers specifically to the movement of Qi, Blood or any body fluid. This slowing or stoppage of the flow of circulating substances is caused by blockages which may result in localized pain. Stagnation may arise from an External Pathogenic invasion or from an internal change produced by the presence of one or more Pathogens. The External Pathogens are Wind, Cold, Damp and Heat – essentially climatic influences.

Bi syndrome

Bi syndrome comprises a group of symptoms vitally connected with the general health and circulation of the body fluids. The body fluid is in a constant state

Table 1.2 A traditional Chinese medicine view of the Brain

Region	Function	Meridians	Useful points	Notes
Lower Brain	Survival Respiration Digestion Sleep	Lung Large Intestine Stomach Spleen	GB 39 GV 15 GV 16	Basic survival functions Brain and Marrow points Same-side treatment
Mid Brain	Movement and interaction	Heart Small Intestine Urinary Bladder Kidney	GB 10 GB 11 GB 34 GB 39 Kid 1	Getting to know yourself and the world Treat contralaterally
Upper Brain	Differentiation, personality	Pericardium Sanjiao (TE) Gallbladder Liver	PE 8 TE 3 GV 20	Judgements and evaluations, the ability to change Sensory organs Same-side treatment

After Jacob (10).

of movement, whether Blood flowing in blood vessels or the interstitial fluid moving slowly between the structures and under the skin or the more precisely defined Jin Ye fluids.

When Pathogenic factors invade the body they enter the most superficial meridians, particularly the Urinary Bladder and Small Intestine, and cause a general slowing of the flow. This affects both Qi and Blood. When fluids are slowed they tend to thicken, stagnate and become sticky. This process is the beginning of the formation of what is defined in TCM as Phlegm (Figure 1.3).

Each of the External Pathogenic factors, Wind, Cold, Damp and Heat, produces characteristic symptoms and this leads to the different classifications of Bi syndrome. It is also sometimes called painful obstruction syndrome and all of the symptoms will affect movement to some degree.

Wind invasion

This is characterized by symptom mobility; the resulting pain tends to be acute and move randomly from one area of the body to another. The muscles and joints are sore, but the quality of pain can change quickly, sometimes manifesting as numbness or at other times as a sharp pain. In terms of neurological illness any type of tremor or uncoordinated muscle movement is associated with Wind.

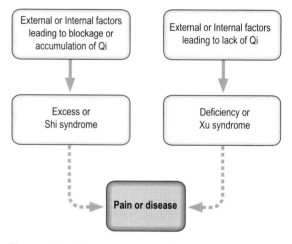

Figure 1.3 ● Origin of pain from Bi syndrome.

Since Wind is a Yang Pathogen it tends to affect the upper part of the body, often typified by an upward movement. The symptoms can appear and disappear very suddenly. This type of Bi is known as wandering Bi or migratory Bi.

The patient will usually express a fear of wind or describe an increase in discomfort in windy weather. It is rare that only Wind is involved: there will usually be elements of Damp and Cold as well, but Wind is predominant. There can be sweating due to the opening of the pores by the invading Wind.

Wind Bi suggested points

- BL 12 Fengmen
- GV 14 Dazhui
- BL 18 Ganshu
- GB 31 Fengshi
- BL 17 Geshu

All points to clear wind except BL 17 and BL 18, which nourish blood in order to expel the Pathogen.

Cold invasion

This is characterized by severe pain and limitation of movement and is often called painful Bi. It is usually unilateral. The pain is often described as deep and 'gnawing'. The cold is perceived as being capable of freezing the tissues, contracting and blocking the meridian. Any blockage of the meridian causes pain. The pain with cold has a constant site, and is frequently accompanied by a loss of joint movement, mainly due to the accompanying blood stagnation. This may be found in neurological conditions where muscle atrophy has led to wasting and contractures.

This type of pain is always improved by warmth and movement but made worse by cold and rest and described as being worse in cold weather. Although an accepted physiotherapy treatment for some arthritic conditions, cryotherapy would not be recommended for the pain produced by this type of pathogenic invasion.

Cold Bi suggested points

- ST 36 Zusanli
- CV 6 Qihai
- BL 10 Tianzhu
- GV 14 Dazhui
- GV 3 Yaoyangguan
- BL 23 Shenshu

Use Moxibustion as a source of heat.

Damp invasion

This is characterized by soreness and swelling in the muscles and joints with a feeling of heaviness and numbness in the limbs. It is worse in damp weather. It generally has a slow onset. It is sometimes referred to as fixed Bi, because it is very localized. Where wandering or Wind Bi tends to affect the upper part of the body, this tends to sink to the lowest level as liquid would. There is a feeling of heaviness, tiredness and inertia in the limbs and the affected parts are often swollen. The pain is heavy and dull in nature and onset is gradual. The skin is often affected, becoming thickened and slightly discoloured. Patients feel worse when the weather conditions are humid, damp or foggy. Clearly this type of situation is associated with neurological problems where lower-limb movement has become difficult or impossible.

Damp Bi suggested points

- SP 9 Yinlingquan
- SP 6 Sanyinjiao
- GB 34 Yanglingquan
- ST 36 Zusanli
- BL 20 Pishu

All points clear Damp and aid in the movement of Qi.

Heat Bi

This can be either the invasion of the body by an external Heat Pathogen or it can arise from an invasion by the other Pathogens, Wind, Cold and Damp, that has already occurred. It presents a complex picture when arising as a superficial syndrome since it will often show symptoms characteristic of the other pathogens. Some authorities describe this situation as the result of Wei Qi opposing invading pathogens.

The patient will have red, swollen and painful joints. There will be marked loss of movement as in acute inflammatory arthritic conditions. The patient is also likely to show some signs of systemic illness, with fever, a hot sensation in the affected tissue, irritability, nervousness or restlessness, thirst and a dry mouth. Further heat of any kind makes the patient uncomfortable. This is included for completeness but rarely found in neurological conditions.

There is a TCM saying: 'better Cold than Heat'. This is a useful guide to treatment priorities: it is nearly always better to clear Heat first. This is primarily because it is more difficult to clear Heat than provide Heat. Also if the Cold condition is treated first by applying Heat, perhaps in the form of moxibustion, the Heat condition would be made worse, perhaps increasing the pain.

Heat Bi suggested points

- LI 11 Quchi
- LI 4 Hegu
- GV 14 Dazhui

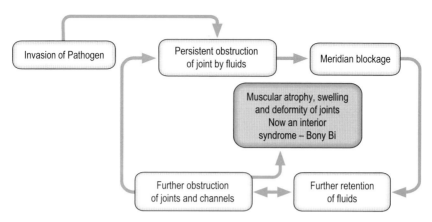

Figure 1.4 • Progression of Bi syndrome from external to internal. (Reproduced with permission from Hopwood V. Acupuncture in Physiotherapy. Oxford: Butterworth Heinemann: 2004.)

Use meridian end points, Spring, Well and Stream points.

All the forms of Bi syndrome discussed so far represent an acute type of condition, with the potential for leading to an excess internal syndrome (Figure 1.4).

Bony Bi

This is the end result of the slowing and congealing of the body fluids and subsequent Phlegm in the joint spaces. The deformity of the joints that results is seen as an accumulation of solidified Phlegm. There is often severe pain and a marked loss of range of movement. The patient complains of heaviness and numbness in the affected limb. Bony spurs around the joint margins can be seen on X-ray.

This situation is strongly linked with the Kidney. The connection between Kidney and bone formation is cited but this type of Bi syndrome takes a long time to evolve and is usually associated with the advent of old age and the general weakening of Kidney energies. It may be complicated by osteoporosis. It is often common after long-standing neurological damage.

Bony Bi suggested points

- ST 40 Fenglong
- BL 23 Shenshu
- BL 11 Dashu
- GB 39 Xuanzhong

These points are used to clear Phlegm and strengthen Kidney and bone.

The preceding forms of Bi syndrome are those encountered in normal clinical practice. However it must be understood that the changes leading to these joint problems and observed symptoms are not confined to the joints. Bi syndrome can be interpreted as a blockage of Qi and Blood capable of attacking any of the body systems. This is often seen as a progression from involvement of a tissue to involvement of one or several of the major Zang Fu organs.

The links obey the laws of TCM Zang Fu theory:

- Tendon Bi can lead to problems with the liver.
- Vascular Bi can lead to heart problems.
- Muscle Bi will have an impact on the spleen.
- Skin Bi will affect the lung.
- Bone Bi is closely linked with Kidney Bi.

Bi syndrome associated with Zang Fu organs

Tendon/Liver Bi

This is of particular interest to physiotherapists since it is always linked to pain and weakness in muscles and joints. These joints tend to flexion contracture as in Dupuytren's contracture, resisting passive extension. Previous physical trauma may contribute to this condition, as in the case of chronic whiplash syndrome. This situation may also be associated with the kind of chronic contractures seen in the late stages of MS or stroke.

Frequent urination may be a symptom along with a marked increase in appetite. The patient often complains of a feeling of cold within the tendons. There may be a degree of irritability and other mental symptoms indicating the involvement of the liver. Sciatica is sometimes considered as a form of tendon Bi.

Local points will be most successful to warm and free the channels and relax the tendons but distal points, particularly Shu Stream points, are also helpful. The Liver will need support from BL 18 Ganshu or GB 34 Yanglingquan.

Vascular/Heart Bi

This is most commonly identified by numbness and pins and needles accompanied by pain and soreness in the affected area and is often found as a neurological symptom. The pain itself is stabbing and fixed, often worse at night, typical of that caused by blood stagnation. The pulse will be weak or may even disappear, indicating the blockage and resulting emptiness of the blood vessels. It has been compared to arteritis in Western medicine.

The fact that this is linked to general circulation disturbances means that there may be accompanying symptoms such as skin changes, light rashes and a feeling of fullness in the body giving rise to general unease and malaise. Since the Shen or Spirit is disturbed by the involvement of the Heart there may be marked anxiety and distress, continuous sighing and overbreathing. This may lead to a form of late-onset asthma.

This problem is linked directly with smoking and an overindulgent lifestyle. The link made between smoking and arterial disease in Western medicine is too obvious for comment here. Internal Heat produced by the excess food and alcohol can be responsible for the decrease of Yin and Qi, leading to easy invasion by the Wind, Cold and Damp.

The following points may be used to relieve blood stasis:

- LI 4 Hegu
- LI 10 Shousanli
- TE 6 Zhigou
- CV 12 Zhongwan
- SP 10 Xuehai
- SP 6 Sanyinjiao
- ST 36 Zusanli
- ST 40 Fenglong

Some of the above points could also be added to the local points used for the painful joint.

It is difficult to separate the circulation disturbances from abnormal blood pressure. Where acupuncture has been shown to decrease mean blood pressure significantly, it would seem a logical use of the intervention in this type of case [11]. A recent review investigating the actions of many complementary therapies in reducing high blood pressure came to the conclusion that acupuncture may have some value [12].

Antihypertensive drug therapy is efficient and reduces morbidity and mortality; however it is expensive and causes undesirable side-effects in some patients. Acupuncture effectively lowered both systolic and diastolic blood pressure after 6 weeks of TCM acupuncture in a recent study; however the effect did not outlast the duration of the treatment [13]. More work is anticipated in this field.

Muscle/Spleen Bi

The characteristic signs of muscle Bi are stiffness and coldness in the particular muscle group. It is not really the function of the muscle, rather the muscle bulk, which is affected. This means that there may be a degree of muscle atrophy and loss of strength due to that. There will be generalized weakness and easy fatigue with only small effort, with excessive sweating.

The Zang Fu function of the Spleen is to maintain muscle bulk from the transformation of food so there is a direct TCM link to the digestive process and the patient may have symptoms of indigestion. Overindulgence at the table is implicated as a partial cause of the Spleen problems. The Spleen symptoms may also include shortness of breath, a tight feeling in the chest, an occasional productive cough, loss of appetite and poor digestion. Examination of the tongue will be helpful; the characteristic tooth-marked body of the tongue will indicate the involvement of the Zang Fu, in particular the Spleen and the Kidney.

Selection of Jing River points will be important as these points give rise to an overflow of Qi into the surrounding muscle tissue, the so-called 'muscle sinews' or 'tendinomuscular meridians'.

As in the other categories, local and distal points to the affected joints are used.

Skin/Lung Bi

The characteristic symptoms of this syndrome are a cold sensation and often numbness of the skin. This will often be described in conditions such as MS. The link with the Lung, since the skin is governed by the Lungs, may mean that there is shortness of breath, manifested in rapid superficial panting. The Wei Qi, produced by the Lungs, should circulate just below the skin and this is prevented in Skin Bi. This sort of syndrome is thought to occur more commonly when the patient is grieving or seriously worried about something.

Points to support the Lungs and strengthen the Wei Qi could be useful with Yintang (Ex HN3) to raise the spirits. The cause of the grief or anxiety should be addressed, if possible. If it is depression associated with the disease process then it will be hard to cure but may respond to the supraspinal effects of acupuncture.

Bone/Kidney Bi

The characteristic symptoms of soreness and pain in the joints are usually accompanied by stiffness and lack of mobility. Patients occasionally complain of heaviness in the affected limb. Kidney energies are said to decrease with advancing age so the fact that the joints and the spine tend to become stiff and limited in movement, resulting in the need to walk with some kind of artificial aid in this syndrome, tallies quite clearly with the universal picture of old age. There are many similarities between these symptoms and those of Parkinson's disease (see Chapter 7). As is the way in most medicine, although some symptoms can be collected together in clear groups to form the syndromes, patients rarely present with such a clear pattern.

The Bi syndrome is a very interesting concept, based on the general idea that full body health is only possible if the Qi or vital energy found in the meridians and organs is able to move freely, flowing to where it is needed most and away from areas of pathological stagnation and concentration [14].

Wei Bi or atrophy syndrome

This is a definition of a neurological condition found in ancient Chinese writings. Wei is translated as 'withered' and implies the loss of muscle bulk or wasting as the direct cause of loss of movement. A loss of muscle condition due to the failure of the Qi to nourish the muscles and tendons is understood to lead to limp, feeble limbs and the eventual inability to walk or move independently.

This can also be described as 'Wei Bi' where Bi indicates an inability to walk because the foot cannot be lifted adequately.

Atrophy or Wei syndrome is characterized by a weakness of the four limbs, often uneven in nature, leading eventually to paralysis. It is often seen as a description of MS, although MS also has other definitive symptoms. It is also used to describe infantile poliomyelitis.

The theories informing a diagnosis of atrophy syndrome involve the invasion of Pathogenic Heat in the initial stages. This Heat dries up the body fluids and by doing so injures both the muscles and tendons. The original invasion also involves both the skin and the Lungs and manifests as a febrile disease (Figure 1.5).

Atrophy syndrome usually results directly from concentration of Exterior Heat in the Lungs, causing injury to body fluid. The general treatment principle will be to tonify Yin and Jin Ye or fluid balance. Most used are the Yang Ming meridians [15]. Stomach points are used for the lower limb and Large Intestine points for the upper limb. Qi deficiency of the Spleen and Stomach, often exacerbated by irregular food intake, can produce similar symptoms, such as weakness of the limbs, with movement impaired but still present. Often there will be indigestion with bloating and faecal frequency. The patient will dislike being cold and have a pale complexion. This can often be seen after a long debilitating illness.

Common TCM syndromes associated with Wei Bi

Deficiencies of Liver and Kidney
Liver Yin Xu
In this syndrome Yin becomes too weak to control Yang, resulting in symptoms of Heat in the upper part of the body and Cold and deficiency in the lower part. This is strongly associated with Kidney Yin Xu. It is linked to hypertension, nervous disorders, chronic eye problems and menstrual problems.

The symptoms include depression, dizziness, afternoon fever and flushed cheeks, dry eyes and blurring of vision. The patient may have warm palms and soles, headache or tinnitus. There may be tremors in the muscles and fragile flaking nails. Also seen is disturbance of menstrual patterns, general irritability and nervous tension.

Treatment
* Tonify Liver and Kidney Yin.
* LR 2 Xingjian. Fire point disperses. Fire in the Liver.

Figure 1.5 • Origin of Wei syndrome patterns. (After Ross J. Zang Fu, The Organ System of Traditional Chinese Medicine. Edinburgh: Churchill Livingstone, 1984.)

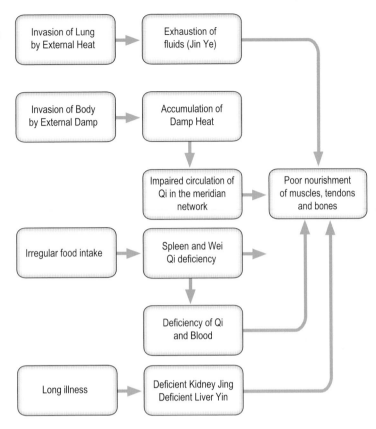

- LR 3 Taichong. Liver source point.
- SP 6 Sanyinjiao. Tonifies Spleen, balances Liver and regulates Blood.
- LR 13 Zhangmen. Front Mu point for the Spleen.
- LR 8 Ququan. Water source point, tonifies Yin.
- KI 3 Taixi. Tonifies Kidney Yin and Yang.
- GB 25 Jingmen. Front Mu point for the Kidney.
- KI 7 Fuliu. Tonifies Kidney. Metal point.

Liver Qi and Yang Xu

Liver Qi Xu occurs first but is often followed by a combination of the two syndromes. This combination may occur in chronic fatigue syndrome, myalgic encephalomyelitis (ME) or MS. Symptoms include mood swings, poor digestion, problems in the eyes and tendons and muscle spasms. There may be a stifling sensation in the chest, bloating in the abdomen and irregular bowels with either constipation or loose stools. The patient may complain of sadness, fear and difficulty making decisions with a feeling of inner cold, severe heartburn and acid reflux.

Treatment

- Strengthen Liver Qi and tonify Kidney and Spleen.
- LR 3 Taichong. Liver Source point. Balances Liver, moves Qi.
- BL 18 Ganshu. Back Shu point for the Liver.
- KI 7 Fuliu. Tonifies both Kidney and Liver.
- SP 6 Sanyinjiao. Tonifies Spleen, balances Liver and regulates Blood.
- GB 34 Yanglingquan. Cools damp Heat anywhere in the body.
- LR 14 Qimen. Front Mu point for the Liver.

General deficiencies of Liver and Kidney may also be seen. These include:

- old age, or general debility following illness
- hyposensitivity of extremities leading to weakness, leading to paralysis
- sore lower back, dysmenorrhoea, premature ejaculation
- dizziness, vertigo, fatigue

- pale tongue
- deep, thready and weak pulse

The treatment here would be to tonify the Kidney Jing and the Liver (for muscles and tendons).

Blood stagnation

This often occurs after a stroke or some kind of tissue trauma. In Chinese terms it indicates that Phlegm remains in the channels, obstructing the smooth flow of Qi. Treatment is primarily to promote Blood circulation. The symptoms can include weakness, leading to numbness and possible spasm leading to paralysis. There may be a purple tongue and a choppy thready pulse.

Feng syndromes

In TCM all involuntary muscular tremor, quivering or unintentional movement is attributed to the stirring of internal Wind. This is a more profound change than that produced by an invasion of external Wind.

These tremors may be associated with Parkinson's disease, cerebellar disease, frontal lobe tumours, benign essential (familial) tremor, alcohol and caffeine toxicity and drug use or withdrawal. Patients who are very anxious are also seen as being more prone to disturbances of internal Wind. Older people with symptoms of Yin deficiency, Phlegm, Pathogenic Heat and Liver Yang rising are also vulnerable to Wind stroke. Often the onset of such symptoms will be apparently sudden, but tremors can also appear in more chronic situations.

Clinical manifestations of internal Wind are many and frequently associated with neurological diseases. As well as tremors and tics, numbness, severe dizziness and vertigo, in more severe cases convulsions, unconsciousness and even opisthotonus (an extreme tetanic arching of the spine) may be seen.

An attack of Wind or Cold on the YangMing or ShaoYang meridians can result in localized symptoms; in particular accumulation of Wind Phlegm in the channels can produce muscle tic or twitch, often seen in facial paralysis (Bell's palsy).

It is interesting that all these symptoms would be considered by Western medicine as evidence of damage to either the central or autonomic nervous systems but, by identifying the early stages of Wind or Feng influences, it may be possible to treat these and prevent the later, more catastrophic effects.

Table 1.3 Points for Feng syndromes	
Point	Comment
LI 4 Hegu	Upper quadrant
LI 11 Quchi	Upper quadrant
LI 20 Yinxiang	Face
GB 20 Fengchi	Neck and shoulder
GB 21 Jianjing	Neck and shoulder
GB 31 Fengshi	Lower limb
GB 41 Zulinqi	Lower limb
BL 12 Fengmen	General
BL 62 Shenmai	Link to central nervous system/extra meridians
GV 20 Baihui	Link to central nervous system/extra meridians

The four main signs of a potential Feng syndrome are clearly shown in the tongue. Wind tends to produce stiffness, deviation, movement or quivering or a combination of all four. Fire makes the tongue red in colour and blood stasis makes the tongue a reddish purple colour. Phlegm in the system produces a swollen tongue with a sticky coating.

Some acupuncture authorities advise that any elderly person with numbness of the fingers, slightly slurred speech and a tongue showing any of the previously described colours should take immediate steps to avoid overwork, excessive stress and a poor diet. A short-term preventive measure would be direct Moxibustion on GB 39 Xuanzhong and ST 36 Zusanli [16].

Similar points to dispel wind, as in the case of wind Bi, mentioned earlier, can also be chosen. Some of the more effective are listed in Table 1.3.

Summary

The three groups of syndromes are all associated with neurological illness to a greater or lesser degree. It would be reasonable to combine these ideas and perhaps suggest a 'neurological syndrome' informed by the theories of pathogens and Zang Fu. The points recommended are frequently repeated.

When neurological diseases are analysed symptom by symptom, the problems experienced by the patient include a wide range of changes and deficits, most of which are common to all the identified conditions, although differing in severity. All of these can be directly related to the malfunction of part of the nervous system, as we currently understand it. Taken in the broadest possible sense, and in no particular order, the following are symptoms which one could expect to find in a patient with severe MS:

- decreased mobility
- autonomic changes
- fatigue
- muscle spasm
- contractures
- cognitive damage
- communication problems
- emotional lability
- breathing and coughing problems
- bladder symptoms
- visual symptoms.

Very few patients are unlucky enough to suffer from all these problems but the nature of nerve damage implicit in the diagnosis of the condition means that they are all possible. Neurological conditions are often difficult to distinguish (with the possible exception of a straightforward stroke), because they have a great deal in common with one another. Table 1.4 shows the symptoms described above and how they relate to some of the diseases commonly treated by neurophysiotherapists.

The full selection is rarely found in each specified disease but the potential remains. The perceived physiological reason may also differ but the end result for the patient is the same. The double symbols indicate some of the defining diagnostic symptoms. When these symptoms are considered from the vantage point of TCM theory they fall into patterns or syndromes suggesting their treatment.

It becomes evident that the treatment of cerebrovascular accident will not be dissimilar to that of MS, apart from the obvious problem of laterality, because the basic physiological functions within the body will need to be stimulated in similar ways. This is heresy to a neurology physiotherapist and quite possibly to a traditional acupuncturist too. However the staging proposed by Blackwell and MacPherson (see Chapter 8), will apply across the range of neurological problems, with minor adjustments, because it is firmly rooted in Zang Fu theory, which in itself regards organ physiology as function [17].

Table 1.4 Neurological symptoms

Symptom	Multiple sclerosis	Cerebrovascular accident	Parkinson's disease	Motor neurone disease
Decreased mobility	○	○	○	○
Fatigue	○ ○	X	○	○
Respiratory problems	○	○	X	○ ○
Muscle spasm	○	○	○	○
Contractures	○	○	○	○
Autonomic changes	○	○	○ ○	○
Cognition/mood	○	○	○	X
Communication	○	○	○ ○	○
Bladder problems	○	○	X	○
Visual problems	○	○	X	X

○ ○ diagnostic symptom; ○ symptom often present; X symptom rarely present.

References

[1] Worsley JR. Talking about Acupuncture in New York. England: Worsley; 1982.

[2] Rosen MR. The heart remembers: clinical implications. Lancet 2001;357:468–71.

[3] Larre C, Rochat de La Vallee E. The Secret Treatise of the Spiritual Orchid. London: Monkey Press; 2003. p. 69.

[4] Maciocia G. The Foundations of Chinese Medicine. New York: Churchill Livingstone; 1989.

[5] Beinfeld H, Korngold E. Between heaven and earth. New York: Ballantine Books; 1992.

[6] Spiritual Pivot or Ling Shu. [Wu Jing-Nuan, Trans.]. Honolulu: University of Hawaii Press; 2002.

[7] Dey T. Soothing the troubled mind. Brookline, Massachusetts: Paradigm Publications; 1999.

[8] McMillin DL, Richards DG, Mein EA, et al. The Abdominal Brain and Enteric Nervous System. J Altern Complementary Med 1999;5(6):575–86.

[9] Ross J, Zang Fu. The Organ System of Traditional Chinese Medicine. Edinburgh: Churchill Livingstone; 1984.

[10] Jacob JH. The Acupuncturist's Clinical Handbook. 5th ed. New York: Integrative Wellness; 2003.

[11] Yin C, Seo B, Park HJ, et al. Acupuncture, a promising adjunctive therapy for essential hypertension: a double-blind, randomized, controlled trial. Neurol Res 2007;29(Suppl. 1): S98–S103.

[12] Nahas R. Complementary and alternative medicine approaches to blood pressure reduction: An evidence-based review. Can Fam Physician 2008;54(11):1529–33.

[13] Flachskampf FA, Gallasch J, Gefeller O, et al. Randomized trial of acupuncture to lower blood pressure. Circulation 2007;115 (24):3121–9.

[14] Hopwood V. Acupuncture in Physiotherapy. Oxford: Butterworth Heinemann; 2004.

[15] Xu H, Ni Y, Liu Y, et al. Diseases of Internal Medicine. Acupuncture Treatment of Common Diseases Based upon Differentiation of Syndromes. Beijing: The Peoples Medical Publishing House; 1988. p. 243–50.

[16] Maciocia G. Wind-stroke. The Practice of Chinese Medicine. Edinburgh: Churchill Livingstone; 1994. p. 665–84.

[17] Blackwell R, MacPherson H. Multiple Sclerosis. Staging and patient management. Journal of Chinese Medicine 1993;42:5–12.

Researching a complex intervention

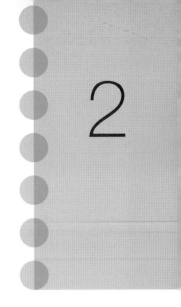

2

CHAPTER CONTENTS

KEY POINTS

- Establishing acupuncture within modern medicine has been problematic.
- A historical blindness to the wider effects of acupuncture has caused confusion in the physiotherapy profession.
- There is a degree of uncertainty about the mechanisms of acupuncture but there is also uncertainty as to whether this actually matters in clinic.
- The definition of Western medical acupuncture does not entirely rule out the use of points with a Chinese background.
- There is certainly confusion about these facts in acupuncture research, principally in regard to the usefulness of a placebo intervention.
- Clear research protocols are needed to attract realistic funding.

Introduction

Acupuncture as an adjunctive technique has been widely accepted within the physiotherapy profession and has now been established for more than 25 years. Initially, interest was shown in the potential pain-relieving properties of the technique and it was mostly adopted in chronic pain situations. Since this was where most of the early research was concentrated, the idea of a strong evidence base lent support to wider use.

Western medical practitioners have had a hard time accepting the traditional Chinese medicine (TCM) philosophies and theories, often failing to see that this is a complete medical paradigm and not just an isolated technique. It is also worth noting that physiotherapists have never been short of useful treatments for their patients and often chose to learn additional techniques without intending that their general practice would change very much. This meant that the somewhat simplified acupuncture techniques, similar to those used by the 'barefoot doctors' after the Chinese Revolution, gained an enthusiastic audience among physiotherapists in the early years. The research available 25 years ago was unsophisticated and only really investigated simple pain relief. Those taking a full TCM training course found themselves in the minority and had a difficult job defending some of their practice. This particular early emphasis on acupuncture exclusively for pain control only served to isolate further those therapists prepared to undertake other forms of treatment and for many years this was discouraged.

It seems odd now, when we consider that the effect of acupuncture is at least partially mediated through the nervous system, that this stricture was widely applied within the physiotherapy profession. It can be argued that it was partly because, as the research techniques became more sophisticated and the randomized controlled clinical trials (RCTs) began to show negative (or, at any rate, less positive) results, physiotherapy practitioners lost some faith in the technique and were less prepared to tackle any condition not on the pain list or even on the National Institutes of Health list [1], although that did include conditions that would have been classified as neurological.

National Institutes of Health List 1998

A claim was made for promising results in the following conditions:

- adult postoperative and chemotherapy nausea and vomiting
- postoperative dental pain
- stroke rehabilitation
- headache
- menstrual cramps
- tennis elbow
- fibromyalgia
- myofascial pain
- osteoarthritis
- low-back pain
- carpal tunnel syndrome
- asthma.

This is an interesting, if eclectic, mix which reflects the random quality and quantity of research at the time.

Research concentrated on the physiological effects mediated by the nervous system, with some of the early work by Andersson and Lundeberg [2–6] providing some answers. Their work highlighted the similarities between the physiological effects of acupuncture and the more familiar effects of exercise, reassuring physiotherapists that the results of their acupuncture treatment could be understood within their own profession, although in a limited context.

Some new thinking was required and, since physiotherapists were well versed in neurophysiology, clinical reasoning began to centre on that. Lynley Bradnam was probably the first to offer a useful structure to support clinical decisions and point choices [7–9]. She suggested that if the known pathology was carefully considered then the choice of appropriate points for musculoskeletal pains would automatically become easy. This approach overcomes the credibility gap often found when a therapist chooses points from a Western perspective but finds a need to extend or amplify the effects by reverting to poorly understood TCM choices, because the simple formulae do not offer much by way of progression when patient improvement slows or stalls. Once the physiological mechanisms are better understood, there is no conflict. This approach also serves as a useful foundation for clinical reasoning when moving beyond treating just pain and considering the wider implications of treating neurological patients.

Although generally less concerned with the specific application of acupuncture in neurology, medical doctors in the UK and around the world have begun to concentrate on what is termed Western medical acupuncture, claiming that acupuncture is increasingly understood through scientifically plausible mechanisms. White, in the journal *Acupuncture in Medicine*, states that there is 'evidence from systematic reviews that acupuncture is superior to placebo for treating nausea, chronic back and knee pain, tension headache and postoperative pain' but continues that now phase II studies to determine the optimal acupuncture treatment should be encouraged [10]. He emphasizes that, although acupuncture involves only minimal technology, there are infinite complexities and uncertainties about the mechanisms involved.

It is useful to quote the definition of Western medical acupuncture in full as this is the thinking that underscores a great deal, although not all, of this textbook.

> Western medical acupuncture is a therapeutic modality involving the insertion of fine needles. It is an adaptation of Chinese acupuncture using current knowledge of anatomy, physiology and pathology and the principles of evidence-based medicine. While Western medical acupuncture has evolved from Chinese acupuncture, its practitioners no longer adhere to concepts such as Yin/Yang and circulation of Qi, and regard acupuncture as part of conventional medicine rather than a complete 'alternative medical system'. It acts mainly by stimulating the nervous system, and its known mode of action includes local antidromic axon reflexes, segmental and extrasegmental neuromodulation, and other central nervous system effects. Western medical acupuncture is principally used by conventional health practitioners, most commonly in primary care. It is mainly used to treat musculoskeletal pain, including myofascial trigger point pain. It is also effective for postoperative pain and nausea. Practitioners of Western medical acupuncture tend to pay less attention than classical acupuncturists to

choosing one point over another, though they generally choose classical points as the best places to stimulate the nervous system. The design and interpretation of clinical studies is constrained by lack of knowledge of the appropriate dosage of acupuncture, and the likelihood that any form of needling used as a usual control procedure in 'placebo-controlled' studies may be active. Western medical acupuncture justifies an unbiased evaluation of its role in a modern health service [11].

Clinical reasoning and acupuncture

Evidence-based medicine

Evidence-based medicine is defined as 'the conscientious, explicit and judicious use of current best evidence in making decisions about the care of individual patients' [12]. It has been argued that evidence-based approaches represent a narrow reductionism that ignores clinical judgement and experience and encourages a slavish reliance on statistical methodology, in particular a dogmatic support of the RCT [13]. It is nonetheless essential that we attempt to use what is still considered best evidence, even though not all of the current research work is of compelling quality.

There are two types of evidence that inform acupuncture practice. The standard RCT certainly has a place and information from these trials has slowly accumulated, making some choices of points or technique more valid than others. However, it must be remembered that the therapeutic encounter in all its richness is very poorly represented by most medical research protocols.

To counter this we also have access to the empirical evidence provided by historical sources, a form of consensus medicine. This has been reproduced since the first written records in a question/answer dialogue, offering a form of intellectual debate, although the terms and concepts are often unfamiliar to a Western health professional. Single case studies are widely published in the East and are also a valuable source of information, although ranked very low in the scale of 'good' evidence.

It is a truism that all medicine is now exhaustively researched before it is applied to a patient and the process for the discovery and subsequent release of new drugs tends to follow a well-worn pattern. The thrust of acupuncture research has been different to that for new drugs and treatments.

This is generally because acupuncture is already in use. Indeed, it has been in use for at least 1000 years in parts of the world and shows no signs of dying out. This has been recognized by the World Health Organization, which has supported it in several ways, recommending minimum training standards, discussing terminology and assembling definitive point locations to make research methodologies more accurate [14]. Now, with definitive locations of acupuncture points agreed in the main by the major acupuncture nations, China, Korea and Japan, the possibility of having precisely repeatable treatment protocols incorporated into research projects is a real one [15]. This will naturally link in with the move to record and report all acupuncture intervention details in a scientific paper, as set out in the Standards for Reporting Interventions in Controlled Trials of Acupuncture (STRICTA) guidelines [16].

Good reporting is essential and, in addition to the STRICTA guidelines, adherence to the advice given by the Consolidated Standards for Reporting of Trials (CONSORT) organization, particularly that for non-pharmacologic interventions [17], will assist in gaining and maintaining scientific credibility for all acupuncture trials.

Nonetheless, the early work done when introducing a new drug on to the market usually begins with an investigation into the mechanism, followed by studies set up to look at the initial effectiveness and, provided the results are promising, efficacy and then safety. The progression of acupuncture research has often appeared to be reversed because the most immediately important factor has been seen as safety, since it is already widely used. Initially, studies were set up to see how it was being used and whether there were associated risks [18, 19].

This has had an effect on the acceptance of acupuncture by the medical community at large. The two major studies published in 2001 [18, 19] were very positive and provided excellent confirmation of the safety of this intervention. A total of 66 000 treatment episodes in the two studies provided very few adverse events, 'the most common minor adverse events being bleeding, needling pain, and aggravation of symptoms; however, aggravation was followed by resolution of symptoms in 70% of cases. There were 43 significant minor adverse events reported, a rate of 14 per 10 000, of which 13 (30%) interfered with daily activities' [18]. No serious adverse events were reported in the study by MacPherson et al. either [19]. The results gave rise to the editorial comment in the *British Medical*

Journal that: 'While the risks of acupuncture cannot be discounted, it certainly seems, in skilled hands, one of the safer forms of medical intervention' [20].

The issue of safety having been dealt with, the way was opened for the RCTs and the results should have justified the inclusion of acupuncture in normal/orthodox medical practice a long time ago. Nothing is that easy however and the results have been equivocal. For every resounding success there have been several trials where the numbers were too few, the protocols too vague, the controls not adequate and the general impression given that acupuncture was not working.

Sometimes this impression was produced by the fact that the acupuncture selected for the condition was hopelessly inadequate, consisting of few treatments or limited points. This arose when the researchers were not acupuncturists and had little understanding of the clinical application of the intervention under scrutiny. A study which unfortunately became a source of much amusement in acupuncture circles [21] claimed that acupuncture had no place in the treatment of rheumatoid arthritis. On careful reading, the intervention proved to have been a single acupuncture point, Liv 3, Taichong, used on five occasions and retained only for 4 minutes each time. This conformed to neither TCM nor Western medical good acupuncture practice. The paper was subsequently heavily criticized but the damage was done [22]. Appearing, as it did, in an influential medical journal, it probably set the use of acupuncture by physiotherapists in this field back by a good 10 years.

Currently there is an increase in research into the mechanisms, including much functional magnetic resonance imaging work examining the effect of acupuncture on the brain, principally by Napadow and his group [23, 24]. Langevin et al., working in parallel, investigated the effect of needle manipulation on connective tissue, looking for a mechanical effect [25].

This change in focus is partly because, as the research community has worked through this process, it has become plain that the entire mechanism is not yet understood. We have parts of the picture but there are still many questions to be asked of what is now recognized as a complex intervention. Also the important German RCTs (Modellvorhaben Akupunktur), where both the true acupuncture and the sham control showed significant effects over normal care, have emphasized the problem of finding an inert placebo for the complex intervention that is acupuncture [26].

It is clear that the traditional construction of an RCT requires the use of a placebo control in order to be considered as first-class evidence but it is debatable whether this is the most appropriate way to investigate an intervention like acupuncture. If we do not fully understand all the neural pathways and mechanisms, how can we be sure that any placebo has no effect? Some researchers are exploring this issue and their early work seems to indicate that there is an additional response in the brain to real acupuncture, as compared to the sham procedures [27]. The different strands for acupuncture research are shown in Table 2.1.

Table 2.1 Useful summary of brain imaging correlates

Evidence	Sources
Patient's expectations of positive acupuncture effect (response to non-invasive sham acupuncture) causes greater brain activation than no expectation of effect (response to skin prick)	Pariente et al. (27)
Brain activity in response to acupuncture is distinct from activity in response to sharp pain	Hui et al. (49)
Acupuncture-induced clinical improvements in chronic pain and carpal tunnel syndrome correlate with changes in brain activity	Harris et al. (50), Newberg et al. (51), Napadow et al. (52)
Whether traditional indications of acupuncture point function, e.g. improvement of sight or hearing, predict acupuncture-induced changes in specific brain regions, e.g. visual or auditory cortices, remains controversial; both positive and negative findings	Positive findings Cho et al. (53), Li et al. (54) Negative findings Gareus et al. (55), Hu et al. (56)

From Hammerschlag et al. (57).

Another major problem has been the research carried out in mainland China. Ostensibly excellent, with very large numbers included in all the trials and a medical community accustomed to using this type of technique on a population equally familiar with needles, it has been largely ignored by Western researchers. This is primarily because most studies did not include a group not receiving acupuncture. Looked at from the Chinese perspective this was quite straightforward as it was perceived to be unethical to withhold a modality that worked. Unfortunately from the perspective of the Western scientific community, if there was no control group that did not receive acupuncture, the comparison of one type of acupuncture technique with another, which was what most trials did, was simply invalid.

Clinical reasoning supporting the use of acupuncture

The process of clinical reasoning as it pertains to everyday practice is rather more than the application of theory to practice. It is defined as a cognitive process of critical analysis and reflection that supports decision-making. The purpose of this process is the well-being of the patients. The treatments are tailored to meet their individual needs, skills and priorities. Applying treatments on the basis of diagnosis only is something done by 'technicians' while those engaging in clinical reflection in order to make techniques directly relevant to their clients' lives are demonstrating 'professionalism' [28].

Clinical reasoning as understood in physiotherapy is a blend of theoretical knowledge, research evidence and experiential knowledge, with meaning and context provided by clients or patients themselves. The problem-solving process includes assessment of the situation, planning the intervention, the intervention itself, some kind of evaluation, preferably an objective outcome measure and then modification if necessary.

An integral part of this approach to therapies is the development and acquisition of treatment models and the following considerations will add up to a reasonable framework, applicable to most conditions, very close to that evolved by Bradnam [9].

Since acupuncture is at least partly mediated by the nervous system it is important to ascertain the nerve supply to the painful site and the surrounding area. Acupoints are always associated with either cutaneous nerves or muscular nerves. Those close to

muscular nerves tend to become tender more quickly than those associated with smaller nerves. As long as the practitioner is familiar with the muscular anatomy Table 2.2 indicates the associated nerve roots.

Linked with the nerve root are the dermatome, myotome and sclerotome sharing that supply. In order to locate dermatomes a body map will be useful but it must be remembered that the areas designated are not precise; small variations frequently occur (Figure 2.1). Nonetheless, when selecting points to needle, those within the segment will often have a more powerful effect. The mechanical needling of sensory nerve endings within a muscle also stimulates the corresponding motor neurons to send signals to relax the tight muscles. It appears that the mechanical movements of the needle in, out and/or rotatory are important. It pulls, moves and stretches all the broken or damaged fibres and leads to a softening of tissue around the needle [29]. This mechanical movement of connective tissue may have a far-reaching effect and has been extensively investigated by Langevin et al. [25].

The approach to the orthodox healing process will vary according to the stage the patient has reached, and that with acupuncture is no different. Whether the situation is acute or chronic will influence the soft-tissue changes that may be present. Interestingly, this idea is closely mirrored within meridian acupuncture, where the activity of the Wei Qi is influenced by the duration of the problem and the involvement of the musculotendinous meridians [30].

Simple segmental needling has been found to be most effective in acute pain. If electroacupuncture (EA) is used, high frequency, 100 Hz or more, low intensity, just perceptible to the patient, is most effective. This is the technique that works best for nociceptive pain, but in an acute situation fewer needles should be used in the segment itself.

In chronic pain more needles can be used in the segment, together with supraspinal techniques and point choices. These would include Back Shu or Huatuojiaji points, having their effect through the dorsal rami. Chronic pain produces ongoing stress which limits the healing process and this can be tackled with acupuncture, whether the pain is physiological or psychological.

Clinical reasoning must take into account the most likely mechanisms involved in the condition to be treated. In the case of pain, the common causes have been defined as nociceptive, neuropathic and centrally evoked. While this book is not exclusively concerned with treatment of pain alone, the

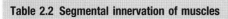

Table 2.2 Segmental innervation of muscles

Upper limb

Muscle	Spinal innervation				
Trapezius	C3	C4			
Levator scapulae		C4	C5		
Rhomboid major and minor		C4	C5	C6	
Latissimus dorsi				C6	C7	C8
Pectoralis major				C6	C7	C8	T1
Serratus anterior			C5	C6	C7	C8
Pectoralis minor					C8	T1
Deltoid		C4	C5	C6	C7
Coracobrachialis			C5	C6	C7	C8
Biceps brachii			C5	C6
Teres major			C5	C6
Triceps brachii				C6	C7	C8
Supraspinatus		C4	C5	C6
Infraspinatus		C4	C5	C6
Teres minor		C4	C5	C6	C7
Brachialis			C5	C6
Brachioradialis			C5	C6
Pronator teres			C5	C6	C7
Pronator quadratus				C6	C7	C8	T1
Palmaris longus				C6	C7	C8	T1
Supinator			C5	C6	C7
Extensor carpi radialis brevis			C5	C6	C7	C8
Extensor carpi			C5	C6	C7	C8
Extenor carpi ulnaris				C6	C7	C8
Extensor digitorum				C6	C7	C8
Extensor indicis				C6	C7	C8	T1
Extensor digiti minimi				C6	C7	C8	T1
Extensor pollicis longus				C6	C7	C8	T1
Extensor pollicis brevis				C6	C7	C8
Flexor carpi ulnaris					C7	C8	T1

Table 2.2 Segmental innervation of muscles—cont'd

Upper limb

Muscle	Spinal innervation			
Flexor carpi radialis	C6	C7	C8	
Flexor pollicis brevis	C6	C7	C8	T1
Flexor digiti minimi brevis	C6	C7	C8	T1
Abductor pollicis	C6	C7	C8	T1
Flexor digitorum superficialis	C6	C7	C8	T1
Flexor digitorum profundus		C7	C8	T1
Flexor pollicis longus	C6	C7	C8	T1
Lumbricales	C6	C7	C8	T1
Abductor brevis	C6	C7	C8	T1
Abductor digiti minimi	C6	C7	C8	T1
Dorsal and palmar interossei			C8	T1
Opponens pollicis	C6	C7	C8	T1
Opponens digiti minimi		C7	C8	T1
Adductor pollicis			C8	T1

Lower limb

Muscle	Spinal innervation				
Pectineus	L2	L3	L4		
Tensor fasciae latae			L4	L5	S1
Adductor brevis	L2	L3	L4	L5	
Rectus femoris	L2	L3	L4	L5	
Vastus lateralis	L2	L3	L4	L5	
Vastus medialis	L2	L3	L4	L5	
Vastus intermedius	L2	L3	L4	L5	
Sartorius	L2	L3	L4		
Adductor longus	L2	L3	L4		
Adductor magnus	L2	L3	L4	L5	
Gluteus maximus			L4	L5	S1	S2	S3
Semimembranosus			L4	L5	S1	S2	S3
Semitendinosus				L5	S1	
Biceps femoris			L4	L5	S1	S2	S3

Continued

Table 2.2 Segmental innervation of muscles—cont'd

Lower limb

Muscle	Spinal innervation					
Gluteus medius			L4	L5	S1	S2	
Gracilis	L2	L3	L4	L5			
Gluteus minimus			L4	L5	S1		
Quadratus femoris			L4	L5	S1		
Piriformis					S1	S2	S3
Gastrocnemius			L4	L5	S1	S2	S3
Soleus			L4	L5	S1	S2	S3
Flexor hallucis longus			L4	L5	S1	S2	S3
Flexor digitorum longus			L4	L5	S1	S2	
Peroneus longus			L4	L5	S1	S2	
Peroneus brevis			L4	L5	S1	S2	
Tibialis posterior			L4	L5	S1	S2	
Tibialis anterior			L4	L5	S1	S2	
Extensor digitorum longus			L4	L5	S1	S2	
Extensor hallucis longus			L4	L5	S1	S2	
Flexor hallucis brevis				L5	S1		
Flexor digitorum brevis				L5	S1		
Plantar and dorsal interossei					S1	S2	
Extensor digitorum brevis			L4	L5	S1	S2	

From Hopwood (58).

definitions will be helpful, involving as they do the pain transmission process and responses.

Nociceptive pain only occurs where the nervous system is intact and relies on nociceptor stimulation. This stimulation can be mechanical, ischaemic or inflammatory. It is usually associated with tissue injury and acute pain. Acupuncture treatment is usually effective in this type of case.

Neuropathic pain usually arises from a segment of nerve or the dorsal root ganglion due to axon damage. It is characterized by allodynia, defined as pain arising from non-injurious contact with the skin, and hyperalgesia, a generally exaggerated sense of pain. Synthesis of cholecystokinin, an antagonist to endogenous opioids, increases, usually cancelling out the effect of the acupuncture. This may well arise after damage incurred as a result of one of the neurological conditions described in this book.

Finally, centrally evoked pain is produced by prolonged central sensitization long after the original injury has healed, leading to a chronic pain situation with atypical and unpredictable pain behaviours. There is often a poor response to medication. The sympathetic nervous system is involved via the lateral sympathetic horn or a centrally mediated autonomic response. There are often visible sympathetic signs, redness, enlarged pores and sometimes swelling. Distal acupuncture may be successful.

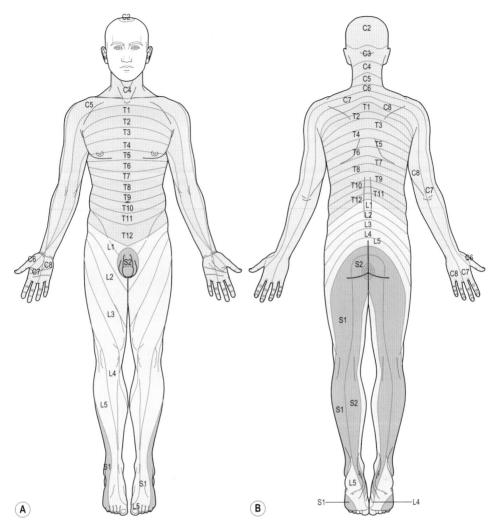

Figure 2.1 • Adult dermatome patterns. (Modified from Abrahams P, Hutchings R, Marks S. McMinn's Color Atlas of Human Anatomy, 4th edn. London: Mosby, 1997.)

Sympathetic or parasympathetic activity cannot be ignored and, before arriving at the nerve supply for the area, careful palpation is recommended. If the aim is to treat relatively superficial injuries, high-frequency, low-intensity acupuncture will aid blood flow to the area by reducing sympathetic tone [31].

If healing damaged tissue is the main aim of the treatment then maximizing local effects will be most important. This can be achieved in several ways but the simple insertion of the needle into the painful tissue remains the most direct. If under-lying symptoms such as loss of sleep, anxiety and general loss of impetus for rehabilitation are to be treated then the picture becomes more complex

and mostly supraspinal responses should be sought. There is now considerable support for the use of acupuncture in insomnia [32].

Neuronal correlates of acupuncture stimulation in the human brain have been investigated by functional neuroimaging. The preliminary findings suggest that acupuncture at analgesic points involves the pain-related neuromatrix and may have acupoint–brain correlation. Wu et al. [33] concluded that the hypo-thalamus–limbic system was significantly modulated by EA at acupoints rather than at non-meridian points, while visual and auditory cortical activation was not a specific effect of treatment-relevant acu-points and requires further investigation of the underlying neurophysiological mechanisms. Real EA elicited significantly higher activation than sham EA over the hypothalamus and primary somatosensory motor cortex and deactivation over the rostral segment of anterior cingulate cortex.

Although the preceding clinical reasoning processes have mostly dealt with Western medical ideas, there is a place for the consensus medicine handed down in the TCM tradition. Points at the corresponding segmental level for the internal organs, in TCM theory the Zang Fu organs, can be accessed via the inner Urinary Bladder line. The points usually chosen will relate to the Spleen, the Lung and the thymus in order to promote production of T lymphocytes and NK cells in order to optimize the healing process.

The only research we have to support this is that by Hsu et al., but the clear effects on the circulatory system demonstrated by BL 15 indicate that other Back Shu points may also be as useful [31]. The designated 'big' points on the hands and feet that have a strong effect on the hypothalamus and regulate autonomic flow can be incorporated. Ear points can also be used.

It is clear that the reasoning process delineated above will form a major part of clinical decisions when selecting acupuncture as part of the treatment of a musculoskeletal condition. It is equally clear, however, that therapists treating other conditions and diseases will also be able to build up their case in this way.

The distinction between TCM and scientific reasoning is diminishing year by year. The recent work by Dorsher et al. [34] indicating a 91% correlation between the distributions of known trigger point regions' referred pain patterns and acupuncture meridians indicates that trigger points most likely represent the same physiological phenomenon as acupuncture points in the treatment of pain disorders. They state: 'It is implausible that trigger point regions and classical acupuncture points would by chance correlate so strongly – anatomically, physiologically (referred-pain patterns and meridians), clinically in pain treatment, and clinically in treating somatovisceral disorders – unless they represented the same phenomenon.'

Maybe this could mean that how the points are chosen depends on the practitioner and a choice guided by TCM theory could be as useful as any other, particularly if it includes points in the area of influence of a known nerve root and also some of the major distal points.

Problems with research protocols

A research methodology depends entirely on the correct question being asked and being answered in some way. With the historical difficulty within acupuncture of being able to define firstly the mechanism and secondly the complex nature of the intervention, placing this within the context of an RCT has been problematic [35]. A major step forward has been the recent publication of a textbook examining the problems associated with rigorous research into acupuncture [36].

Many of the key issues are discussed and the overwhelming conclusion reached is that acupuncture is not yet fully understood. It is a complex non-pharmacological intervention with many facets and does not fit easily into the conventional drug trial format. This problem has also been discussed in detail in a previous book [37] but the most frequent problem is that of finding an adequate control.

The sham needles, those with a shaft that collapses into the handle like a stage dagger, have some value but still excite the C or touch fibres when used [38]. Also the researchers cannot be unaware that these needles are being used; the technique requires some care to avoid dropping the needles or failing to keep them adequately stuck to the skin surface [39].

Ingenious new needles, designed to maintain operator blindness to those receiving the sham needle, are now available but not yet in widespread use [40, 41]. These involve insertion into some soft substance inside the opaque applicator tube for the sham needle while the real one will be longer and enter the tissues. Most acupuncturists are convinced they could tell the difference but more research needs to be done with this.

RCTs are still recommended for evaluating acupuncture and are still perceived by the scientific community as being the best way to separate the specific from the non-specific effects of acupuncture. Those non-specific aspects rely on several factors, including context, patient–practitioner relationship and co-interventions, and are further complicated by spontaneous change or regression to the mean.

It is not really possible to indicate how much of the total effect may be represented by each of the components suggested in Table 2.3 but it is probable that spontaneous changes vary from condition to condition while the associated or context effects

Table 2.3 Component parts of total acupuncture effect

Spontaneous change	Associated/context effects				Attributable therapy effect
	Meaning	Co-interventions	Practitioner effect	Direct effects of consultation process	

After Linde (59).

may vary depending on the type of consultation taking place. It is also probable that the practitioner is the most important variable [42]. Clearly where there is both an element of ritual and an extensive clinical interview, the placebo effect of the intervention will be substantially reinforced and may be both practitioner- and dose-dependent [43, 44].

Minimal acupuncture, frequently used as a control, has been shown to be an active placebo and far from inert in a physiological sense. While it is possible that the varying responses to 'verum' and sham acupuncture are dependent on the cause of the pain, there is enough doubt about the validity of sham needling to suggest that it may be unfair to judge the effect of acupuncture in this way [45]. Depending on the aetiology of the problem the response to acupuncture is varying. Lundeberg et al. recommend that the evaluated effects of acupuncture could be compared with those of standard treatment, also taking the individual response into consideration, before its use or non-use is established [46].

It is indeed difficult to use an intervention resembling acupuncture in all essentials which will convince the patient and, hopefully, the operator but offer no sensory stimulus other than visual to confound the results. Work continues on trying to find the ideal but the answers so far have been neither adequate nor inexpensive.

Table 2.4 gives an indication of the varieties of approach required if the investigation into any relatively unfamiliar treatment/intervention is to be comprehensive. Very few studies so far can be cited as excellent examples of any approach.

Particular problems researching neurological conditions

Finally, the difficulties encountered when researching any neurological condition apply equally to any acupuncture research in this field. There is a fundamental problem with finding homogeneous groups of sufferers; the neurological damage is rarely easily comparable from one patient to another. The damage in the nerve network or the higher centres is infinitely variable in nature and also in effect. This means that finding large enough groups of patients to be able to do appropriate power calculations is a difficulty and is also likely to prove expensive. If the final group is too small, as many have been historically, than the results will be invalid or, at the very least, open to challenge because it is impossible to be sure that the results are not just random.

Most neurological conditions – stroke, Parkinson's disease and multiple sclerosis (MS) – do not offer a complete recovery; indeed, some, like motor neurone disease, are progressive illnesses over short periods of time without any favourable outcome. These conditions have attracted a limited amount of research funding over the years but a lot of this has been supported by specific charities rather than major government initiatives. To be fair, stroke prevention has received a lot of support recently, linked as it often is with cardiovascular disease, but dealing with the sequelae of stroke is a lot less glamorous, with many variables to confound the outcomes. The NHS has funded one major study of acupuncture and stroke [47], but, with the exception of the study by Park et al. [48], most of the other work has been done abroad. The MS Society is often helpful, financing smaller projects, but the logistics of setting up a study with a reasonably homogenous group of subjects with comparable MS disabilities is daunting, with very large numbers required.

Another issue is consent. When a patient has just suffered a serious and potentially catastrophic event such as a stroke it can be ethically difficult to offer an unknown or previously little-researched intervention. The response from relatives, 'Leave them alone, they've suffered enough!' is not uncommon. If members of the family have previously had successful acupuncture for a minor problem, it may

Table 2.4 Developing a framework to accommodate the complexities of investigating acupuncture

Research phase	Usual methods
Theoretical development Practitioner world view Underlying assumptions Historical use Possible mechanisms involved	Individual case studies Reflective practice Laboratory work Reviewing existing literature
Modelling Distinguishing key components Defining actual intervention Defining outcomes Developing methodology/protocol	Delphi process gaining professional consensus on best practice Case series Clinical outcomes data Qualitative research Quantitative research
Exploratory trial Testing all aspects of the protocol from recruitment and blinding to outcomes assessment Treatment effect (power calculations) Adapting trial design	$n = 1$ study Pilot study Small RCT Pragmatic RCT
Definitive RCT	Double-blind RCT Pragmatic RCT
Long-term implementation Real world Long-term benefits Cost Compliance Safety	Pragmatic RCT Clinical outcomes data Patient/practitioner surveys Qualitative research Observational studies

After McIntyre (60).
RCT, randomized controlled trial.

be much easier to gain consent, so with the general increase of acupuncture availability in both the NHS and the wider community, there is cause for hope that this situation may improve.

Funding for this type of research is hard to raise, unless it can be linked with a demonstrable diminution of the general financial care burden on the NHS, in both primary and secondary care.

This means that the research methodologies must be quite complex and, of necessity, involve long time periods in order to make a fair judgement on economic validity. There is no reason to suppose this to be impossible but further impetus must now come from demonstrable clinical results and the publication of careful case studies is increasingly important.

References

[1] NIH consensus development panel on acupuncture. Acupuncture. JAMA 1998;280(17):1518–24.

[2] Andersson S, Lundeberg T. Acupuncture from empiricism to science: functional background to acupuncture effects in pain and disease. Med Hypotheses 1995; 45(3):271–81.

[3] Andersson S. Physiological mechanisms in acupuncture. In: Hopwood V, Lovesey M, Mokone S, editors. Acupuncture and Related Techniques in Physiotherapy. London: Churchill Livingstone; 1997. p. 19–39.

[4] Carlsson C. Acupuncture mechanisms for clinically relevant

long-term effects. Acupunct Med 2002;20(2–3):82–99.

[5] Lundeberg T. A comparative study of the pain alleviating effect of vibratory stimulation, transcutaneous electrical nerve stimulation, electroacupuncture and placebo. Am J Chin Med 1984;XII(1–4):72–9.

[6] Lundeberg T, Hurtig T, Lundeberg S, et al. Long term results of acupuncture in chronic head and neck pain. Pain Clinic 1988;2(1):15–31.

[7] Bradnam L. A proposed clinical reasoning model for western acupuncture. New Zealand Journal of Physiotherapy 2003;31(1):40–5.

[8] Bradnam L. A physiological underpinning for treatment progression of western acupuncture. Journal of Acupuncture Association of Chartered Physiotherapists 2007;25–33.

[9] Bradnam L. A proposed clinical reasoning model for western acupuncture. Journal of the Acupuncture Association of Chartered Physiotherapists 2007;21–30.

[10] White A. Editorial. Acupunct Med 2009;27(1):1–2.

[11] White A. Western medical acupuncture: a definition. Acupunct Med 2009;27(1):33–5.

[12] Sackett DL, Rosenberg WMC, Muir Gray JA. Evidence-based medicine: what it is and what it isn't. BMJ 1996;(312):71–2.

[13] Ross EG. If not evidence, then what? Or does medicine really need a base. J Eval Clin Pract 2002;8(2):113–9.

[14] WHO Western Pacific Region. WHO Standard Acupuncture Point Locations. Geneva: World Health Organization; 2008.

[15] Hopwood V. A new bronze man!. Journal of the Acupuncture Association of Chartered Physiotherapists 2007;59–60.

[16] MacPherson H, White AR, Cummings M, et al. Standards for Reporting Interventions in Controlled Trials of Acupuncture: the STRICTA recommendations. Acupunct Med 2002;20(1):22–5.

[17] Boutron I, Moher D, Altman DG, et al. Extending the CONSORT statement to randomized trials of nonpharmacologic treatment: explanation and elaboration. Ann Intern Med 2008;148(4):295–309.

[18] White A, Hayhoe S, Hart A, et al. Adverse events following acupuncture: prospective survey of 32 000 consultations with doctors and physiotherapists. BMJ 2001;323:485–6.

[19] MacPherson H, Thomas K, Walters S, et al. The York acupuncture safety study: prospective survey of 34 000 treatments by traditional acupuncturists. BMJ 2001;323:486–7.

[20] Vincent C. The safety of acupuncture. BMJ 2001; (323):467–8.

[21] David J, Townsend S, Sathanathan R, et al. The effect of acupuncture on patients with rheumatoid arthritis: a randomised, placebo-controlled crossover study. Rheumatology 1999;38:864–9.

[22] Tukmachi E. Acupuncture and rheumatoid arthritis. Rheumatology 2000;39:1153–65.

[23] Napadow V, Makris N, Liu J, et al. Effects of electroacupuncture versus manual acupuncture on the human brain as measured by fMRI. Hum Brain Mapp 2004; 24(3):193–205.

[24] Napadow V, Dhond R, Park K, et al. Time-variant fMRI activity in the brainstem and higher structures in response to acupuncture. Neuroimage 2009;47:289–301.

[25] Langevin HM, Bouffard NA, Churchill DL, et al. Connective tissue fibroblast response to acupuncture: dose-dependent effect of bidirectional needle rotation. J Altern Complement Med (New York, N Y) 2007;13 (3):355–60.

[26] Cummings M. Modellvorhaben Akupunktur – a summary of the ART, ARC and GERAC trials. Acupunct Med 2009;27(1):26–30.

[27] Pariente J, White P, Frackowiak RSJ, Lewith G. Expectancy and belief modulate the neuronal substates of pain treated by acupuncture. Neuroimage 2005;25(4):1161–7.

[28] Richardson B. Professional development. 2 Professional knowledge and situated learning in the workplace. Physiotherapy 1999;(85):467–74.

[29] Ma Y-T, Ma M, Cho ZH. Biomedical Acupuncture for Pain Management. St Louis: Elsevier (USA); 2005.

[30] Pirog JE. Meridian sinews and the treatment of musculoskeletal pain. The Practical Application of Meridian Style Acupuncture 1996;219–39.

[31] Hsu CC, Weng CS, Liu TS, et al. Effects of electrical acupuncture on acupoint Bl15 evaluated in terms of heart rate variability, pulse rate variability and skin conductance response. Am J Chin Med 2006;34(1):23–6.

[32] Bosch PMPC, van den Noort MWM. Schizophrenia, Sleep and Acupuncture. Göttingen: Hogrefe & Huber; 2008.

[33] Wu M, Sheen J, Chuang K, et al. Neuronal specificity of acupuncture response: a fMRI study with electroacupuncture. Neuroimage 2002;16(4):1028.

[34] Dorsher PT, Fleckenstein J. Trigger points and classical acupuncture points: part 3: relationships of myofascial referred pain patterns to acupuncture meridians. Deutsche Zeitschrift für Akupunktur 2009;52(1):9–14.

[35] Hopwood V, Lewith G. Acupuncture trials and methodological considerations. Clinical Acupuncture and Oriental Medicine 2003;3(4):192–9.

[36] MacPherson H, Hammerschlag R, Lewith G, et al. Acupuncture Research. Edinburgh: Churchill Livingstone, Elsevier; 2008.

[37] Hopwood V. Acupuncture trials and methodological considerations. Acupuncture in Physiotherapy. Oxford: Butterworth Heinemann; 2004.

[38] Park J, White A, Stevinson C, et al. Validating a new non-penetrating sham acupuncture device: two randomised controlled trials. Acupunct Med 2002;20(4):168–74.

[39] White P, Lewith G, Hopwood V, et al. The placebo needle, is it a valid and convincing placebo for use in acupuncture trials? A randomised, single-blind,

cross-over pilot trial. Pain 2003;106:401–9.

[40] Takakura N, Yajima H. A double-blind placebo needle for acupuncture research. Biomed Central 1–15. 2007.

[41] Takamura N. Not yet known. Medical Acupuncture 2008;20 (3):169–74.

[42] Paterson C, Dieppe P. Characteristic and incidental (placebo) effects in complex interventions such as acupuncture. BMJ 2005;330:1202–5.

[43] Kaptchuk T, Kelley JM, Conboy LA, et al. Components of placebo effect: randomised controlled trial in patients with irritable bowel syndrome. BMJ 2008;336(7651):999–1003.

[44] Kaptchuk TJ, Stason WB, Davis RB, et al. Sham device v inert pill: randomised controlled trial of two placebo treatments. BMJ 2006;332(7538):391–7.

[45] Lund I, Naslund J, Lundeberg T. Minimal acupuncture is not a valid placebo control in randomised controlled trials of acupuncture: a physiologist's perspective. Chinese Medicine 2009;4(1):1.

[46] Lundeberg T, Lund I, Sing A, et al. Is placebo acupuncture what it is intended to be? eCAM 2009; nep049.

[47] Hopwood V, Lewith G, Prescott P, et al. Evaluating the efficacy of acupuncture in defined aspects of stroke recovery: a randomised, placebo controlled single blind study. J Neurol 2008;255(6):858–66.

[48] Park J, White AR, James MA, et al. Acupuncture for subacute stroke rehabilitation. Arch Intern Med 2005;165:2026–31.

[49] Hui KK, Liu J, Makris N, et al. Acupuncture modulates the limbic system and subcortical gray structures of the human brain: evidence from fMRI studies in normal subjects. Hum Brain Mapp 2000;9(1):13–25.

[50] Harris RE, Gracely RH, McLean SA, et al. Comparison of clinical and evoked pain measures in fibromyalgia. J Pain 2006;7 (7):521–7.

[51] Newberg AB, Lariccia PJ, Lee BY, et al. Cerebral blood flow effects of pain and acupuncture: a preliminary single-photon emission computed tomography imaging study. J Neuroimaging 2005;15(1):43–9.

[52] Napadow V, Kettner N, Liu J, et al. Hypothalamus and amygdala response to acupuncture stimuli in carpal tunnel syndrome. Pain 2007;130:254–66.

[53] Cho ZH, Chung SC, Jones JP, et al. New findings of the correlation between acupoints and corresponding brain cortices using functional MRI. Proc Natl Acad Sci U S A 1998;95 (March):2670–3.

[54] Li G, Liu HL, Cheung RT, et al. An fMRI study comparing brain activation between word generation and electrical stimulation of language-implicated acupoints. Hum Brain Mapp 2003;18(3):233–8.

[55] Gareus IK, Lacour M, Schulte AC, et al. Is there a BOLD response of the visual cortex on stimulation of the vision-related acupoint GB 37? J Magn Reson Imaging 2002;15 (3):227–32.

[56] Hu KM, Wang CP, Xie HJ, et al. Observation on activating effectiveness of acupuncture at acupoints and non-acupoints on different brain regions. Zhongguo Zhen Jiu 2006;26(3):205–7.

[57] Hammerschlag R, Langevin H, Lao L, et al. Physiologic dynamics of acupuncture: correlations and mechanisms. In: MacPherson H, Hammerschlag R, Lewith G, et al., Acupuncture Research. Strategies for Establishing an Evidence Base. Edinburgh: Churchill Livingstone; 2008. p. 188.

[58] Hopwood V. Acupuncture in Physiotherapy. Oxford: Butterworth Heinemann; 2004.

[59] Linde K. The specific placebo effect. Bundesgesundheitsblatt Gesundheitsforchung Gesundheitsschutz 2006;49 (8):729–35.

[60] McIntyre M. Report to Ministers from the Department of Health Steering Group on the Statutory Regulation of practitioners of acupuncture, herbal medicine, traditional Chinese medicine and other traditional medicine systems practised in the UK. Annex 1. Aberdeen: Department of Health; 2008.

Current context: neurological rehabilitation and neurological physiotherapy

3

CHAPTER CONTENTS

KEY POINTS

- Neurological conditions are common, affecting around 10 million people in the UK, and causing a major health burden worldwide.
- Neurological conditions are often complex, requiring support from a range of specialist services over many years.
- Physiotherapists are an integral part of the multidisciplinary team supporting people with neurological conditions.
- Interventions focus around patients' goals and aim to maximize their functional ability, prevent secondary complications and enhance self-efficacy.

Introduction

Neurological conditions are those conditions which affect parts of the nervous system. The causes of these conditions are varied and may include trauma,

Table 3.1 Examples of common neurological conditions

Central nervous system	Peripheral nervous system
Stroke – cerebral or spinal	Guillain–Barré syndrome
Multiple sclerosis	Peripheral neuropathy
Parkinson's disease	Chronic inflammatory
Traumatic brain injury	demyelinating polyneuropathy
Spinal cord injury	
Cerebral palsy	
Brain or spinal tumours	
Meningitis or encephalitis	

vascular disruption, infection, tumour or degeneration of the nervous system. Conditions may affect the central nervous system, consisting of the brain and spinal cord, or the peripheral nervous system, consisting of the peripheral nerves (Table 3.1). Neurological conditions are often complex, and people with these conditions may require support from many different services. Acupuncture may provide benefits for people with neurological conditions, but it represents just one possible option among many. An awareness of the important aspects of a comprehensive service for people with neurological conditions is important. This chapter aims to outline the various components that are required for effective management of people with neurological conditions.

Prevalence and incidence of neurological conditions

Neurological conditions are common. Around 10 million people in the UK live with a neurological condition which substantially affects their life [1]. Stroke is by far the commonest neurological condition. Each year, around 125 000 people in the UK, 700 000 in the USA and 1 million in the European Union have a stroke [2]. In the UK, of those individuals with neurological conditions, around 350 000 require help for most of their daily activities, and over 1 million require assistance with some daily tasks [1]. Each year 1% of the UK population are newly diagnosed with a neurological condition and 19% of hospital admissions are for a neurological problem requiring treatment from a neurologist or neurosurgeon [1].

Models of health care

Medical model

The medical model assumes that all illnesses are explained by disease and that the treatment of disease will restore the individual to health [3]. This model was originally developed in the late 19th and early 20th centuries following the scientific discoveries of infectious disease by Pasteur and cellular pathology by Virchow [4]. The medical model is based on reductionism and a dualistic notion of the mind and body. It evaluates individuals in isolation from their environment and takes no account of the social, psychological or behavioural aspects of illness or the patient's experience of that illness [5, 6]. It was originally developed for the management of severe medical conditions. In these situations treatment of the disease may indeed result in substantial improvements in health. However, with the growing prevalence of chronic disease, the inadequacies of this model are highlighted. The model cannot explain symptoms for which there is no underlying pathology. It also fails to appreciate the complex interaction of social, psychological and environmental factors and their impact on the overall experience of illness by the individual.

Biopsychosocial model

The biopsychosocial model considers individuals as well as their health problem and the social context. It recognizes that health, disease, illness and disability result from complex interactions of biological, emotional, cognitive, social and environmental factors. It recognizes that psychological and social factors influence the person's perceptions and actions, and therefore the experience of illness. This model suggests that effective treatment of the disease may not automatically result in the resolution of illness and disability. This model has been adopted by the World Health Organization as the basis for the *International Classification of Function* (ICF) [7].

Presentation of neurological conditions and ICF

Neurological conditions may result in a wide range of difficulties. These may include problems with physical ability, sensation, cognition, communication,

Figure 3.1 • Example of *International Classification of Function* applied to an individual with multiple sclerosis.

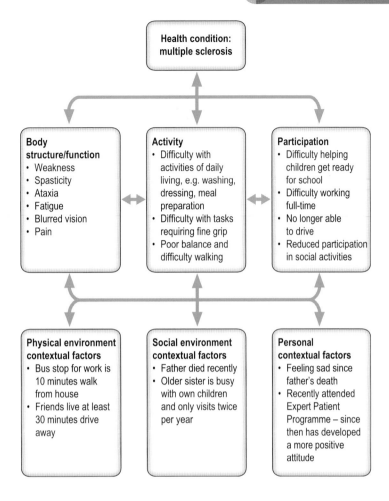

behaviour and psychological functioning. The ICF developed by the World Health Organization [7] provides a useful framework to classify the consequences of disease (Figure 3.1) [8]. It is based on the biopsychosocial model of disability and supports the consideration of an individual's situation within the context of biological factors and also the social and physical environment.

Management of neurological conditions

Neurological conditions may represent a one-off event followed by resolution and no further needs. However, neurological conditions often cause long-lasting difficulties which require management over the lifetime of the individual. These types of long-term

neurological conditions broadly fall into one of four categories:

1. sudden-onset conditions
2. intermittent and unpredictable conditions
3. progressive conditions
4. stable neurological conditions, but with changing needs due to development or ageing [9].

People with neurological conditions often need to access a wide range of services such as those provided by health services, social services and charitable organizations. They will need information and education about their condition as well as support regarding finance and employment.

Key priorities for effective management include:

- prompt initial diagnosis and treatment
- emergency admission if required
- specialist rehabilitation

- effective symptom management
- prevention of secondary complications
- provision of relevant equipment
- adaptations to home environment
- support to remain in their own home
- vocational rehabilitation
- support for families and carers
- access to palliative care if required
- regular review and ability to re-access services in a timely manner [9].

General principles of rehabilitation

Rehabilitation has been defined as: 'the use of all means aimed at reducing the impact of disabling and handicapping conditions and at enabling people with disabilities to achieve optimal social integration' [10]. Rehabilitation is a continuous and coordinated process which starts at the onset of an illness or injury and aims to support individuals to achieve roles in society consistent with their aspirations [8]. Many individuals with neurological conditions will require access to rehabilitation services. Support needs to be provided for individuals throughout their life. Clear mechanisms for

individuals to re-access relevant services are required (Figure 3.2). In addition palliative care is required to support individuals coming to the end of their lives [11].

Key aspects of effective rehabilitation

Person-centred service

The person should be at the centre of the service provided. Individuals should be provided with sufficient information about treatment options to allow them to be actively involved in all decisions regarding their management [9]. Information provided needs to take account of any communication difficulties that the individual may have. Attention should be paid to the person's emotional needs as well as practical needs. Support should also be provided to family members and carers [9].

Specialist multidisciplinary team

Access to a coordinated specialist rehabilitation team is an important factor in effective management of the wide range of difficulties an individual may

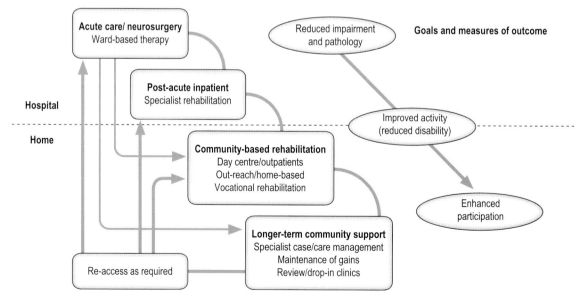

Figure 3.2 • The 'slinky' model of the phases of rehabilitation. (From RCP, BRSM. Rehabilitation following acquired brain injury: national clinical guidelines. London: Royal College of Physicians; British Society of Rehabilitation Medicine, 2003. with kind permission.)

report [12, 13]. The specialist team members should include a doctor, nurse, physiotherapist, occupational therapist, speech and language therapist, clinical psychologist and social worker. Access to the expertise of other services is also important. Such services include dietetics, continence advisory service, orthotics, chiropody, pain management and spasticity management services, ophthalmology and liaison psychiatry.

Goal-setting

Goal-setting is an integral part of rehabilitation and allows the person and the specialist team to focus on key aspects identified as important by the individual [14]. Goals are specific time-bound measurable outcomes relating to a desired or expected future state. Goals are set by the individual, with support from the relevant team members. They guide and inform therapy, as well as providing a structure for the individual regarding future targeted outcomes [15]. Goals need to be challenging but achievable and include long-term (weeks/months) and short-term goals (days/weeks) [12].

Outcome measures

Outcome measures provide information regarding the outcome for an individual following rehabilitation. The use of validated standardized outcome measures is required within rehabilitation services to provide information on individual outcomes, as well as to allow service evaluation [16]. A wide range of outcomes measures have been validated, and they include those that reflect the perspective of the person as well as the clinician [17].

Evidence-based practice

Management programmes for people with neurological conditions need to be based on best available evidence. Evidence-based practice involves the integration of individual clinical expertise with the findings from the best available research [18]. A range of clinical guidelines have been developed to support improved care of people with conditions such as stroke or multiple sclerosis. Guidelines have been based on an extensive review of available research evidence combined with expert opinion [12, 13, 19, 20].

Chronic disease management

Chronic disease

Chronic diseases are diseases of long duration and usually slow progress. They are the leading cause of death and disability worldwide [21]. Many neurological conditions are chronic diseases requiring management over time. These diseases often have a range of persistent symptoms with no cure and the potential for significant impact on the individual's quality of life [22]. Successful management requires an effective collaboration between the person and relevant health and social care professionals.

The 'expert patient'

Over time individuals with chronic conditions develop considerable knowledge and experience about their condition and how it affects their life. This expertise has not always been utilized fully within management decisions. There is now a shift in emphasis to support these individuals to be key decision-makers in collaboration with health care professionals [23]. Self-management programmes are supporting this process of the development of 'expert patients' [24].

Chronic disease self-management programmes

Self-management programmes aim to equip people with chronic diseases with the skills to manage problems that they frequently encounter. These programmes have been developed over the last 20 years and are delivered in countries across the globe [21]. Many programmes are generic whilst some are specific to a particular chronic condition. The programmes are led by teams of trained volunteers all living with a long-term condition. Evidence indicates that these programmes can help to reduce severity of symptoms, improve life control and resourcefulness, and improve activity levels and life satisfaction [24]. The programmes aim to support people to develop the following skills:

- disease-related problem-solving
- managing medications
- exercise

- cognitive symptom management, e.g. relaxation, reframing
- management of emotions, e.g. fear, self-doubt
- communication skills, e.g. within family, with health professionals
- use of community resources.

An important aspect of the programme is to enhance the individual's perceived self-efficacy. Self-efficacy denotes confidence in one's ability to accomplish a particular goal. Evidence shows that those with higher levels of self-efficacy are more effective in managing their condition [25].

Health and clinical governance

Health governance is a global concept which relates to the actions and means by which a society organizes itself for the promotion and protection of the health of its population [26]. In the UK this has been labelled 'clinical governance' and defined as 'a framework through which National Health Service organizations are accountable for continuously improving the quality of their services and safeguarding high standards of care by creating an environment in which excellence in clinical care will flourish' [27]. It was introduced as part of health service reform and aimed to address inequalities in quality of service provision across the country. An intrinsic aspect of clinical governance is the establishment of clinical standards against which performance can be measured. Clinical guidelines for people with neurological conditions have been developed, such as those relating to stroke, Parkinson's disease, multiple sclerosis, motor neurone disease and acquired brain injury [12, 13, 19, 20, 28, 29].

Consent and capacity

Patients must consent to treatments that they receive. Valid consent will depend upon the individual having the capacity to make a decision, as well as ensuring they are not acting under duress. In addition they must have received sufficient information about the intended benefits and possible risks of the proposed procedure [30]. The Mental Capacity Act 2005 for England and Wales came fully into force in October 2007. This provides a statutory framework to empower and protect any person who may lack capacity [31]. Every individual is presumed to have capacity unless it is proved otherwise. People with brain injury or disease may have impaired capacity and therefore may be unable to consent. When patients do lack capacity, any acts or decisions made under the Act on their behalf must be carried out in their best interests.

Key principles of neurological physiotherapy

The physiotherapist is an important member of the multidisciplinary team supporting people with neurological conditions. Physiotherapy is defined as a 'health-care profession concerned with human function and movement and maximizing potential. It uses physical approaches to promote, maintain and restore physical, psychological and social well-being, taking account of variations in health status' [32]. Physiotherapy input follows the general principles of rehabilitation outlined earlier, such as using a person-centred approach, use of goals and outcome measurement and the principles of chronic disease management.

Historical development of neurological physiotherapy

Neurological physiotherapy has undergone substantial changes over the past century. During the first half of the 20th century, treatments focused on individual muscle strengthening, bracing or surgery [33]. New treatment methods emerged during the 1950s and 1960s. These were based on the understanding of neurophysiology at that time, and assumed that abnormal movement patterns could be changed by applying afferent stimulation [34]. These 'neurofacilitation' approaches were developed by Rood (1956), Kabat (1961), the Bobaths (1965), Brunnstrom (1966) and Knott and Voss (1968). More recently, approaches based on insights from the fields of motor control and learning, biomechanics, muscle biology, brain imaging and cognitive psychology have been developed [34–37].

Physiotherapy within the multidisciplinary team

Physiotherapists work closely with other members of the multidisciplinary team. The physiotherapist's particular expertise lies within the assessment, analysis and treatment of movement disorders, which are limiting the function of the individual [34]. The physiotherapist will also liaise with colleagues to gain additional information, such as information from the speech and language therapist on the person's ability to understand language, as well as information from the occupational therapist and psychologist regarding the person's cognitive ability and emotional status.

Neurological physiotherapy assessment

Neurological physiotherapy involves individualized assessment of movement dysfunction and related functional difficulties. Assessment and subsequent management are guided by the priorities identified by the individual. Evaluation of relevant aspects of the ICF classification will be completed as necessary.

Body structure/function

Assessment may include evaluation of sensation, proprioception, muscle function, including ability to activate muscles, sustain activation of muscles and coordinate movements, muscle power, muscle tone, including presence of hypotonia, spasticity, dystonia, athetosis, chorea, rigidity, tremor and ataxia, flexibility of joints and muscles, praxis, perceptual ability and cardiorespiratory fitness [34]. Additional assessments may include review of visual and vestibular systems [38] and neurodynamics [39]. Problematic symptoms such as pain or fatigue will also be evaluated.

Activity

Functional activities will be assessed. This may include reviewing the person's ability to move from one position to another and to maintain balance in the new position during functional tasks, for example, whilst getting out of bed. Other functional activities, such as walking or using the hands to pick up and carry objects, will also be assessed. The relationships between activity and body structure and function will be explored as a basis for effective management.

Participation

Assessment of participation will usually occur within the individual's own environments such as home or work, and will consider how the person is able to fulfil his or her usual roles in life. Activities important to

the individual will be considered and may include reviewing the person's ability to complete tasks such as preparing a meal at home for the family, completing a full day of work without excessive fatigue or climbing into and out of a local swimming pool.

Context

The personal context of individuals, including their expectations and attitudes to their situation, will be considered. Relevant physical environments will be assessed and their social environment reviewed. Some of these assessments may be carried out in conjunction with the occupational therapist.

Interventions

Interventions will be determined by the stated aims of the person in conjunction with findings on assessment. Broad categories of interventions are outlined in Figure 3.3 and discussed below. Interventions will be modified when required to ensure effective participation by those individuals with cognitive, communicative or behavioural difficulties.

Influence sensorimotor system

People with neurological conditions may present with a wide range of different sensory and motor

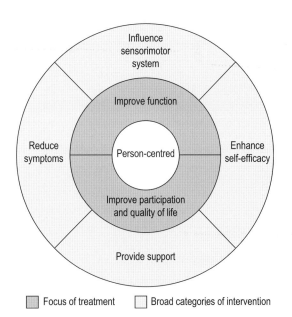

Figure 3.3 • Focus of treatment and broad categories of intervention in neurological physiotherapy.

impairments which compromise functional ability [34]. Key principles of treatment will be to maximize remaining functional ability and to minimize secondary complications [40, 41]. Important therapeutic options will now be outlined.

Maximize functional ability

Movement is an essential component of functional ability and is therefore a prime target for intervention [34]. Treatments will be task-oriented and broadly aimed towards enhancing sensorimotor control as a basis for improved posture, balance and mobility including walking, upper-limb function and orofacial function [42–44]. Treatments aim to help individuals achieve their goals and may include intensive task-specific training, for example, treadmill training or constraint-induced movement therapy [34, 40, 44, 45]. In addition, interventions such as muscle strengthening and aerobic conditioning will be utilized as required [42]. The individual will be encouraged to participate actively throughout the rehabilitation process.

Minimize secondary complications

Complications such as adaptive shortening of muscles may occur secondary to primary impairments such as weakness [46]. These secondary complications may have a profound effect on the individual and need to be minimized as far as possible. Those individuals with complex and severe disability may require effective postural management over the 24-hour period, including comfortable but supported sleeping postures and customized support within their wheelchair [41, 47]. Those who are more able may benefit from targeted activity and stretch of 'at-risk' muscles such as gastrocnemius and soleus [40]. Passive muscle length may be improved by serial casting [48]. Spasticity may be problematic for some individuals and may contribute to loss of muscle length, as well as difficulties with postural management [41]. Useful interventions to manage spasticity may include oral medication, focal botulinum toxin injections or intrathecal baclofen [49].

Reduce symptoms

Individuals with different neurological conditions commonly report high levels of problematic symptoms such as pain and fatigue as well as sleep and mood disturbance [50–52]. These symptoms are commonly overlooked and undertreated [53, 54]. Physiotherapy options for these symptoms may include education regarding self-management as well as the use of exercise and acupuncture.

Pain

Pain is commonly a target for physiotherapeutic intervention. Treatment options may include exercise, re-education of movement control, manual or manipulative therapy, education about self-management, graded exposure to problematic activities and pacing of activity level [55]. Pain-relieving modalities used may include transcutaneous electrical nerve stimulation (TENS) or acupuncture [56]. These pain management options may be valuable to people with neurological conditions. There are indications that TENS may be of value for pain associated with spasticity in multiple sclerosis [57]. Neuromuscular stimulation via implanted electrodes may be a useful option to reduce shoulder pain in hemiplegia [58]. A few studies have evaluated the impact of acupuncture on pain in neurological conditions (see Chapter 4).

Fatigue

Fatigue is described as an overwhelming sense of tiredness, lack of energy or exhaustion and is very common in many different neurological conditions [59, 60]. It is a complex symptom with possible contributions from muscle weakness, general physical deconditioning, cognitive impairment, mood disturbance and poor sleep [61, 62]. Active exercise programmes have resulted in reduced fatigue for people with multiple sclerosis [63, 64]. Exercise programmes for other conditions such as stroke have revealed the benefits of increased cardiovascular fitness, but not clear effects on fatigue [65]. Preliminary studies indicate the value of acupuncture for cancer-related fatigue and in fibromyalgia [66, 67]. There are anecdotal reports of improved energy levels and reduced fatigue in neurological conditions following acupuncture but no formal studies.

Sleep disturbance

Sleep disturbance or insomnia includes difficulty falling asleep, staying asleep or non-restorative sleep [68]. In neurological conditions sleep quality is commonly reduced and may be affected by pain, anxiety, muscle spasms in limbs, periodic limb movements or nocturia [69]. Lack of sleep may contribute to daytime fatigue and mood disturbance and commonly coexists with anxiety or depression. Non-pharmacological management includes education regarding good sleep hygiene practices and relaxation. Exercise has long been suggested as an option to enhance sleep quality, but studies evaluating clinical populations are not common [70]. King et al. [71] noted benefits on sleep in older adults following moderate-intensity exercise. Physical exercise using a bicycle ergometer was found to be as effective as dopaminergic agents for sleep disturbed by periodic limb movements in spinal cord injury [72]. Improved sleep quality has been reported by individuals with multiple sclerosis following aerobic and strengthening exercises [73]. Acupuncture may provide reduction of insomnia in a range of psychiatric and medical conditions, although more randomized controlled trials are required [74]. Benefits from acupuncture for sleep quality have been noted in people with Parkinson's disease and stroke [75, 76].

Mood disturbance

Mood disturbances such as anxiety and depression are highly prevalent in neurological conditions and commonly coexist with pain, fatigue and insomnia. Numerous studies have highlighted the benefits of exercise for depression and anxiety within a wide range of conditions, although large studies of greater rigour are still required [77, 78]. The positive benefits from exercise have also been noted in people with neurological conditions [79]. The evidence for acupuncture in mood disorder is inconclusive, although there have been some positive studies [80]. There are no major studies assessing the impact of acupuncture in neurological conditions, although anecdotal reports and case reports indicate benefit [81]. More research is needed.

Enhance self-efficacy

Self-efficacy in neurological conditions

Many studies have highlighted the impact of low self-efficacy in neurological conditions. In spinal cord injury low self-efficacy was strongly associated with lower self-assessed quality of life [82]. Individuals were also at higher risk of experiencing debilitating pain. In Parkinson's disease individuals with low balance self-efficacy were able to walk shorter distances than those with higher

self-efficacy [83]. In stroke, lower levels of self-efficacy were associated with higher levels of depression, poorer walking ability, poorer function, poorer quality of life, increased disability and greater dissatisfaction with community integration [84–87].

Options to enhance self-efficacy

Self-efficacy may be enhanced by a number of processes. These include helping the individual to experience success when completing a chosen task, the observation of others completing similar tasks, as well as verbal affirmation from others, including health care professionals or peers. These opportunities may be built into standard rehabilitation programmes. Effective goal-setting, based around the individual's own priorities, with regular review, allows the repeated experience of achievement as successive short-term goals are achieved. Treatment of patients within a group context may provide additional opportunities for the experience of success coupled with peer support. Those with particularly low levels of self-efficacy may benefit from targeted support, especially at times of transition such as discharge from inpatient services [88]. Self-efficacy is an important target for treatment. Treatment programmes focusing on physical ability need to incorporate strategies to enhance self-efficacy to ensure that gains for the individual are maximized.

Provide support

Neurological conditions commonly result in substantial difficulties for the individual. An event such as a stroke, spinal cord injury or traumatic brain injury will change the person's life forever. A relapse of multiple sclerosis is likely to mean that some functional ability may be lost and not regained. The development of Parkinson's disease marks the beginning of a process of gradual deterioration of function. Active physiotherapy treatments and education aim to make the best of people's remaining abilities, but they cannot replace that which is lost. Therefore part of the physiotherapist's role lies in supporting patients in coming to terms with the ways in which their body, their life and their possibilities for the future have changed [89]. This support provides the background context for all other encounters with the person.

Acupuncture within neurological physiotherapy

Acupuncture has a wide range of possible applications for people with neurological conditions. Anecdotal reports indicate a diverse range of benefits, including improved sensorimotor function, reduced pain and fatigue, improved sleep quality and energy levels as well as improved mood. These improvements may also allow the person to participate more effectively with other interventions, for example a person with less fatigue may be able to gain more benefit from attending an education programme on self-management. Acupuncture is easily integrated with other treatment options. Rigorous trials evaluating the effects of acupuncture for people with neurological conditions are few, and are mainly confined to stroke. Additional studies using appropriate outcome measures are required.

Conclusion

This chapter has discussed the many and varied options to support people with neurological conditions. It has highlighted the need for long-term support with regular review and periods of intensive rehabilitation if required. Acupuncture may be a useful option to consider for people with these conditions, particularly within the context of a specialist neurological rehabilitation team.

References

[1] Neurological Alliance. Neuro Numbers: A Brief Review of the Numbers of People in the UK with a Neurological Condition. London: Neurological Alliance; 2003.

[2] Pendlebury ST. Worldwide underfunding of stroke research. Int J Stroke 2007;2(2):80–4.

[3] Wade DT, Halligan PW. Do biomedical models of illness make for good healthcare systems? BMJ 2004;329(7479):1398–401.

[4] Waddell G. Biopsychosocial analysis of low back pain. Baillières Clin Rheumatol 1992;6(3):523–57.

[5] Engel GL. The need for a new medical model: a challenge for biomedicine. Science 1977;196(4286):129–36.

[6] Waddell G. Preventing incapacity in people with musculoskeletal disorders. Br Med Bull 2006;77–78(1):55–69.

[7] World Health Organization. Towards a common language for functioning, disability and health: ICF. Geneva: World Health Organization; 2002.

[8] Gutenbrunner C, Ward AB, Chamberlain MA. White book on physical and rehabilitation medicine in Europe. J Rehabil Med 2007;39(S45):1–48.

[9] Department of Health. The National Service Framework for Long-term Conditions. London: Department of Health; 2005.

[10] Martin J, Meltzer H, Eliot D. Report 1: The prevalence of disability among adults. Office of Population, Census and Surveys, Social Survey Division; OPCS surveys of disease in Great Britain, 1988–89; 1988.

[11] RCP. The National Council for Palliative Care, BSRM. Long-term neurological conditions: management at the interface between neurology, rehabilitation and palliative care. London: Royal College of Physicians; 2008.

[12] RCP. National clinical guideline for stroke. London: Royal College of Physicians; 2008.

[13] NICE. Multiple sclerosis: National clinical guidelines for diagnosis and management in primary and secondary care. London: National Institute for Clinical Excellence/National Collaborating Centre for Chronic Conditions; 2003.

[14] Wade DT. Evidence relating to goal planning in rehabilitation. Clin Rehabil 1998;12(4):273–5.

[15] Holliday RC, Ballinger C, Playford ED. Goal setting in neurological rehabilitation: patients' perspectives. Disabil Rehabil 2007;29(5):389–94.

[16] Freeman JA, Hobart JC, Playford ED, et al. Evaluating neurorehabilitation: lessons from routine data collection. J Neurol Neurosurg Psychiatry 2005;76(5):723–8.

[17] Skinner A, Turner-Stokes L. The use of standardized outcome measures in rehabilitation centres in the UK. Clin Rehabil 2006;20(7):609–15.

[18] Sackett DL, Rosenberg WM, Gray JA, et al. Evidence based medicine: what it is and what it isn't. BMJ 1996;312(7023):71–2.

[19] RCP BRSM. Rehabilitation following acquired brain injury: national clinical guidelines. London: Royal College of Physicians; British Society of Rehabilitation Medicine; 2003.

[20] National Collaborating Centre for Chronic Conditions. Parkinson's disease; national clinical guideline for diagnosis and management in primary and secondary care. London: Royal College of Physicians; 2006.

[21] World Health Organization. Preventing chronic diseases: a vital investment: WHO global report. Geneva: World Health Organization; 2005.

[22] Holman H, Lorig K. Patient self-management: a key to effectiveness and efficiency in care of chronic

disease. Public Health Rep 2004;119(3):239–43.

[23] Lorig K. Partnerships between expert patients and physicians. Lancet 2002;359(9309):814–5.

[24] Department of Health. The expert patient: a new approach to chronic disease management for the 21st century. London: Department of Health; 2001.

[25] Marks R, Allegrante JP, Lorig K. A review and synthesis of research evidence for self-efficacy-enhancing interventions for reducing chronic disability: implications for health education practice (part I). Health Promot Pract 2005;6(1):37–43.

[26] Dodgson R, Lee K, Drager N. Global health governance: a conceptual review. Geneva: WHO; 2002.

[27] Department of Health. Clinical governance: in the new NHS. London: Department of Health; 1999.

[28] BSRM. Job Centre Plus, RCP. Vocational assessment and rehabilitation after acquired brain injury: inter-agency guidelines. London: Royal College of Physicians; 2004.

[29] Motor Neurone Disease Association. Standards of care to achieve quality of life for people affected by motor neurone disease. Motor Neurone Disease Association; 2000.

[30] CSP. Core standards of physiotherapy practice. London: Chartered Society of Physiotherapy; 2005.

[31] Department of Health, Public Guardianship Office. Mental capacity act 2005 - summary, Department of Health; Public Guardianship Office; 2007. Available online at: http://www. dh.gov.uk/en/SocialCare/ Deliveringadultsocialcare/ MentalCapacity/ MentalCapacityAct2005/ DH_064735. 10-1-0009.

[32] Chartered Society of Physiotherapy. Curriculum framework for qualifying programmes in physiotherapy. London: Chartered Society of Physiotherapy; 2002.

[33] Gordon J. Assumptions underlying physical therapy intervention: theoretical and historical perspectives. Movement science; foundations for physical therapy in rehabilitation. Maryland: Aspen; 2000. p. 1–31.

[34] Shumway-Cook A, Woollacott M. Motor control: translating research into clinical practice. Philadelphia: Lippincott, Williams & Wilkins; 2007.

[35] Woollacott MH, Shumway-Cook A. Changes in posture control across the life span – a systems approach. Phys Ther 1990;70(12):799–807.

[36] Carr JH, Shepherd RB. A Motor Relearning Programme for Stroke. 2nd ed. London: Heinemann; 1987.

[37] Carr J, Shepherd R. Stroke Rehabilitation:Guidelines for Exercise and Training to Optimize Motor Skill. Edinburgh: Elsevier; 2003.

[38] Boyer FC, Percebois-Macadre L, Regrain E, et al. Vestibular rehabilitation therapy. Neurophysiol Clin 2008;38(6): 479–87.

[39] Butler DS. The sensitive nervous system. Adelaide: Noigroup; 2000.

[40] Carr J, Shepherd R. Movement science; foundations for physical therapy in rehabilitation. 2nd ed. Maryland: Aspen; 2000.

[41] Pope PM. Severe and complex neurological disability: management of the physical condition. Edinburgh: Elsevier; 2007.

[42] Refshauge K, Ada L, Ellis E. Science-based rehabilitation: theories into practice. Edinburgh: Elsevier; 2005.

[43] Vanswearingen J. Facial rehabilitation: a neuromuscular reeducation, patient-centered approach. Facial Plast Surg 2008;24(2):250–9.

[44] Schmidt RA, Wrisberg CA. Motor Learning and Performance: A Situation-Based Learning Approach. 4th ed. Illinois: Human Kinetics; 2008.

[45] Wolf SL, Winstein CJ, Miller JP, et al. Retention of upper limb function in stroke survivors who have received constraint-induced movement therapy: the EXCITE randomised trial. Lancet Neurol 2008;7(1):33–40.

[46] Ada L, O'Dwyer N, O'Neill E. Relation between spasticity, weakness and contracture of the elbow flexors and upper limb activity after stroke: an observational study. Disabil Rehabil 2006;28(13/14): 891–7.

[47] Holmes KJ, Michael SM, Thorpe SL, et al. Management of scoliosis with special seating for the non-ambulant spastic cerebral palsy population – a biomechanical study. Clin Biomech 2003; 18(6):480–7.

[48] Singer BJ, Jegasothy GM, Singer KP, et al. Evaluation of serial casting to correct equinovarus deformity of the ankle after acquired brain injury in adults. Arch Phys Med Rehabil 2003;84(4):483–91.

[49] Barnes MP, Johnson GR. Upper motor neurone syndrome and spasticity. Cambridge: Cambridge University Press; 2008.

[50] Simuni T, Sethi K. Nonmotor manifestations of Parkinson's disease. Ann Neurol 2009;64(S2): S65–S80.

[51] Brown RF, Valpiani EM, Tennant CC, et al. Longitudinal assessment of anxiety, depression, and fatigue in people with multiple sclerosis. Psychol Psychother 2009;82:41–56.

[52] Leppavuori A, Pohjasvaara T, Vataja R, et al. Insomnia in ischemic stroke patients. Cerebrovasc Dis 2002;14(2):90–7.

[53] Ludwig J. Parkinson disease: do we need to improve treatment strategies that focus on nonmotor complications such as pain? Nat Clin Pract Neurol 2008; 4(9):478–9.

[54] Korostil M, Feinstein A. Anxiety disorders and their clinical correlates in multiple sclerosis patients. Mult Scler 2007;13 (1):67–72.

[55] Gifford L, Thacker M, Jones MA. Physiotherapy and pain. In: McMahon SB, Koltzenburg M, editors. Wall and Melzack's

textbook of pain. Philadelphia: Elsevier; 2006. p. 603–17.

[56] Barlas P, Lundeberg T. Transcutaneous electrical nerve stimulation and acupuncture. In: McMahon SB, Koltzenburg M, editors. Wall and Melzack's textbook of pain. Philadelphia: Elsevier; 2006. p. 583–90.

[57] Miller L, Mattison P, Paul L, et al. The effects of transcutaneous electrical nerve stimulation (TENS) on spasticity in multiple sclerosis. Mult Scler 2007; 13(4):527–33.

[58] Chae J, Yu DT, Walker ME, et al. Intramuscular electrical stimulation for hemiplegic shoulder pain: a 12-month follow-up of a multiple-center, randomized clinical trial. Am J Phys Med Rehabil 2005; 84(11):832–42.

[59] Schepers VP, Visser-Meily AM, Ketelaar M, et al. Poststroke fatigue: course and its relation to personal and stroke-related factors. Arch Phys Med Rehabil 2006; 87(2):184–8.

[60] Belmont A, Agar N, Hugeron C, et al. Fatigue and traumatic brain injury. Ann Readapt Med Phys 2006;49(6):283–4.

[61] Leocani L, Colombo B, Comi G. Physiopathology of fatigue in multiple sclerosis. Neurol Sci 2008;29(0):241–3.

[62] Barat M, Dehail P, de Seze M. Fatigue after spinal cord injury. Ann Readapt Med Phys 2006; 49(6):277–9.

[63] Fragoso YD, Santana DL, Pinto RC. The positive effects of a physical activity program for multiple sclerosis patients with fatigue. NeuroRehabilitation 2008;23(2):153–7.

[64] Dodd KJ, Taylor NF, Denisenko S, et al. A qualitative analysis of a progressive resistance exercise programme for people with multiple sclerosis. Disabil Rehabil 2006;28(18):1127–34.

[65] Macko RF, Ivey FM, Forrester LW, et al. Treadmill exercise rehabilitation improves ambulatory function and cardiovascular fitness in patients with chronic stroke: a randomized, controlled trial. Stroke 2005;36(10):2206–11.

[66] Martin DP, Sletten CD, Williams BA, et al. Improvement in fibromyalgia symptoms with acupuncture: results of a randomized controlled trial. Mayo Clin Proc 2006;81(6):749–57.

[67] Molassiotis A, Sylt P, Diggins H. The management of cancer-related fatigue after chemotherapy with acupuncture and acupressure: A randomised controlled trial. Complement Ther Med 2007; 15(4):228–37.

[68] Roth T. Insomnia: definition, prevalence, etiology, and consequences. J Clin Sleep Med 2007;3(5 Suppl.):S7–110.

[69] Stanton BR, Barnes F, Silber E. Sleep and fatigue in multiple sclerosis. Mult Scler 2006; 12(4):481–6.

[70] Driver HS, Taylor SR. Exercise and sleep. Sleep Med Rev 2000; 4(4):387–402.

[71] King AC, Pruitt LA, Woo S, et al. Effects of moderate-intensity exercise on polysomnographic and subjective sleep quality in older adults with mild to moderate sleep complaints. J Gerontol A Biol Sci Med Sci 2008;63(9):997–1004.

[72] de Mello MT, Esteves AM, Tufik S. Comparison between dopaminergic agents and physical exercise as treatment for periodic limb movements in patients with spinal cord injury. Spinal Cord 2004;42(4):218–21.

[73] Smith C, Hale L, Olson K, et al. How does exercise influence fatigue in people with multiple sclerosis? Disabil Rehabil 2008;1–8.

[74] Kalavapalli R, Singareddy R. Role of acupuncture in the treatment of insomnia: a comprehensive review. Complement Ther Clin Pract 2007;13(3):184–93.

[75] Kim YS, Lee SH, Jung WS, et al. Intradermal acupuncture on shen-men and nei-kuan acupoints in patients with insomnia after stroke. Am J Chin Med 2004; 32(5):771–8.

[76] Shulman LM, Wen X, Weiner WJ, et al. Acupuncture therapy for the symptoms of Parkinson's disease. Mov Disord 2002;17(4):799–802.

[77] Daley A. Exercise and depression: a review of reviews. J Clin Psychol Med Settings 2008;15(2):140–7.

[78] Martinsen EW. Physical activity in the prevention and treatment of anxiety and depression. Nord J Psychiatry 2008;62(Suppl. 47): 25–9.

[79] Macko RF, Benvenuti F, Stanhope S, et al. Adaptive physical activity improves mobility function and quality of life in chronic hemiparesis. J Rehabil Res Dev 2008;45(2):323–8.

[80] Karst M, Winterhalter M, Munte S, et al. Auricular acupuncture for dental anxiety: a randomized controlled trial. Anesthesia Analgesia 2007;104(2): 295–300.

[81] Donnellan CP. Acupuncture for central pain affecting the ribcage following traumatic brain injury and rib fractures – a case report. Acupunct Med 2006; 24(3):129–33.

[82] Middleton J, Tran Y, Craig A. Relationship between quality of life and self-efficacy in persons with spinal cord injuries. Arch Phys Med Rehabil 2007;88 (12):1643–8.

[83] Mak MKY, Pang MYC. Balance self-efficacy determines walking capacity in people with Parkinson's disease. Mov Disord 2008;23 (13):1936–9.

[84] Robinson-Smith G, Johnston MV, Allen J. Self-care self-efficacy, quality of life, and depression after stroke. Arch Phys Med Rehabil 2000;81(4):460–4.

[85] LeBrasseur NK, Sayers SP, Ouellette MM, et al. Muscle impairments and behavioral factors mediate functional limitations and disability following stroke. Phys Ther 2006;86(10):1342–50.

[86] Pang MYC, Eng JJ, Miller WC. Determinants of satisfaction with community reintegration in older adults with chronic stroke: role of balance self-efficacy. Phys Ther 2007;87(3): 282–91.

[87] Bonetti D, Johnston M. Perceived control predicting the recovery of individual-specific walking behaviours following stroke: testing psychological models and constructs. Br J Health Psychol 2008;13(Pt 3): 463–78.

[88] Jones F, Partridge C, Reid F. The Stroke Self-Efficacy Questionnaire: measuring individual confidence in functional performance after stroke. J Clin Nurs 2008;17(7B):244–52.

[89] Toombs SK. Healing and incurable illness. In: Fulford KWM, Dickenson DL, Murray TH, editors. Healthcare ethics and human values: an introductory text with readings and case studies. Massachusetts: Blackwell; 2002. p. 125–32.

Western medical acupuncture in neurological conditions

4

CHAPTER CONTENTS

KEY POINTS

- Acupuncture clinical reasoning in neurological conditions may be approached from a Western medical standpoint.
- Application of acupuncture requires an understanding of symptoms common in neurological conditions.
- Awareness of other treatments indicated for each presentation helps identify the place of acupuncture within the overall management plan for the patient.
- Evidence from studies indicates a range of applications of acupuncture for sensory, motor, visceral and generalized disorders.
- Few studies have specifically examined the efficacy of acupuncture in neurological conditions.
- Uncontrolled studies, case reviews and case reports suggest interesting possible applications of acupuncture in neurological conditions.
- Complex symptom patterns are the norm in neurological patients and medication interactions in these situations can be problematic.
- Acupuncture may offer an additional treatment option in some cases.
- Acupuncture is a valuable option within the toolbox of practitioners working within neurological rehabilitation.

Introduction

Acupuncture may be useful in the treatment of people with neurological conditions. The approach to treatment of pain lends itself to the application of Western medicine principles with the consideration of local, segmental and extrasegmental effects. The approach to other symptoms is perhaps less obvious at first glance. At this point many practitioners choose to consider Chinese medical principles to guide treatment. This chapter aims to explore the possibility of applying Western medical acupuncture in neurological conditions. The following chapter will explore the practical application of acupuncture in these presentations.

Application of acupuncture in neurological conditions

People with neurological conditions report a wide range of problematic symptoms. The first step is to identify which of these features might be influenced by acupuncture. Acupuncture will not restore function that has been lost due to the disease or injury process. However, it may be able to modify activity in those systems that are still functioning to some extent. In general it is more likely to influence 'positive' symptoms, which relate to 'over'- or 'hyper'-functioning of a system, where modulation may be possible. It is likely to have less impact on 'negative' features such as severe sensory loss or paralysis.

Presenting symptoms may be broadly categorized as: (1) sensory symptoms; (2) motor symptoms; (3) visceral symptoms; and (4) generalized symptoms such as mood disturbance. The development of clearly reasoned treatments for patients based on Western science requires some understanding of these presentations and an awareness of current literature. This chapter will explore these presentations and consider possible treatment options, including acupuncture.

Basic mechanisms of action of acupuncture

White et al. [1] have clearly summarized the main mechanisms underlying the effects of acupuncture. These include: (1) local effects; (2) segmental effects; (3) extrasegmental and central regulatory effects; and (4) effects relating to myofascial trigger points.

Local effects

Inserting a needle through the skin will cause firing of small-diameter fibres A-δ, C-fibres and group II/III fibres. Firing of these nerve endings will contribute to the sensation of Deqi often described by the patient as aching, fullness or warmth. Needling will cause local effects of increased blood flow in the skin and the muscle due to release of neuropeptides.

Segmental effects

Impulses from nerve fibres stimulated in the skin and muscle are transmitted into the dorsal horn of the spinal cord tissues via somatic nerves. The spinal cord receives converging information from the periphery, including skin, muscles, joints, bones and at some levels viscera. The spinal cord is also influenced by descending impulses from the brainstem and higher centres. Therapeutic effects from acupuncture may be gained by considering the segmental nerve supply of the target tissue, e.g. a painful ankle or an overactive bladder (OAB). Needling according to the segmental nerve supply provides the potential to modulate activity in the spinal cord, for example causing inhibition of the transmission of nociceptive information through the dorsal horn.

Extrasegmental and central regulatory effects

Inserting an acupuncture needle into the body will influence structures in the brainstem such as the periaqueductal grey area, as well as higher centres such as structures of the limbic, endocrine and autonomic systems. These may provide more global effects on the body such as generalized pain relief, improvement of sleep quality or mood. It is difficult to predict exactly which points will elicit these effects but major points such as LI4, LR 3, SP6 and ST36 are likely to support these responses in many patients.

Effects relating to myofascial trigger points

Needling myofascial trigger points has the potential to reduce pain and contribute to improved muscle function.

Part 1: Sensory function

Absent or impaired sensation

Damage to sensory pathways within the nervous system may lead to impairments in sensation. The degree of impairment will depend on the site and extent of the lesion. Sensation and proprioceptive deficits may lead to considerable difficulties with balance and mobility as well as functioning of the upper limbs [2]. The loss of sensory information due to lesions within the pathways has a substantial effect on cortical responsiveness and topographical organization of the primary sensory cortex [3].

Prevalence of impaired sensation in neurological conditions

Sensory deficits are common in neurological conditions, with an estimated prevalence of up to 65% in stroke [4], 80–90% of those with multiple sclerosis [5] and most individuals with spinal cord injury. Sensory features are also prominent in peripheral neuropathies involving the sensory nerves, such as alcoholic peripheral neuropathy and the acute motor and sensory axonal neuropathy subtype of Guillain–Barré syndrome [6, 7].

Acupuncture for impaired sensation

We are unaware of any studies specifically using acupuncture to improve sensation, although studies by Napadow et al. [8] indicate that modifications of the primary sensory cortex may be induced by acupuncture. Many studies in neurorehabilitation have used various types of sensory stimulation, but these usually measure the outcome in terms of improved motor function rather than commenting on sensory function [9]. Perhaps this is an area that merits further exploration.

Abnormal sensations, including paraesthesia and pain

Pain is common and problematic in neurological conditions (Table 4.1). Effective management is needed and acupuncture may be of value in this situation. It is important to understand the nature of the pain presentation to guide acupuncture intervention and expected outcomes.

Is the pain nociceptive or neuropathic?

'Nociceptive pain' refers to pain which results from activation of nociceptors in the tissues, for example by injury, inflammation, ischaemia or degeneration [10]. It is commonly described as dull or aching and may affect the musculoskeletal system or the viscera. This type of pain is very common and often responds well to simple interventions such as analgesics, exercise, transcutaneous electrical nerve stimulation (TENS) or acupuncture (Tables 4.2 and 4.3).

'Neuropathic pain' refers to pain which arises as a direct consequence of a lesion or disease affecting the somatosensory system [10]. As such it is common in neurological conditions. This type of pain

may develop spontaneously or may be evoked by various stimuli, which are normally innocuous. It is commonly described as burning, shooting, pricking or throbbing. Neuropathic pain may affect the peripheral or central neural pathways (Tables 4.2 and 4.3). It is challenging to treat and may require the use of medications such as amitriptyline or gabapentin, psychological therapies such as cognitive-behavioural therapy and physiotherapy [11]. Refractory cases may require consideration for spinal cord stimulation or deep brain stimulation.

Mechanisms of neuropathic pain in neurological conditions

Peripheral neuropathy

Peripheral focal or generalized neuropathies involve loss of myelin and/or axonal damage of peripheral nerves. Neuropathic pain may arise from molecular changes in the area of injured or degenerating axons [12]. Hypersensitivity in the peripheral nervous system will then drive the development of hypersensitivity in the spinal cord and central pain transmission pathways.

Table 4.1 Prevalence of pain in common neurological conditions

Condition	Nociceptive pain	Neuropathic pain
Stroke	No data	9% 25% (lateral medullary infarction)
Traumatic brain injury	58–93% have chronic pain – nature not specified Headache in 31–88%	
Parkinson's disease	Up to 70%	10%
Cerebral palsy (adult)	82%	No data
Multiple sclerosis	No data	28%
Spinal cord injury	59% (musculoskeletal) 35% (visceral)	Up to 41%
Guillain–Barré syndrome	55% (acute phase)	28–49%

References: MacGowan et al. (147); Moulin et al. (148); Weimar et al. (149); Siddall et al. (150); Jahnsen et al. (151); Kogos et al. (152); Nampiaparampil (153); Ruts et al. (154); Beiske et al. (155); Osterberg & Boivie (5).

Table 4.2 Definitions of nociceptive and neuropathic pain

Type of Pain	IASP* Definition, 2008	Subdivisions of pain
Nociceptive pain	Pain arising from stimulation of nociceptors	**Somatic nociceptive pain** Pain arising from nociceptors located in skin and musculoskeletal system, e.g. muscles, tendons, ligaments, joints
		Visceral nociceptive pain Pain arising from visceral organs, e.g. bladder, bowel, uterus
Neuropathic pain	Pain arising as a direct consequence of a lesion or disease affecting the somatosensory system	**Peripheral neuropathic pain** Pain arising from a lesion or disease affecting the peripheral somatosensory system
		Central neuropathic pain Pain arising from a lesion or disease affecting the central somatosensory system

*IASP, International Association for the Study of Pain.[10]

Table 4.3 Clinical examples of nociceptive and neuropathic pain

Nociceptive pain	Neuropathic pain
Somatic nociceptive pain 1. Simple nociceptive pain Pain experienced by the general population, including those with neurological conditions 2. Pain directly associated with a neurological condition For example, muscle pain due to spasticity in stroke or multiple sclerosis, or due to rigidity, e.g. in Parkinson's disease; also pain secondary to trauma, e.g. in traumatic spinal cord or brain injury 3. Pain secondary to neurological condition For example, low-back pain due to prolonged sitting in wheelchair in multiple sclerosis; shoulder pain due to propelling wheelchair in spinal cord injury; hip pain due to abnormal gait in adult cerebral palsy	**Peripheral neuropathic pain** Pain due to peripheral neuropathy, Guillain–Barré syndrome, brachial plexus lesion, trigeminal neuralgia
Visceral nociceptive pain This may occur in the general population; however visceral dysfunction may be specifically related to neurological condition. Examples might include pain associated with urinary tract infection, urinary retention or constipation in spinal cord injury, multiple sclerosis, traumatic brain injury, stroke or adult cerebral palsy	**Central neuropathic pain** Pain due to multiple sclerosis, spinal cord injury (below lesion), stroke, traumatic brain injury, Parkinson's disease, syringomyelia

Stroke, traumatic brain injury, spinal cord injury, multiple sclerosis

In stroke, traumatic brain injury, spinal cord injury and multiple sclerosis functional impairment of the spinothalamocortical tract conveying pain and temperature sensation from the periphery to the cortex seems crucially important in the development of neuropathic pain [5, 13–15]. In spinal cord injury evidence suggests that those individuals with more extensive reorganization of the primary somatosensory cortex experience more severe ongoing pain [16].

Parkinson's disease

The disturbance of central processing of nociceptive information by the basal ganglia is likely to have a role in the development of central neuropathic pain in Parkinson's disease [17, 18]. In addition dysfunction of nociceptive processing at spinal cord level is also involved [19].

Evidence for use of acupuncture for pain in neurological conditions

Peripheral neuropathy

Studies have evaluated the use of acupuncture for peripheral neuropathy of various aetiologies (Table 4.4). These reveal some positive results, particularly the finding that acupuncture improved nerve conduction in tibial and sural nerves [20]. Further prospective research is needed.

Spinal cord injury

Studies in spinal cord injury are small. They provide hints that acupuncture may be useful for nociceptive and neuropathic pain (Table 4.5).

Multiple sclerosis

No large-scale trials have been conducted. Descriptive case reports suggest benefit from electroacupuncture at 50 Hz for painful trigeminal neuralgia [21], as well as body and ear acupuncture for leg pain and dysaesthesia affecting the hands [22, 23].

Stroke, traumatic brain injury, Parkinson's disease and adult cerebral palsy

Descriptive case reports indicate benefits from acupuncture for central neuropathic pain in stroke [24], for nociceptive shoulder pain in stroke [25] and for central neuropathic pain in traumatic brain injury [26]. Implanted percutaneous electrical nerve stimulation (PENS) reduced chronic hemiplegic shoulder pain [27]. No large-scale studies have been conducted.

Paraesthesia and dysaesthesia

At this point it is worth mentioning abnormal sensations which are commonly reported in neurological conditions. 'Paraesthesia' refers to abnormal sensations which are not described as unpleasant [28]. This may include sensations such as tingling, prickling, pins and needles, burning, aching and tightness. 'Dysaesthesia' is defined as an unpleasant abnormal sensation and includes the more specific categories of allodynia and hyperalgesia. It is therefore included in the category of neuropathic pain [28]. Paraesthesia and dysaesthesia may represent a pure sensory phenomenon such as in cortical strokes affecting the postcentral gyrus, or may be accompanied by motor signs such as tonic spasms in multiple sclerosis [29, 30]. Paraesthesia and dysaesthesia may be spontaneous or evoked. They arise from abnormal activity in the nervous system such as ectopic impulse activity in the central or peripheral nerves, or ephaptic transmission between physically adjacent neurones in areas of demyelination [31]. These sensations cause substantial distress to some individuals. Management of these sensations follows the recommendations for neuropathic pain.

Acupuncture for paraesthesia and dysaesthesia

Carpal tunnel syndrome is an entrapment neuropathy of the median nerve causing paraesthesia and pain. Napadow [8, 32] reported improvements in these symptoms following a course of acupuncture (Table 4.6). Functional magnetic resonance imaging indicated changes in cortical representation as well as reduced activation of the limbic system. These changes accompanied reports of improvement from the patients. It may also be worth attempting needling with patients with dysaesthesia from central sensory lesions. No research has been conducted on this population.

Part 2: Motor function

Motor dysfunction

Motor symptoms are extremely common in neurological conditions. These range from complete paralysis through to excessive muscle activity such as spasticity or dyskinesia. Each of these presentations will be considered.

Table 4.4 Acupuncture for pain in peripheral neuropathy

Authors and year	n	Design and inclusion criteria	Assessment	Interventions	Results
Shlay et al. 1998 (122)	250	RCT 2 × 2 factorial design HIV-related peripheral neuropathy	Pain intensity diary Global pain relief 39-item self-rated QOL assessment	Acupuncture and amitriptyline compared with sham acupuncture and placebo amitriptyline Points needled were SP 6, SP 7, SP 9, Bafeng, KI 2, KI 3 Sham points were three points in the calf Points needled for 20–25 minutes twice weekly for 6/52; once weekly for 8/52	All groups noted small reduction in pain – no significant difference between the groups
Abuaisha et al. 1998 (123)	44	Pretest, posttest study Diabetic neuropathy with Neuropathy Disability Score of more than 2; painful symptoms for at least 6 months	Graphical 0–10 rating scale for two most problematic symptoms, e.g. pain, difficulty sleeping	Six acupuncture treatments of 20 minutes over 10 weeks; points used were LR 3, SP 6, SP 9, ST 36	77% noted improvement, including pain relief and improved sleep 21% noted complete pain relief 32% stopped all pain medications
Phillips et al. 2004 (124)	21	Pretest, posttest study HIV-related peripheral neuropathy	0–10 VAS for current pain and for least and worst pain over last 24 hours Subjective Peripheral Neuropathy Screen (SPNS) (includes pain, paraesthesia and numbness)	10 individualized acupuncture treatments over 5 weeks; treatments lasted 35–40 minutes Ear points: Neurogate, Sympathetic, Heart, Lungs Body points: HT 7, SP 6, KI 3, PC 6, LU 9, LI 4, LI 11, TE 5, ST 36, ST 41, Bafeng	Significant reduction in VAS and SPNS Reduction in pain, burning in hands and arms and numbness in hands
Wong & Sagar 2006 (125)	5	Case series Chemotherapy-induced peripheral neuropathy (CIPN) with WHO grade at least II	WHO peripheral neuropathy grade (includes assessment of paraesthesia, pain, weakness and tendon reflexes)	6 weekly treatments, 4 weeks rest, further 6 weekly treatments CV 6 and bilateral ST 36, LI 11, Bafeng, Baxie Jing points on hands or feet for severe numbness and dysfunction of fingers and toes Points needled for 30–45 minutes with no stimulation	All patients reported reduced pain, numbness and tingling as reflected by improved WHO peripheral neuropathy grade Improved sensation in response to Jing point needling Reduced use of analgesics
Schröder et al. 2007 (20)	47	Retrospective case review Peripheral neuropathy of unknown aetiology Neuropathy confirmed by nerve conduction studies (NCS)	Self-rated pain, paraesthesia and numbness NCS of tibial and sural nerves assessing velocity and amplitude of sensory and motor responses	10 acupuncture treatments over 10 weeks for 20 minutes Points mainly on ST and LI meridians and included ST34 Also used Bafeng and Qiduan (EX-LE 12: on tips of toes)	In acupuncture group (n = 20) 76% improved on self-rated scales and NCS and none deteriorated In non-acupuncture group 15% noted similar improvement, whilst 36% noted a deterioration

RCT, randomized controlled trial; HIV, human immunodeficiency virus; QOL, quality of life; VAS, Visual Analogue Scale; WHO, World Health Organization.

Table 4.5 Acupuncture for pain in spinal cord injury

Authors and year	n	Design and inclusion criteria	Assessment	Interventions	Results
Nayak et al. 2001 (126)	22	Pretest, posttest study Traumatic spinal cord injury Pain for at least 6 months Pain severity of at least 5/10	Pain 0–10 NRS 0–10 scale for pain impact 0–10 scale of 5 most bothersome symptoms, e.g. sleep problems Self-report 20-item CES Depression Scale Anxiety Index (STAI-S), General Wellbeing Scale	15 acupuncture treatments of 20 minutes over 7.5 weeks 6–14 points selected from a list All participants were needled at GV 14, Huatuojiaji points at the level of their spinal lesion and either BL 10 or BL 40 Other points selected according to patient's pain from Bafeng, KI 3, BL 60, LR 3, GB 34, SP 6, ST 36, Baxie, SI 3, HT 3, PC 6, TE 5, LU 7, LI 4 as well as Ah-shi points and ear points	Substantial pain relief in 46% 35% reported continuing relief at 3 months whilst 27% reported increased pain at 3 months Factors indicating better response were nociceptive pain, pain above spinal lesion, incomplete spinal lesions 42% with central neuropathic pain reported pain relief
Rapson et al. 2003 (127)	36	Retrospective case review of patients with below-lesion central neuropathic pain for 1 month to 15 years Spinal cord injury $n = 22$ Other cases included Guillain–Barré syndrome, multiple sclerosis, CIDP, syringomyelia	0–10 VAS for pain	Up to 26 scalp acupuncture treatments; initial treatments provided 5 days/week; frequency reduced as effects became cumulative GV 18, GV 20, GV 21 and Yintang needled for 30 minutes with electroacupuncture at 1 Hz	24 patients reported reduced pain Those who gained benefit responded by treatment 4 and many responded after first treatment More favourable response in those with bilateral, symmetrical, continuous burning pain
Dyson-Hudson et al. 2007 (156)	17	RCT Spinal cord injury Musculoskeletal shoulder pain for more than 3 months	Wheelchair User's Shoulder Pain Index (WUSPI) 0–10 NRS for pain intensity	10 acupuncture treatments of 20–30 minutes over 5 weeks Points from a list were needled, including 6 local, 2 distal and Ah-shi points as required Compared with superficially invasive sham acupuncture at sites at least 1 cm away from real points	WUSPI and NRS scores significantly improved in both groups Benefits still noted at 5-week follow-up No difference between treatment groups

NRS, numerical rating scale; STAI-S, State-Trait Anxiety Inventory; CES, Centre for Epidemiologic Studies; CIDP, chronic inflammatory demyelinating polyneuropathy; VAS, Visual Analogue Scale; RCT, randomized controlled trial;

Weakness and paralysis

Damage within central or peripheral pathways controlling movement may cause weakness or complete paralysis. Weakness is very common in stroke, traumatic brain injury, multiple sclerosis and peripheral neuropathies.

Acupuncture for weakness and paralysis

Many studies have assessed the impact of acupuncture on motor recovery in stroke. Fewer studies have assessed weakness in other populations (Table 4.7).

Table 4.6 Acupuncture for paraesthesia and dysaesthesia

Authors and year	n	Design and inclusion criteria	Assessment	Interventions	Results
Napadow et al. 2007 (8)	25	Experimental longitudinal neuroimaging study n = 13 mild to moderate carpal tunnel syndrome with pain and/or paraesthesia for 3 months or more n = 12 age- and sex-matched healthy adults	fMRI Nerve conduction studies of median nerve Grip strength Sensation with Semmes Weinstein monofilaments Phalen's and Tinel's sign Boston Carpal Tunnel Syndrome Questionnaire	13 acupuncture treatments over 5 weeks 10 minutes EA at 2 Hz at TE 5 and PC 7 followed by manual needling of 3 points selected from HT 3, PC 3, SI 4, LI 5, LI 10, LU 5; needles stimulated for Deqi	Acupuncture group noted significant improvements in paraesthesia, dysaesthesia, grip strength and median nerve sensory latencies; fMRI revealed close representation of index and middle finger on primary sensory cortex before acupuncture; following acupuncture increased separation between index and middle-finger representation

fMRI, functional magnetic resonance imaging; EA, electroacupuncture.

Table 4.7 Acupuncture for motor paralysis or paresis

Authors and year	n	Design and inclusion criteria	Assessment	Interventions	Results
Wong et al. 2003 (128)	100	RCT Acute traumatic spinal cord injury	Neurological scores of sensory and motor function (ASIA scale) Functional Independence Measure (FIM)	Transcutaneous electrical stimulation at 75 Hz to SI 3 and BL 62 combined with needling of 4 ear acupuncture points × 5/week from admission to discharge Treatment started in the emergency room or soon after spinal surgical intervention Control group received no TENS and acupuncture Both groups received standard rehabilitation	Significant improvements in sensory and motor function and FIM scores in acupuncture group as well as a greater percentage recovering to a higher ASIA impairment grade
Alexander et al. 2004 (129)	32	Pilot RCT Acute stroke resulting in hemipareisis Recruited within 60 days of stroke onset	Fugl–Meyer Assessment (FMA): total score, upper- and lower-limb subscales FIM	Manual acupuncture selected from list of 29 points according to patient presentation Control group received no intervention	All patients improved in FMA and FIM Significant improvement in Fugl–Meyer lower-limb subscale and in 'tub/shower transfer' component of FIM in acupuncture group

Continued

Table 4.7 Acupuncture for motor paralysis or paresis—cont'd

Authors and year	n	Design and inclusion criteria	Assessment	Interventions	Results
Wayne et al. 2005 (130)	33	RCT First stroke (8 months–24 years poststroke) Some upper-limb ability, i.e. able to raise impaired arm on to a table while seated Ability to stand and walk independently	FMA upper-limb component Modified Ashworth Scale (MAS) Dynamometer for grip strength Range of active assisted arm movement ADL, QOL and mood questionnaires	Manual and EA to body points selected from list of over 40 points Manual scalp acupuncture to sensory and motor lines on side over affected brain Body and scalp acupuncture alternated on weekly basis Up to 20 treatments over 11 weeks for 20–30 minutes Sham group received non-invasive placebo acupuncture to body or scalp	No significant differences on ITT analysis Per-protocol analysis indicated improvement in FMA arm score, MAS for wrist and shoulder and active wrist movement in acupuncture group
Liu et al. 2008 (131)	10	Cross-over study – each intervention × 2/week for 6 weeks Stroke (2–31 years poststroke) MAS of 3 or more at wrist Fugl–Meyer upper-limb score ranged from 16 to 59/66	Isometric strength of wrist flexors and extensors on Biodex Active ROM for wrist and index finger extension FMA upper-limb score Assessment of muscle response to different velocity stretch	Intervention 1 EA at 2 Hz to LI 4, LI 10, LI 11, LI 15, SI 3, TE 5 for 40 minutes followed by 30–45 minutes of wrist-strengthening exercises on Biodex machine Intervention 2 30–45 minutes of wrist-strengthening exercises on Biodex machine	Significant improvement in combined intervention group for: • active range of wrist extension • active finger extension which increased by 30° in those 2 participants who had some finger extension at baseline • modest increase in FMA upper-limb score by 5 points • muscle response to stretch (i.e. less 'spasticity') No changes in strength in either group

RCT, randomized controlled trial; ASIA, American Spinal Injuries Association; TENS, transcutaneous electrical nerve stimulation; EA, electroacupuncture; ADL, activities of daily living; QOL, quality of life; ITT, intention to treat; ROM, range of motion. FMA, Fugl Meyer Assessment.

These studies suggest some benefits from a range of interventions, including body, ear and scalp acupuncture, as well as in combination with a strengthening programme. However these studies also raise questions about acupuncture study design, particularly regarding the upper limb. None of the acupuncture studies assessing arm function in stroke had exclusion criteria according to motor ability in the fingers or wrist. Research indicates that the ability to extend the fingers is a powerful prognostic factor for eventual arm function in stroke [33]. Other studies stipulate this ability as minimal entry level to studies, for example in constraint-induced movement therapy [34]. Interestingly, in Liu's study [35], those individuals with some active finger extension before the acupuncture intervention gained an additional 30° with combined acupuncture and strength training. Design of studies with more defined entry criteria might provide useful information about the effects of acupuncture for motor recovery in specific subpopulations.

Spasticity

Spasticity is a movement disorder observed in individuals with lesions of the upper motor neurone pathways, for example, in stroke, multiple sclerosis or spinal cord injury. Spasticity is classically defined as a motor disorder characterized by a velocity-dependent increase in tonic stretch reflexes [36]. It is accompanied by a range of other features such as weakness and loss of dexterity [37]. The neurophysiology of spasticity is complex but involves abnormalities in proprioceptive, cutaneous and nociceptive reflexes. Persistent spasticity may lead to adaptive changes such as soft-tissue contracture. The impact of spasticity on functional ability is unclear but for many individuals spasticity is problematic [38].

Prevalence of spasticity

The prevalence of spasticity varies according to condition, with over 90% of those with cerebral palsy [39], 84% of people with multiple sclerosis [40], 65–78% of people with spinal cord injury [41] but only around 17% of people with stroke presenting with spasticity [42]. Some people with traumatic brain injury develop severe and chronic spasticity but prevalence figures are not reported [43].

Management of spasticity

Effective management of spasticity is dependent on detailed assessment. Provoking factors such as ill-fitting splints, constipation or pain need to be addressed since these have the potential to increase spasticity. Oral medications such as baclofen may be used for generalized spasticity, whilst focal treatments such as botulinum toxin injections or phenol nerve blocks would be considered when spasticity was more localized. Insertion of an intrathecal baclofen pump might be considered for cases of severe regional spasticity, for example affecting both lower limbs. Physiotherapy to improve movement control, balance and strength, as well as stretches for specific muscles, is helpful [44]. Occupational therapists can advise on many useful aids or adaptations, such as an appropriate wheelchair with suitable cushion [38].

Acupuncture for spasticity

Spasticity is notoriously difficult to quantify. Electrophysiological tests such as the H-reflex, H_{max}/M_{max} ratio and F-wave may provide information about the excitability of the spinal motorneurone pool. These tests are moderately reliable. However, they do not always correlate with clinical assessments of spasticity. In addition commonly used assessments, such as the Modified Ashworth Scale (MAS), provide information about contracture as well as spasticity [45]. Therefore interventions directed at the dynamic component of spasticity may not result in a change in the MAS score. These methods of assessment have been used in acupuncture studies (Table 4.8).

These studies suggest that acupuncture may influence the excitability of spinal motor neurones. This effect is usually an inhibitory effect, but may be facilitatory, as in the Fink study. It is worth remembering that all individuals in these studies demonstrated cerebral spasticity. Responses in these situations may not be identical to those presenting with spasticity from spinal lesions such as spinal cord injury and multiple sclerosis. More detailed evaluation is required.

Parkinsonian dyskinesia

Dyskinesias are abnormal involuntary movements which may appear as jerking, twisting or writhing of parts of the body. This type of movement abnormality is very common in Parkinson's disease and may result from the disease process itself or as a side-effect of levodopa medication used to treat symptoms. Dyskinesias may be present when drugs have worn off, such as first thing in the morning ('off'-medication dyskinesia) or during the day when the medication is working ('on'-medication dyskinesia) [46].

The most common types of dyskinesia in Parkinson's disease are chorea, ballism, dystonia and myoclonus. Although these movement disorders are problematic, many individuals would prefer being 'on' with dyskinesia rather than 'off' without dyskinesia [47]. Studies have indicated that dyskinesia and pain commonly coexist and some authors suggest that they may share common pathophysiological mechanisms [48].

Prevalence of parkinsonian dyskinesia

Between 22% and 40% of people with Parkinson's disease present with 'on'-medication dyskinesias after 5 years on levodopa medication. This rises to around 62% after 9 years [47]. 'Off'-medication dyskinesia occurs in about 16% of people with Parkinson's disease [46].

Table 4.8 Acupuncture for spasticity

Authors and year	n	Design and inclusion criteria	Assessment	Interventions	Results
Yu et al. 1995 (132)	16	Observational study of stroke (16) and controls (11) Stroke with spastic hemipareisis (1–18 months poststroke)	H-reflex recovery time	Manual acupuncture to GB 34, GB 31, BL 57, BL 60 for 15–20 minutes	H-reflex recovery time was longer in stroke limbs after acupuncture Suggests a reduction in spinal motor neurone excitability following acupuncture
Fink et al. 2004 (133)	25	RCT Stroke with chronic leg spasticity (7–180 months poststroke)	2-minute walk test and other motor assessments Modified Ashworth Scale (MAS) H-reflex and H_{max}/M_{max} ratio VAS pain Clinical Global Impressions (CGI) scale Questionnaires regarding QOL	Verum manual acupuncture to GB 34, GB 39, ST 36, ST 40, SP 6, SP 9, KI 3, KI 6, BL 62, LR 3, LR 9, LI 4, LI 10, LU 9, GV 20 for 30 minutes; no stimulation (maximum 15 needles) compared to non-invasive placebo needles in non-acupoints 8 treatments over 4 weeks	No change in MAS CGI significantly worse in verum group at end of treatment H_{max}/M_{max} ratio higher, suggesting greater excitability of motor neurone pool in verum group at end of treatment
Mukherjee et al. 2007 (134)	7	Cross-over study – each intervention × 2/week for 6 weeks Stroke (2.5–31 years poststroke) MAS of 3 or more at wrist	Quantitative assessment of muscle response to different velocity stretch (to give an indication of spasticity) MAS for wrist and index finger flexors and extensors	Intervention 1 EA at 2 Hz to LI 4, LI 10, LI 11, LI 15, SI 3, TE 5 for 40 minutes followed by 30 minutes of wrist-strengthening exercises on Biodex machine Intervention 2 30–45 minutes of wrist-strengthening exercises on Biodex machine	No immediate effects After 6 weeks a significant reduction on MAS and in velocity sensitivity of average speed-dependent reflex – torque noted in combined acupuncture and strengthening group
Zhao et al. 2009 (135)	131	RCT Stroke (mean 17 months poststroke)	MAS Fugl–Meyer Assessment (FMA) Barthel Index (BI) Electromyogram of affected limb	Daily treatment for 30 days Control group PC 6, SP 6, GV 26, HT 1, LU 5, BL 40, GB 20 Treatment group Addition of BL 9, BL 10 and 4 equidistant points (to stimulate surface projection zone of the decussation of the pyramid) Daily treatment in both groups for 20 minutes	Significant improvements in treatment group on MAS, BI, FMA total score Significant reduction in F-wave amplitude and F/M ratio, suggesting reduction in excitability in motor neurone pool

RCT, randomized controlled trial; VAS, Visual Analogue Scale; QOL, quality of life; EA, electroacupuncture.

Acupuncture for Parkinson's disease

Studies evaluating the use of acupuncture in Parkinson's disease have generally used measures assessing the global effect of acupuncture on individuals with Parkinson's disease rather than considering specific impairments such as dyskinesia or pain (Table 4.9).

The studies by Shulman et al. [49] and Cristian et al. [50] demonstrate a trend towards improvement in the acupuncture group, including improved sleep, but the evidence is not clear. It is worth noting that both studies are small and the Cristian study used an active control procedure. Chae's team [51] have provided an interesting insight into the effects of needling GB 34 on motor function and

Table 4.9 Acupuncture for Parkinson's disease

Authors and year	n	Design and inclusion criteria	Assessment	Interventions	Results
Shulman et al. 2002 (49)	20	Pretest/posttest study Idiopathic Parkinson's disease on stable dose of medications	Outcome measures, including: Sickness Impact Profile (SIP) Unified Parkinson's Disease Rating Scale (UPDRS) Beck Anxiety Index (BAI) and Beck Depression Index (BDI)	10–16 acupuncture treatments received over a 5–8 weeks period (treatments × 2/week) Body points: LI 4, GB 34, ST 36 plus KI 3, KI 7, SP 6, SI 3, TE 5 Scalp points: 9 needles in chorea control area Treatment lasted for 1 hour	Significant benefit on sleep component of SIP No other significant findings on large range of outcome measures 85% of patients reported improvement in symptoms on a non-validated questionnaire
Cristian et al. 2005 (50)	14	RCT Idiopathic Parkinson's disease on stable medication regime	Outcome measures including: UPDRS, Parkinson's Disease Questionnaire-39 (PDQ-39 & PDQ-8 summary index), Geriatric Depression Scale	5 treatments of 20 minutes over 2 weeks; electroacupuncture of 4 Hz to bilateral KI 3 and KI 10 Manual acupuncture to bilateral BL 60, LR 3, ST 41, ST 36, GB 34, Bafeng, PC 6, LI 4, and GV 20 'Control' group received subcutaneous acupuncture in areas with 'no known acupuncture points' in arms, legs and scalp – exact sites not stated	No significant differences between groups Trend towards significance in true acupuncture groups on PDQ
Chae et al. 2009 (51)	10	Observational study Mild idiopathic Parkinson's disease No Parkinson's disease medications for at least 12 hours	fMRI – random-order block design Finger-tapping test of motor function	Verum acupuncture at GB 34 compared with overt and covert sham needling at the same point Verum or sham needle 'inserted' and stimulated at 1 Hz for 1 minute then withdrawn	Verum acupuncture led to increased activation of putamen and primary motor cortex; this increase was significantly correlated with enhanced motor function Placebo (covert) needling led to increase in activation of anterior cingulate gyrus and other regions

RCT, randomized controlled trial; fMRI, functional magnetic resonance imaging.

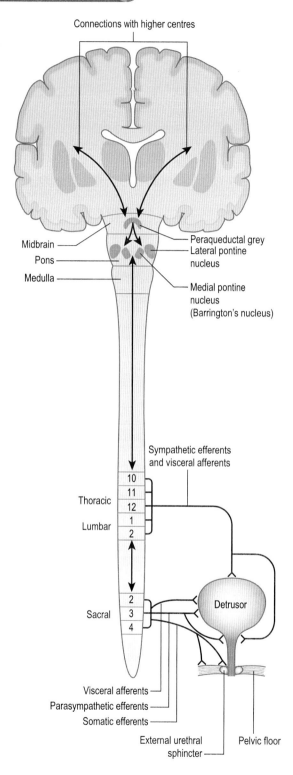

brain activation in experimental conditions. There is a clear need for well-designed, clinically relevant studies to examine this question further.

Part 3: Visceral function

Bladder dysfunction

The bladder has two main functions: storage of urine and voiding of urine. Problems can arise from a disruption of either of these functions, leading to a range of problems such as stress incontinence, urge incontinence or a mixture of these presentations [52]. Urinary incontinence is defined as 'any involuntary leakage of urine'. The combination of urgency, urge incontinence, daytime frequency and nocturia is termed Overactive Bladder Syndrome (OAB) and reflects hyperactivity of the detrusor [52].

Neural control of the bladder is complex, involving autonomic and somatic pathways linking the spinal cord, brainstem and higher brain centres (Figure 4.1). Control of bladder function in the spinal cord is localized in two main regions (Table 4.10).

Prevalence of urinary problems in neurological disease

Bladder dysfunction is common in neurological conditions. Estimated prevalence is more than 80% in those with multiple sclerosis [53], most people with spinal cord injury, 54% of patients with acute stroke and 32% of those at 1 year poststroke [54], up to 39% of those with Parkinson's disease [55], and around 27% of those with Guillain–Barré syndrome [56].

Figure 4.1 • Diagrammatic representation of neural control of bladder. Arrows indicate connections between different areas that are important in control of bladder activity. *Lateral pontine nucleus*: important for storage of urine. *Medial pontine nucleus*: important for micturition. *Periaqueductal grey*: important area for integrating information about bladder control from the spinal cord as well as from higher centres such as anterior cingulate cortex, prefrontal cortex, sensorimotor cortex, insula, basal ganglia, thalamus and cerebellum; projects on to medial and lateral pontine nuclei.

Table 4.10 Spinal cord control of bladder function

Spinal cord level	Pathways	Effect
Thoracic 10–lumbar 2	Visceral afferents	Conveys information regarding bladder distension and contraction
	Sympathetic efferents	Relaxation of detrusor Contraction of internal urethral sphincter
Sacral 2–4	Visceral afferents	Conveys information regarding bladder distension and contraction
	Parasympathetic efferents	Contraction of detrusor Relaxation of internal urethral sphincter
	Somatic efferents	Contraction of external urethral sphincter Contraction of pelvic floor

Key patterns of urinary dysfunction in neurological conditions

Urinary symptoms vary according to the site of the lesion within the neural pathways (Table 4.11).

The primary problems seen are overactivity of the bladder (detrusor hyperreflexia), underactivity of the bladder (detrusor areflexia or hypocontractility) or incoordination of activity between the bladder and the urethral sphincters (detrusor-sphincter dyssynergia).

Table 4.11 Urodynamic patterns according to level of lesion in nervous system

Level of lesion in nervous system	Conditions	Urodynamic patterns	Symptoms
Suprapontine	Stroke, hydrocephalus, intracerebral neoplasm, traumatic brain injury, Parkinson's disease, multiple sclerosis, cerebral palsy	Detrusor hyperreflexia	Urgency, urge incontinence, daytime frequency, nocturia
Pontine	Pontine stroke Multiple sclerosis	Detrusor hypocontractility Some cases of detrusor hyperreflexia and detrusor-sphincter dyssynergia (DSD)	Bladder overdistension with inadequate emptying Incomplete emptying of bladder
Suprasacral spinal cord	Spinal cord injury in cervical, thoracic or lumbar spinal cord Multiple sclerosis plaques in suprasacral spinal cord (incomplete spinal cord lesion)	Detrusor areflexia in period of spinal cord injury spinal shock DSD Detrusor hyperreflexia	No bladder emptying in period of spinal shock Incomplete emptying of bladder Urgency, urge incontinence, daytime frequency, nocturia
Sacral spinal cord	Spinal cord injury or multiple sclerosis plaques in sacral spinal cord	Detrusor hypocontractility Often intact external urethral sphincter	Bladder overdistension with inadequate emptying
Peripheral somatic or autonomic nerves	Guillain–Barré syndrome, chronic inflammatory demyelinating polyneuropathy	Detrusor hypocontractility Detrusor hyperreflexia	Bladder overdistension with inadequate emptying Urgency, urge incontinence, daytime frequency, nocturia

Management of urinary dysfunction

Management of urinary dysfunction is based on effective assessment and may include the use of bladder diaries, urine testing, postmicturition residual volumes and, when necessary, urodynamic studies [52, 57]. Different types of incontinence will require different management strategies but treatment options may include a combination of advice, education, pelvic floor exercises, bladder retraining, lifestyle modification such as adequate fluid intake and reduction of caffeine intake, as well as use of medications such as antimuscarinics, for example, oxybutynin or tolterodine. Some people may need intermittent catheterization or use of an indwelling catheter. Surgical options may be appropriate for some patients [52].

Electrical stimulation for urinary dysfunction

Electrical stimulation of pelvic floor muscles may be considered for those with stress incontinence who are unable actively to contract their pelvic floor muscles [52]. Various types of sacral nerve and posterior tibial nerve stimulation have been suggested for OAB and for urinary retention. PENS provided benefits for OAB in multiple sclerosis and Parkinson's disease [58, 59]. Stimulation was applied to the posterior tibial nerve at the area known in acupuncture as Spleen 6. TENS over sacral dermatomes in multiple sclerosis was not effective [60]. However benefits were noted from TENS applied over the posterior tibial nerve in OAB due to multiple sclerosis, Parkinson's disease, spinal cord injury and stroke [61]. An implanted sacral nerve root stimulator may be useful for individuals with refractory OAB [52]. However in neurological conditions botulinum toxin injections of detrusor would probably be considered first [57].

Acupuncture for bladder dysfunction

Acupuncture for bladder dysfunction has been considered in a variety of studies (Table 4.12). Early studies on spinal cats by Sato et al. [62] highlighted the influence of somatic afferent stimulation on bladder activity. More recently, Tanaka et al. [63] examined electroacupuncture to the sacral segment in rats and noted suppression of detrusor activity which was often also accompanied by changes in electroencephalogram. This suggests that acupuncture may affect the bladder

as well as the sleep arousal system. These would be useful findings for those presenting with nocturia.

These studies (Table 4.12) indicate that stimulation, whether via TENS, manual acupuncture or electroacupuncture, may provide a valuable treatment option to consider in people with neurological conditions who present with urinary dysfunction, particularly OAB. Parasympathetic and sympathetic outflow to the bladder and sphincter may be influenced according to the location of afferent stimulation. Further high-quality studies with larger numbers and appropriate control groups are required.

Bowel dysfunction

The main functions of the distal part of the large intestine or colon are to absorb water and electrolytes, move residual contents through the colon and to store faeces prior to elimination [64]. The colon and rectum are controlled by the enteric nervous system which includes sympathetic and parasympathetic neurones interconnected with local nerve networks. The maintenance of faecal continence requires the coordinated action of these different neural pathways (Figure 4.2). Spinal control of bowel function is outlined in Table 4.13.

Prevalence of bowel problems in neurological conditions

Bowel problems are more common in neurological conditions than in the general population. There is an estimated prevalence of bowel dysfunction, including incontinence and constipation, in up to 73% of those with multiple sclerosis [65], 42–95% of those with spinal cord injury [64], 29–67% in Parkinson's disease [66], up to 56% of those with cerebral palsy [67] and around 30% in patients with stroke [68].

Key patterns of bowel dysfunction in neurological conditions

Reduced activity of the colon with increased colonic transit time is common in many neurological conditions contributing to constipation [64]. Incoordination between the anal sphincter and rectal activity (defecation dyssynergia) may cause obstructed defecation and is found in Parkinson's disease and multiple sclerosis [65, 66]. Chronic constipation in stroke appears to be related to damage of the

Table 4.12 Acupuncture for bladder dysfunction in neurological conditions

Authors and year	n	Design and inclusion criteria	Assessment	Interventions	Results
Cheng et al. 1998 (135)	80	Controlled trial of acupuncture compared to standard bladder training for spinal cord injury with neurogenic bladder	Total days required to achieve 'balanced bladder', i.e. easily able to pass urine, residual urine volume was 100 ml or less and no urinary tract infection	Electroacupuncture compared with conventional bladder training; both groups performed intermittent catheterization as required Electroacupuncture at 20–30 Hz, pulse duration 200 s for 30 minutes, 4–5/week until continent. Points used were CV 3, CV 4, BL 32 bilaterally	Fewer days required to achieve continence in acupuncture group No response to acupuncture in those with complete spinal cord injury with persistent detrusor-sphincter dyssynergia or areflexic bladder
Honjo et al. 2000 (136)	13	Pre- and posttreatment study of acupuncture for detrusor hyperreflexia in spinal cord injury	Urodynamic assessment, bladder diary	Manual acupuncture at BL 33 bilaterally – deep needling so needle tip close to the sacral periosteum. Manual stimulation. Treatment × 1/week for 4 weeks	Incontinence was resolved in 2, reduced by 50% in 6 and minimal change in 5 Significant increase in bladder capacity in those who responded to acupuncture
Keppel Hesselink & Kopsky 2005 (137)	2	Descriptive case reports Two patients with multiple sclerosis with bladder dysfunction (1 × detrusor hyperreflexia; 1 × urinary retention)	Patient reported symptoms	Electroacupuncture at 15 Hz to SP 6, SP 4 for 30 minutes every week, intensity just below pain threshold Use of TENS over same points for home use	Reduction of bladder symptoms during course of treatment TENS also useful
Dorsher et al. 2009 (121)	2	Descriptive case reports Two patients with incomplete spinal cord lesions with urinary incontinence refractory to other treatments	Patient-reported symptoms	Electroacupuncture at 2 Hz to GB 25, BL 23, BL 52 (15 minutes) and BL 31, BL 34 (15 minutes) bilaterally plus stimulation at GV 1 Second patient also received PENS at 30 Hz (25 minutes) bilaterally at spinal levels T9, L1, S1, S2–S4 and suprapubic region; then later at CV 2,3 with 2 Hz (15 minutes)	Improvements in continence, sleep and reduction of pain

TENS, trancutaneous electrical nerve stimulation; PENS, percutaneous electrical nerve stimulation.

dominant cortical area controlling defecation [68]. Faecal incontinence may be noted where there is a lack of anorectal sensation or lack of voluntary control of external anal sphincter and pelvic floor, for example, in spinal cord injury affecting the sacral cord or cauda equina [64].

Management of bowel dysfunction

Full assessment by health care professionals with relevant skills is required to identify the nature of bowel dysfunction and to recommend an appropriate plan [69]. Management options may include

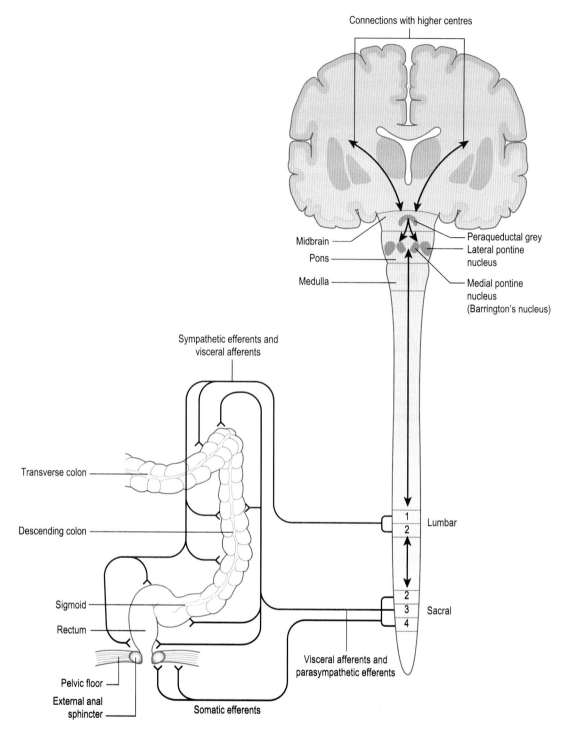

Figure 4.2 • Diagrammatic representation of neural control of distal colon and rectum. Arrows indicate connections between different areas important in control of bowel activity. Medial pontine nucleus (Barrington's nucleus): probable role in coordinating afferent information from distal colon with information from higher centres.

Table 4.13 Spinal cord control of bowel function

Spinal cord level	Pathways	Effect
Lumbar 1–2	Visceral afferents	Convey information on distension and discomfort from distal colon and rectum
	Sympathetic efferents	Reduced motility of distal colon, rectum and upper anal canal Contraction of internal anal sphincter
Sacral 2–4	Visceral afferents	Convey information regarding distension of the distal colon and rectum
	Parasympathetic efferents	Increased motility of distal colon, rectum and upper anal canal Relaxation of internal anal sphincter
	Somatic efferents	Contraction of external anal sphincter Contraction of pelvic floor

Note: distal colon includes distal one-third of transverse colon, descending and sigmoid colon.

advice on diet, fluid intake, exercise and bowel habits, as well as the prescription of various medications. Interventions such as pelvic floor exercises, bowel retraining or biofeedback will be appropriate for some individuals. Discussion of practical issues including access to toilet, mobility, clothing and use of continence products will be relevant in some situations. Sacral nerve stimulation or surgery may be considered for some individuals [69].

Electrical stimulation for bowel dysfunction

Electrical stimulation of pelvic floor muscles has been used for those with faecal incontinence but there is currently insufficient evidence to indicate whether this is useful [70]. Sacral nerve stimulation has been used successfully to manage faecal incontinence and constipation in some patients [71]. Few studies have included people with neurological diseases but a prospective non-randomized study by Jarrett et al. [72] demonstrated a reduction in incontinent episodes in a group of 13 individuals with faecal incontinence due to partial spinal cord injury, with stimulation parameters of a frequency of 15 Hz and pulse duration 200 s [72].

Acupuncture for bowel dysfunction

Acupuncture for bowel dysfunction has received very little attention. No placebo-controlled trials have been conducted. A few small uncontrolled trials have been conducted (Table 4.14). Animal studies demonstrate a modulatory effect of electroacupuncture at 10 Hz to Stomach 36 on the motility of the distal colon. This effect is usually to increase motility in the distal colon, although it may be the reverse in some conditions. The effect seems to be mediated through parasympathetic outflow from the sacral spinal cord as well as involving activity in brainstem nuclei [73, 74].

The small studies by Broide et al. [75] and Scaglia et al. [76] suggest benefits for those with constipation and faecal incontinence. No studies have looked at the impact of acupuncture on bowel dysfunction for those with a specific neurological condition. Anecdotal reports suggest benefit for this population but well-designed research is required to guide practice more effectively.

Part 4: Generalized symptoms

Insomnia

Insomnia relates to the difficulty in falling asleep, staying asleep, waking up too early or sleep that is of poor quality [77]. Symptoms occurring in the absence of any other medical condition are termed primary insomnia whilst secondary insomnia refers to symptoms occurring in relation to another medical or psychiatric disorder. Insomnia is typically a complex condition with many contributing factors [78]. It is thought to be a hyperarousal disorder with

Table 4.14 Acupuncture for bowel dysfunction

Authors and year	n	Design and inclusion criteria	Assessment	Interventions	Results
Klauser et al. 1993 (138)	8	Pre- and posttreatment study Constipation	Stool frequency Colonic transit time of radiopaque markers	Electroacupuncture at 10 Hz for 25 minutes to LI 4, ST 25, LR 3, BL 25 for six treatments over 3 weeks	2 dropped out as constipation worse Remaining 6: no change in colonic function
Broide et al. 2001 (75)	17	Placebo-controlled trial comparing acupuncture and control group Children with constipation for at least 6 months (age range 3–13 years)	Anal manometry at beginning of study Questionnaire about constipation issues Opioid levels in blood plasma	5 weekly sham acupuncture (superficial needling of 'non'-acupuncture points) Followed by 10 weekly acupuncture treatments based on Chinese medical diagnosis –needled LI 4, LR 2 and ST 36 for 20 minutes	Small increase in bowel movement after placebo; greater improvement of bowel movements after true acupuncture Opioid levels lower in constipated children than in controls; opioid levels increased over course of true acupuncture
Scaglia et al. 2009 (76)	15	Pre- and post-treatment study Females with faecal incontinence for at least 1 year	Cleveland Clinic Continence Score Anorectal manovolumetry Follow-up until 18 months	10 weekly 20-minute acupuncture treatments based on Chinese medicine – included CV 3, CV 6, GV 4, BL 23, BL 32, LI 4, ST 36, KI 3	Substantial reduction in Cleveland Clinic Continence Score, i.e. improvement in stool consistency, frequency and regularity Many improved by the third treatment Minimal change in manovolumetric assessments

hyperactivity of the hypothalamic–pituitary axis [77]. Difficulty with sleeping may contribute to daytime sleepiness, fatigue, mood disturbance and poor concentration. In addition, good-quality sleep is important for consolidation of new memories such as new motor skills or declarative knowledge [79, 80].

Prevalence of insomnia in neurological conditions

Prevalence of insomnia is over 50% in stroke [81], up to 51% in people with multiple sclerosis [82], between 46% and 70% of those with traumatic brain injury [83] and between 60% and 98% in Parkinson's disease [84]. These figures are clearly higher than those for the general population, of around 30% [77].

Insomnia in neurological conditions

Normal sleep patterns are generated and modulated by complex neural systems located mainly in the hypothalamus, brainstem and thalamus [85]. People with neurological conditions may develop sleep dysfunction due to primary involvement of these areas [84, 86, 87]. In addition insomnia may be secondary to factors which may predispose the individual to wake, such as pain, anxiety, depression, involuntary limb movements or nocturia [85].

Management of insomnia

Management of insomnia includes the treatment of any precipitating factors, education regarding good sleep habits and the use of medications as necessary. Pharmacological treatments have been widely used for the treatment of insomnia and have included benzodiazepines or other drugs such as zoplicone. These show clear benefits for short-term reduction of sleep disturbance but effects reduce with time [78]. Non-pharmacological options such as cognitive-behavioural therapy provide lasting effects for up to 6 months or longer [78, 83]. However this therapy is not always available and some patients are unwilling or unable to engage in the process.

Acupuncture for insomnia

Anecdotal reports by people with neurological conditions indicate benefits from acupuncture for insomnia [88]. An interesting pretest, posttest study by Spence et al. [89] used polysomnography, nighttime melatonin levels and questionnaires to measure the effect of 10 acupuncture treatments provided over 5 weeks to 18 anxious adults [89]. Results indicated improvements in sleep as recorded by polysomnography, increases in nighttime melatonin secretion and improvements in self-rated fatigue and sleepiness. Points used were not specified. Other studies have considered the use of acupuncture in insomnia. However many of these have been small or poorly designed. Consequently a number of recent systematic reviews have concluded that whilst results are promising there is insufficient evidence to support the use of acupuncture for insomnia [90–92]. Studies evaluating acupuncture in neurological conditions have found a reduction of insomnia in patients with stroke and Parkinson's disease [49, 93]. There is a clear need for large well-designed trials to evaluate this question further.

Fatigue

Fatigue may be defined as feelings of tiredness, exhaustion and lack of physical or mental energy which are abnormal, excessive, chronic, persistent or problematic [94]. In general the type of fatigue reported by people with neurological conditions is disproportionate to the amount of activity carried out and is generally not relieved by resting or sleeping. Fatigue has peripheral and central components. Peripheral fatigue relates to the peripheral neural and musculoskeletal system and results in difficulty performing motor activities. Central fatigue relates to dysfunction of the central nervous system and may cause difficulties in initiating and executing motor or cognitive tasks [95, 96].

Prevalence of fatigue in neurological conditions

Fatigue is reported in many neurological conditions, with prevalence higher than those for the general population. The prevalence of fatigue is reported to be between 39% and 72% of people with stroke [97], 57% of those with spinal cord injury [98], up to 58% of those with Parkinson's disease [99], 60% of people with Guillain–Barré syndrome [100], around 70% of people with multiple sclerosis [101] and up to 73% of those with traumatic brain injury [102].

Fatigue in neurological conditions

Fatigue is complex. An element of peripheral fatigue will be evident in those individuals with muscle dysfunction such as weakness. However a substantial contribution to fatigue in neurological conditions is made by central mechanisms. The role of impaired central muscle activation and altered activation patterns of motor neurones has been reported [103]. Dopamine deficiency is likely to play a role in fatigue noted in Parkinson's disease [96]. A role for proinflammatory cytokines in multiple sclerosis fatigue has been suggested [104]. Dysfunction of pathways involved in cognitive-attentional processes has been highlighted as important in fatigue reported in multiple sclerosis and traumatic brain injury [105, 106]. In addition a range of other factors contribute to the presence of fatigue. These include depression, anxiety, sleep disturbance, chronic pain and medication side-effects [94].

Management of fatigue in neurological conditions

Fatigue management will be tailored according to individualized assessment. Options might include medications such as modafinil or amantadine. Non-pharmacological options will broadly aim to maximize the person's physical ability and minimize fatigue impact. Therapeutic strategies include strengthening and conditioning exercise, education regarding energy conservation and pacing of activities, as well as cognitive-behavioural therapy [94, 107]. Contributory factors such as mood or sleep disturbance also need to be addressed.

Acupuncture for fatigue

A number of studies have evaluated the use of acupuncture for fatigue in fibromyalgia and cancer-related fatigue. Some studies have noted benefits (Table 4.15) whilst other studies have not [108]. No studies have considered acupuncture for fatigue in neurological conditions.

Table 4.15 Acupuncture for fatigue

Authors and year	n	Design and inclusion criteria	Assessment	Interventions	Results
Deluze et al. 1992 (139)	70	RCT Fibromyalgia	Pain threshold, analgesic use, regional pain scores, VAS pain, stiffness and sleep	Six EA treatments at 1–99 Hz over 3 weeks to bilateral LI 4 and ST 36; up to 6 other points used; strong EA stimulation to obtain visible muscle contraction Compared with invasive sham treatment	Significant improvements in 5 out of 8 assessments in acupuncture group compared with sham
Vickers et al. 2004 (140)	37	Before/after study Post-cytotoxic chemotherapy fatigue Fatigue score of 4 or more on Brief Fatigue Inventory (BFI) and HADS depression score of less than 11 were included	BFI	MA for 20 minutes; either 8 treatments over 4 weeks or 6 treatments over 6 weeks Points used included CV 4, CV 6, bilateral ST 36, SP 8, SP 9, KI 3, KI 27; bilateral LI 11 used in most cases (except in cases of axillary lymph node resection)	Mean improvement in BFI from baseline of 31%; of the group, 3 experienced more than 75% improvement; 3 noted exacerbations in fatigue Younger and less depressed patients showed greater improvement, as did those with higher baseline anxiety scores
Martin et al. 2006 (141)	50	RCT Fibromylagia	Fibromyalgia Impact Questionnaire (FIQ) Multidimensional Pain Inventory (MPI)	Six acupuncture treatments for 20 minutes over 2–3 weeks in sitting with view of treatment obscured by screen EA at 2 Hz to bilateral LI 4 and ST 36; MA to LR 2, SP 6, PC 6, HT 7; EA at 10 Hz to BL points in cervical and in lumbar spine; EA at comfortable level of stimulation Control group received 6 non-invasive sham treatments	1 month after treatment significant improvements in acupuncture group in FIQ total score as well as fatigue & anxiety subscales; also significant improvement in pain severity and affective distress on MPI

RCT, randomized controlled trial; VAS, Visual Analogue Scale; EA, electroacupuncture; HADS, Hospital Anxiety and Depression Scale; MA, manual acupuncture.

Mood disturbance

Mood disorders such as depression and anxiety are highly prevalent in people with neurological conditions (Table 4.16).

Depression and anxiety

Depression is characterized by a loss of interest in and enjoyment of ordinary things and experiences, as well as low mood, which is persistent and problematic. It is associated with behavioural and physical symptoms such as tearfulness, irritability and social withdrawal as well as less obvious symptoms of poor sleep, general pain or fatigue. Feelings of worthlessness, low self-confidence and helplessness are common. Cognitive symptoms include poor concentration, reduced attention and mental slowing. In some situations agitation and anxiety are also present [109].

Generalized anxiety disorder is characterized by excessive anxiety and worry about various events or activities. Symptoms such as restlessness, becoming fatigued easily, difficulty concentrating, irritability, muscle tension or disturbed sleep will also be evident [110].

Table 4.16 Prevalence of mood disturbance in neurological conditions

Condition	Depression	Anxiety
Stroke	24–30%	22–25%
Traumatic brain injury	42%	18–60%
Parkinson's disease	4–76%	43%
Multiple sclerosis	31–56%	19%
Spinal cord injury	37%	30%
Guillain–Barré syndrome (acute phase)	67%	82%

References: Hibbard et al. 1998 (157); Kreutzer et al. 2001 (158); Weiss et al. 2002 (116); De Wit et al. 2008 (159); Brown et al. 2009 (160); Migliorini et al. 2009 (161); Simuni & Sethi 2009 (84); Pontone et al. 2009 (161).

Mood disorders in neurological conditions

Mood is regulated by intricate networks of neurones connecting areas such as the anterior cingulate cortex, prefrontal cortex and amygdala. The amygdala coordinates behavioural and autonomic activity in response to sensory information perceived as threatening. Overactivity of this structure has been found in major depression and anxiety [111]. The amygdala is regulated by activity in areas such as the prefrontal cortex and anterior cingulate cortex [112]. Problems with these modulatory circuits may predispose individuals to the development of mood disorders. A number of neurological conditions cause direct damage to these pathways, such as traumatic brain injury and multiple sclerosis [113, 114]. Additionally individuals may develop anxiety and depression as a response to real concerns and fears about how they will cope in their life with the range of difficulties they have developed as a result of their neurological condition.

Management of mood disorders in neurological disorders

Screening for mood disorders should begin early after new diagnosis of a neurological condition and be reviewed on regular basis. This is particularly relevant for those people with communication difficulties who commonly experience anxiety and depression but may be less able to express these concerns [115, 116]. Mild symptoms may respond to the provision of advice and information or the resolution of associated factors such as pain or sleep dysfunction. Symptoms which do not respond to simple measures may require referral to appropriate experts such as clinical psychologists or psychiatrists for specialized assessment. Specific interventions may include medications or psychological therapies such as cognitive-behavioural therapy [117–120].

Acupuncture for mood disturbance

A number of studies have considered the use of acupuncture for mood disorders. Studies evaluating acupuncture in anxiety are reported in Table 4.17, whilst those evaluating acupuncture in depression are listed in Table 4.18.

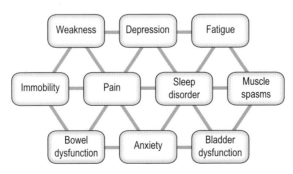

Figure 4.3 • Complex symptom relationships in neurological conditions. Note: the links represent symptoms which may influence each other, for example bladder dysfunction may disturb sleep and this in turn may contribute to fatigue. The symptoms could be arranged in many different ways for different patients.

Table 4.17 Acupuncture for anxiety

Authors and year	n	Design and inclusion criteria	Assessment	Interventions	Results
Wang et al. 2001 (145)	91	RCT Elective ambulatory surgery patients	State-Trait Anxiety Inventory	Ear acupuncture based on Chinese medicine; ear points for Kidney, Heart and Shenmen needled Ear acupuncture for relaxation – ear points Relaxation, Tranquillizer and Master Cerebral points were needled Control group – received ear acupuncture group at 3 points with no documented effect on anxiety All treatments lasted 30 minutes; no stimulation	Significant reduction in anxiety in the 'relaxation' group compared to the control group. Smaller non-significant reduction in anxiety in 'Chinese medicine' group
Karst et al. 2007 (146)	67	RCT Dental extraction	State-Trait Anxiety Inventory, VAS of anxiety, Sedation score, Quality of dental treatment, Physiological status – heart rate and oxygen saturation	Ear acupuncture to Relaxation, Tranquillizer and Master Cerebral points Non-invasive placebo ear acupuncture to 2 points with no documented effect on anxiety Intranasal midazolam No treatment Interventions started 35 minutes before dental treatment; needles remained in place for 25 minutes	Significant reduction in anxiety in ear acupuncture and intranasal midazolam groups compared with non-active groups No adverse effects in acupuncture group; reports of burning sensation from midazolam in some patients

RCT, randomized controlled trial; VAS, Visual Analogue Scale.

There are promising findings among these studies, although more research is needed. No studies have assessed the use of acupuncture for mood disturbance in neurological conditions.

Conclusion

People with neurological conditions present with a wide range of symptoms which commonly interact in complex ways (Figure 4.3). Medications for these symptoms may have unexpected side-effects on other symptoms. Research indicates that acupuncture may be able to contribute to the management of some of these symptoms in some individuals. In general side-effects from acupuncture are low. It therefore represents a useful therapeutic option to consider within the overall management of people with neurological conditions. Findings from the scientific literature provide ideas regarding the application of acupuncture, although more research is required into the specific uses in this population.

Table 4.18 Acupuncture for depression

Authors and year	n	Design and inclusion criteria	Assessment	Interventions	Results
Luo et al. 1985 (142)	47	Clinical trial Hamilton's Depression Rating Scale score over 20	Hamilton Depression Rating Scale, Clinical Global Impression Scale, Antidepressant side-effect rating scale	Electroacupuncture to GV 20, Yintang at 80–90 Hz for 1 hour; stimulation increased until slight muscle twitching evident Total of 30 treatments over 5 weeks Control group received amitriptyline; dose gradually increased; daily dose of 100–200 mg; treatment for 5 weeks	Significant improvement in both groups Fewer side-effects in acupuncture group
Röschke et al. 2000 (143)	70	RCT Major depression according to DSM-III-R	Global Assessment Scale, Bech–Rafaelsen Melancholia Scale, Clinical Global Impressions Scale	Mianserin Mianserin and verum acupuncture Mianserin and 'placebo' acupuncture involving superficial needling 12 acupuncture treatments for 30 minutes over 4 weeks Verum acupuncture at bilateral BL 15, BL 17, BL 18, HT 7, PC 6, ST 40, SP 5, SP 6, LU 1 Placebo needling at non-specific locations near the verum points	Significantly greater improvement in those groups with acupuncture No significant difference between effects of verum and 'placebo' acupuncture
Allen et al. 2006 (144)	151	RCT Major depressive disorder (DSM-IV) Score of 14 or more on Hamilton Rating Scale for Depression (HAM-D)	HAM-D, Beck Depression Inventory (BDI)	Group 1 Individualized acupuncture treatments for depression based on standardized manual Group 2 'Placebo-like' acupuncture using real points not normally used for depression; 12 treatments given over 8 weeks; 10–16 points needled for 20 minutes in each group Group 3 Waiting list control	Significant reduction in depression in all three groups by week 8; significantly greater reduction in both acupuncture groups but no difference between them Continued reduction in depression between weeks 8 and 16 in all groups No significant difference between groups for reduction in depression by week 16

RCT, randomized controlled trial; DSM-III-R, Diagnostic and Statistical Manual, third revision.

Note: The Hamilton Rating Scale for Depression (HRSD) is also known as the Hamilton Depression Rating Scale (HDRS) or HAM-D: these are all the same scale.

References

[1] White A, Cummings M, Filshie J. An introduction to western medical acupuncture. Edinburgh: Churchill Livingstone; 2008.

[2] Thoumie P, Mevellec E. Relation between walking speed and muscle strength is affected by somatosensory loss in multiple sclerosis. J Neurol Neurosurg Psychiatry 2002;73 (3):313–5.

[3] Corbetta M, Burton H, Sinclair RJ, et al. Functional reorganization and stability of somatosensory-motor cortical topography in a tetraplegic subject with late recovery. Proc Natl Acad Sci U S A 2002;99 (26):17066–71.

[4] Winward CE, Halligan PW, Wade DT. Somatosensory recovery: a longitudinal study of the first 6 months after unilateral stroke. Disabil Rehabil 2007;29 (4):293–9.

[5] Osterberg A, Boivie J. Central pain in multiple sclerosis – sensory abnormalities. Eur J Pain 2009; doi:10.1016/j. ejpain.2009.03.003.

[6] Hughes RA, Cornblath DR. Guillain–Barré syndrome. Lancet 2005;366(9497):1653–66.

[7] Koike H, Sobue G. Alcoholic neuropathy. Curr Opin Neurol 2006;19(5):481–6.

[8] Napadow V, Liu J, Li M, et al. Somatosensory cortical plasticity in carpal tunnel syndrome treated by acupuncture. Hum Brain Mapp 2007;28(3):159–71.

[9] Conforto AB, Cohen LG, dos Santos RL, et al. Effects of somatosensory stimulation on motor function in chronic cortico-subcortical strokes. J Neurol 2007;254(3):333–9.

[10] Loeser JD, Treede RD. The Kyoto protocol of IASP Basic Pain Terminology. Pain 2008;137 (3):473–7.

[11] Hansson PT, Attal N, Baron R, et al. Toward a definition of pharmacoresistant neuropathic pain. Eur J Pain 2009;13 (5):439–40.

[12] Baron R. Mechanisms of disease: neuropathic pain – a clinical perspective. Nat Clin Pract Neurol 2006;2(2):95–106.

[13] Hari AR, Wydenkeller S, Dokladal P, et al. Enhanced recovery of human spinothalamic function is associated with central neuropathic pain after SCI. Exp Neurol 2009;216(2):428–30.

[14] Kumar B, Kalita J, Kumar G. Central poststroke pain: a review of pathophysiology and treatment. Anesth Analg 2009;108(5):1645–57.

[15] Ofek H, Defrin R. The characteristics of chronic central pain after traumatic brain injury. Pain 2007;131(3):330–40.

[16] Wrigley PJ, Press SR, Gustin SM, et al. Neuropathic pain and primary somatosensory cortex reorganization following spinal cord injury. Pain 2009;141(1–2): 52–9.

[17] Boivie J. Pain in Parkinson's disease (PD). Pain 2009;141(1–2):2–3.

[18] Chudler EH, Dong WK. The role of the basal ganglia in nociception and pain. Pain 1995;60(1):3–38.

[19] Mylius V, Engau I, Teepker M, et al. Pain sensitivity and descending inhibition of pain in Parkinson's disease. J Neurol Neurosurg Psychiatry 2009;80(1):24–8.

[20] Schröder S, Liepert J, Remppis A, et al. Acupuncture treatment improves nerve conduction in peripheral neuropathy. Eur J Neurol 2007;14(3):276–81.

[21] Rampes H. Treatment of trigeminal neuralgia with electro-acupuncture in a case of multiple sclerosis. Acupunct Med 1994;12 (1):45.

[22] Blackwell R. What are the options available for the treatment of multiple sclerosis by acupuncture?. University of Wales; 2001.

[23] Smith MO, Rabinowitz N. Acupuncture treatment of multiple sclerosis: two detailed clinical presentations. Am J Acupunct 1986;14(2):143–6.

[24] Yen HL, Chan W. An East–West approach to the management of central post-stroke pain.

Cerebrovasc Dis 2003;16 (1):27–30.

[25] Lindfield H. Chronic shoulder pain in stroke. Are we missing the acupoint? Physiother Res Int 2002;7(1):44.

[26] Donnellan CP. Acupuncture for central pain affecting the ribcage following traumatic brain injury and rib fractures – a case report. Acupunct Med 2006;24 (3):129–33.

[27] Chae J, Yu DT, Walker ME, et al. Intramuscular electrical stimulation for hemiplegic shoulder pain: a 12-month follow-up of a multiple-center, randomized clinical trial. Am J Phys Med Rehabil 2005;84 (11):832–42.

[28] IASP Task Force on Taxonomy. Classification of chronic pain. Part III: pain terms, a current list with definitions and notes on usage. Seattle: IASP Press; 1994.

[29] Kim J. Patterns of sensory abnormality in cortical stroke; evidence for a dichotomized sensory system. Neurology 2007;68(3):174–80.

[30] Toru S, Yokota T, Tomimitsu H, et al. Somatosensory-evoked cortical potential during attacks of paroxysmal dysesthesia in multiple sclerosis. Eur J Neurol 2005;12(3):233–4.

[31] Smith K, McDonald W. The pathophysiology of multiple sclerosis: the mechanisms underlying the production of symptoms and the natural history of the disease. Philos Trans R Soc Lond B Biol Sci 1999;354 (1390):1649–73.

[32] Napadow V, Kettner N, Liu J, et al. Hypothalamus and amygdala response to acupuncture stimuli in carpal tunnel syndrome. Pain 2007;130 (3):254–66.

[33] Smania N, Gambarin M, Tinazzi M, et al. Are indexes of arm recovery related to daily life autonomy in patients with stroke? Eur J Phys Rehabil Med 2009;45 (3):349–54.

[34] Taub E, Uswatte G, King DK, et al. A placebo-controlled trial of constraint-induced movement

therapy for upper extremity after stroke. Stroke 2006;37 (4):1045–9.

[35] Liu W, Mukherjee M, Sun C, et al. Electroacupuncture may help motor recovery in chronic stroke survivors: a pilot study. J Rehabil Res Dev 2008;45 (4):587–95.

[36] Lance JW. Symposium synopsis. In: Feldman RG, Young RR, Koella WP, editors. Spasticity: disordered motor control. Chicago: Year Book Medical Publishers; 1980. p. 485–94.

[37] Gracies JM. Pathophysiology of spastic paresis. I: Paresis and soft tissue changes. Muscle Nerve 2005;31(5):535–51.

[38] Barnes MP, Johnson GR. Upper motor neurone syndrome and spasticity. Cambridge: Cambridge University Press; 2008.

[39] Wichers MJ, Odding E, Stam HJ, et al. Clinical presentation, associated disorders and aetiological moments in cerebral palsy: a Dutch population-based study. Disabil Rehabil 2005;27 (10):583–9.

[40] Rizzo MA, Hadjimichael OC, Preiningerova J, et al. Prevalence and treatment of spasticity reported by multiple sclerosis patients. Mult Scler 2004;10 (5):589–95.

[41] Adams MM, Hicks AL. Spasticity after spinal cord injury. Spinal Cord 2005;43(10):577–86.

[42] Lundstrom E, Terent A, Borg J. Prevalence of disabling spasticity 1 year after first-ever stroke. Eur J Neurol 2008;15(6):533–9.

[43] Francisco GE, Latorre JM, Ivanhoe CB. Intrathecal baclofen therapy for spastic hypertonia in chronic traumatic brain injury. Brain Inj 2007;21(3):335–8.

[44] Boyd RN, Ada L. Physiotherapy management of spasticity. In: Barnes MP, Johnson GR, editors. Upper motor neurone syndrome and spasticity. Cambridge: Cambridge University Press; 2008. p. 79–98.

[45] Patrick E, Ada L. The Tardieu scale differentiates contracture from spasticity whereas the Ashworth scale is confounded by it. Clin Rehabil 2006;20 (2):173–82.

[46] Cubo E, Gracies JM, Benabou R, et al. Early morning off-medication dyskinesias, dystonia, and choreic subtypes. Arch Neurol 2001;58(9):1379–82.

[47] Jankovic J. Motor fluctuations and dyskinesias in Parkinson's disease: clinical manifestations. Mov Disord 2005;20(Suppl. 11): S11–6.

[48] Lim SY, Farrell MJ, Gibson SJ, et al. Do dyskinesia and pain share common pathophysiological mechanisms in Parkinson's disease? Mov Disord 2008;23 (12):1689–95.

[49] Shulman LM, Wen X, Weiner WJ, et al. Acupuncture therapy for the symptoms of Parkinson's disease. Mov Disord 2002;17(4):799–802.

[50] Cristian A, Katz M, Cutrone E, et al. Evaluation of acupuncture in the treatment of Parkinson's disease: a double-blind pilot study. Mov Disord 2005;20 (9):1185–8.

[51] Chae Y, Lee H, Kim H, et al. Parsing brain activity associated with acupuncture treatment in Parkinson's diseases. Mov Disord 2009;24(12):1794–802.

[52] NICE. Urinary incontinence: the management of urinary incontinence in women. London: National Institute for Health & Clinical Excellence/National Collaborating Centre for Women's and Children's Health; 2006.

[53] Ciancio SJ, Mutchnik SE, Rivera VM, et al. Urodynamic pattern changes in multiple sclerosis. Urology 2001;57 (2):239–45.

[54] Kolominsky-Rabas PL, Hilz MJ, Neundoerfer B, et al. Impact of urinary incontinence after stroke: results from a prospective population-based stroke register. Neurourol Urodyn 2003;22 (4):322–7.

[55] Winge K, Fowler CJ. Bladder dysfunction in parkinsonism: mechanisms, prevalence, symptoms, and management. Mov Disord 2006;21(6):737–45.

[56] Sakakibara R, Uchiyama T, Kuwabara S, et al. Prevalence and mechanism of bladder dysfunction in Guillain–Barré syndrome. Neurourol Urodyn 2009;28(5):432–7.

[57] Fowler CJ, Panicker JN, Drake M, et al. A UK consensus on the management of the bladder in multiple sclerosis. J Neurol Neurosurg Psychiatry 2009;80(5):470–7.

[58] Kabay SC, Kabay S, Yucel M, et al. Acute urodynamic effects of percutaneous posterior tibial nerve stimulation on neurogenic detrusor overactivity in patients with Parkinson's disease. Neurourol Urodyn 2009;28(1):62–7.

[59] Kabay SC, Yucel M, Kabay S. Acute effect of posterior tibial nerve stimulation on neurogenic detrusor overactivity in patients with multiple sclerosis: urodynamic study. Urology 2008;71(4):641–5.

[60] Fjorback MV, Van Rey FS, Rijkhoff NJ, et al. Electrical stimulation of sacral dermatomes in multiple sclerosis patients with neurogenic detrusor overactivity. Neurourol Urodyn 2007;26 (4):525–30.

[61] Amarenco G, Ismael SS, Even-Schneider A, et al. Urodynamic effect of acute transcutaneous posterior tibial nerve stimulation in overactive bladder. J Urol 2003;169(6):2210–5.

[62] Sato A, Sato Y, Schmidt RF, et al. Somato-vesical reflexes in chronic spinal cats. J Auton Nerv Syst 1983;7(3–4):351–62.

[63] Tanaka Y, Koyama Y, Jodo E, et al. Effects of acupuncture to the sacral segment on the bladder activity and electroencephalogram. Psychiatry Clin Neurosci 2002;56(3):249–50.

[64] Krogh K, Christensen P, Laurberg S. Colorectal symptoms in patients with neurological diseases. Acta Neurol Scand 2001;103(6):335–43.

[65] Wiesel PH, Norton C, Glickman S, et al. Pathophysiology and management of bowel dysfunction in multiple sclerosis. Eur J Gastroenterol Hepatol 2001;13(4):441–8.

[66] Pfeiffer RF. Gastrointestinal dysfunction in Parkinson's disease. Lancet Neurol 2003;2 (2):107–16.

[67] Turk MA, Scandale J, Rosenbaum PF, et al. The health of women with cerebral palsy. Phys Med Rehabil Clin N Am. 2001;12(1):153–68.

[68] Bracci F, Badiali D, Pezzotti P, et al. Chronic constipation in hemiplegic patients. World J Gastroenterol 2007;13 (29):3967–72.

[69] NICE. Faecal incontinence: the management of faecal incontinence in adults. London: National Institute for Health & Clinical Excellence; 2007.

[70] Hosker G, Cody JD, Norton CC. Electrical stimulation for faecal incontinence in adults. Cochrane Database Syst Rev 2007;3: CD001310.

[71] Mowatt G, Glazener C, Jarrett M. Sacral nerve stimulation for faecal incontinence and constipation in adults. Cochrane Database Syst Rev 2007;3:CD004464.

[72] Jarrett ME, Matzel KE, Christiansen J, et al. Sacral nerve stimulation for faecal incontinence in patients with previous partial spinal injury including disc prolapsed. Br J Surg 2005;92(6):734–9.

[73] Iwa M, Matsushima M, Nakade Y, et al. Electroacupuncture at ST-36 accelerates colonic motility and transit in freely moving conscious rats. Am J Physiol Gastrointest Liver Physiol 2006;290(2): G285–92.

[74] Luo D, Liu S, Xie X, et al. Electroacupuncture at acupoint ST-36 promotes contractility of distal colon via a cholinergic pathway in conscious rats. Dig Dis Sci 2008;53(3):689–93.

[75] Broide E, Pintov S, Portnoy S, et al. Effectiveness of acupuncture for treatment of childhood constipation. Dig Dis Sci 2001;46(6):1270–5.

[76] Scaglia M, Delaini G, Destefano I, et al. Fecal incontinence treated with acupuncture – a pilot study. Auton Neurosci 2009;145(1–2): 89–92.

[77] Roth T. Insomnia: definition, prevalence, etiology, and consequences. J Clin Sleep Med 2007;3(5 Suppl.):S7–S10.

[78] Sateia MJ, Nowell PD. Insomnia. Lancet 2004;364(9449):1959–73.

[79] Gais S, Albouy G, Boly M, et al. Sleep transforms the cerebral trace of declarative memories. Proc Natl Acad Sci U S A 2007;104(47):18778–83.

[80] Fischer S, Nitschke MF, Melchert UH, et al. Motor memory consolidation in sleep shapes more effective neuronal representations. J Neurosci 2005;25(49):11248–55.

[81] Bassetti CL. Sleep and stroke. Semin Neurol 2005;25(1):19–32.

[82] Bamer AM, Johnson KL, Amtmann D, et al. Prevalence of sleep problems in individuals with multiple sclerosis. Mult Scler 2008;14(8):1127–30.

[83] Ouellet MC, Morin CM. Efficacy of cognitive-behavioral therapy for insomnia associated with traumatic brain injury: a single-case experimental design. Arch Phys Med Rehabil 2007;88 (12):1581–92.

[84] Simuni T, Sethi K. Nonmotor manifestations of Parkinson's disease. Ann Neurol 2009;64(S2): S65–80.

[85] Jennum P, Santamaria J. Report of an EFNS task force on management of sleep disorders in neurologic disease (degenerative neurologic disorders and stroke). Eur J Neurol 2007;14 (11):1189–200.

[86] Parcell DL, Ponsford JL, Redman JR, et al. Poor sleep quality and changes in objectively recorded sleep after traumatic brain injury: a preliminary study. Arch Phys Med Rehabil 2008;89 (5):843–50.

[87] Zeitzer JM, Ayas NT, Shea SA, et al. Absence of detectable melatonin and preservation of cortisol and thyrotropin rhythms in tetraplegia. Journal of Clinical Endocrinology Metabolism 2000;85(6):2189–96.

[88] Vaghela SA, Donnellan CP. Acupuncture for back pain, knee pain and insomnia in transverse myelitis – a case report. Acupunct Med 2008;26(3):188–92.

[89] Spence DW, Kayumov L, Chen A, et al. Acupuncture increases nocturnal melatonin secretion and reduces insomnia and anxiety: a preliminary report. J Neuropsychiatry Clin Neurosci 2004;16(1):19–28.

[90] Cheuk DK, Yeung WF, Chung KF, et al. Acupuncture for insomnia. Cochrane Database Syst Rev 2007;3:CD005472.

[91] Huang W, Kutner N, Bliwise DL. A systematic review of the effects of acupuncture in treating insomnia. Sleep Med Rev 2009;13(1):73–104.

[92] Yeung WF, Chung KF, Leung YK, et al. Traditional needle acupuncture treatment for insomnia: A systematic review of randomized controlled trials. Sleep Med 2009;10(7):694–704.

[93] Kim YS, Lee SH, Jung WS, et al. Intradermal acupuncture on shen-men and nei-kuan acupoints in patients with insomnia after stroke. Am J Chin Med 2004;32 (5):771–8.

[94] De Groot MH, Phillips SJ, Eskes GA. Fatigue associated with stroke and other neurologic conditions: Implications for stroke rehabilitation. Arch Phys Med Rehabil 2003;84 (11):1714–20.

[95] Levine J, Greenwald BD. Fatigue in Parkinson disease, stroke, and traumatic brain injury. Phys Med Rehabil Clin N Am 2009;20 (2):347–61.

[96] Lou JS, Kearns G, Benice T, et al. Levodopa improves physical fatigue in Parkinson's disease: a double-blind, placebo-controlled, crossover study. Mov Disord 2003;18(10):1108–14.

[97] Colle F, Bonan I, Gellez Leman MC, et al. Fatigue after stroke. Ann Readapt Med Phys 2006;49(6):272–4.

[98] Fawkes-Kirby TM, Wheeler MA, Anton HA, et al. Clinical correlates of fatigue in spinal cord injury. Spinal Cord 2008;46 (1):21–5.

[99] Barone P, Antonini A, Colosimo C, et al. The PRIAMO study: A multicenter assessment of nonmotor symptoms and their impact on quality of life in Parkinson's disease. Mov Disord 2009;24(11):1641–9.

[100] Garssen MP, van KR, van Doorn PA. Residual fatigue is independent of antecedent events and disease severity in Guillain–Barré syndrome. J Neurol 2006;253(9):1143–6.

[101] Zwarts MJ, Bleijenberg G, van Engelen BGM. Clinical neurophysiology of fatigue. Clin Neurophysiol 2008;119(1):2–10.

[102] Belmont A, Agar N, Hugeron C, et al. Fatigue and traumatic brain injury. Ann Readapt Med Phys 2006;49(6):283–4.

[103] Dobkin BH. Fatigue versus activity-dependent fatigability in patients with central or peripheral motor impairments. Neurorehabil Neural Repair 2008;22(2):105–10.

[104] Heesen C, Nawrath L, Reich C, et al. Fatigue in multiple sclerosis: an example of cytokine mediated sickness behaviour? J Neurol Neurosurg Psychiatry 2006;77(1):34–9.

[105] Sepulcre J, Masdeu JC, Goni J. Fatigue in multiple sclerosis is associated with the disruption of frontal and parietal pathways. Mult Scler 2009;15(3):337–44.

[106] Ziino C, Ponsford J. Selective attention deficits and subjective fatigue following traumatic brain injury. Neuropsychology 2006;20(3):383–90.

[107] van Kessel K, Moss-Morris R, Willoughby E, et al. A randomized controlled trial of cognitive behavior therapy for multiple sclerosis fatigue. Psychosom Med 2008;70(2):205–13.

[108] Assefi NP, Sherman KJ, Jacobsen C, et al. A randomized clinical trial of acupuncture compared with sham acupuncture in fibromyalgia. Ann Intern Med 2005;143(1):10–9.

[109] National Collaborating Centre for Mental Health & Royal College of Psychiatrists. Depression: management of depression in primary and secondary care. National clinical practice guideline number 23. London: The British Psychological Society/The Royal College of Psychiatrists; 2004.

[110] McIntosh A, Cohen A, Turnbull N, et al. Clinical guidelines and evidence review for panic disorder and generalised anxiety disorder. Sheffield: University of Sheffield/London: National Collaborating Centre for Primary Care; 2004.

[111] Carter CS, Krug MK. The functional neuroanatomy of dread: Functional magnetic resonance imaging insights into generalized anxiety disorder and its treatment. Am J Psychiatry 2009;166(3):263–5.

[112] Johnstone T, van Reekum CM, Urry HL, et al. Failure to regulate: counterproductive recruitment of top-down prefrontal-subcortical circuitry in major depression. J Neurosci 2007;27(33):8877–84.

[113] Jorge RE, Robinson RG, Moser D, et al. Major depression following traumatic brain injury. Arch Gen Psychiatry 2004;61(1):42–50.

[114] Passamonti L, Cerasa A, Liguori M, et al. Neurobiological mechanisms underlying emotional processing in relapsing-remitting multiple sclerosis. Brain 2009; (in press).

[115] Kauhanen ML, Korpelainen JT, Hiltunen P, et al. Aphasia, depression, and non-verbal cognitive impairment in ischaemic stroke. Cerebrovasc Dis 2000;10(6):455–61.

[116] Weiss H, Rastan V, Mullges W, et al. Psychotic symptoms and emotional distress in patients with Guillain–Barré syndrome. Eur Neurol 2002;47(2):74–8.

[117] Royal College of Physicians. National clinical guideline for stroke. London: Royal College of Physicians; 2008.

[118] Royal College of Physicians and British Society of Rehabilitation Medicine. Rehabilitation following acquired brain injury: national clinical guidelines. London: Royal College of Physicians; British Society of Rehabilitation Medicine; 2003.

[119] National Collaborating Centre for Chronic Conditions. Parkinson's disease; national clinical guideline for diagnosis and management in primary and secondary care. London: Royal College of Physicians; 2006.

[120] NICE. Multiple sclerosis: National clinical guidelines for diagnosis and management in primary and secondary care. London: National Institute for Clinical Excellence/National Collaborating Centre for Chronic Conditions; 2003.

[121] Dorsher PT, Reimer R, Nottmeier E. Treatment of urinary incontinence due to incomplete spinal cord injury with acupuncture and percutaneous electrical nerve stimulation: two cases and literature review. Medical Acupuncture 2009;21(1):21–6.

[122] Shlay JC, Chaloner K, Max MB, et al. Acupuncture and amitriptyline for pain due to HIV-related peripheral neuropathy: a randomized controlled trial. JAMA 1998;280(18):1590–5.

[123] Abuaisha BB, Costanzi JB, Boulton AJM. Acupuncture for the treatment of chronic painful peripheral diabetic neuropathy: a long-term study. Diabetes Res Clin Pract 1998;39(2):115–21.

[124] Phillips KD, Skelton WD, Hand GA. Effect of acupuncture administered in a group setting on pain and subjective peripheral neuropathy in persons with human immunodeficiency virus disease. J Altern Complement Med 2004;10(3):449–55.

[125] Wong R, Sagar S. Acupuncture treatment for chemotherapy-induced peripheral neuropathy – a case series. Acupunct Med 2006;24(2):87–91.

[126] Nayak S, Shiflett SC, Schoenberger NE, et al. Is acupuncture effective in treating chronic pain after spinal cord injury? Arch Phys Med Rehabil 2001;82(11):1578–86.

[127] Rapson LM, Wells N, Pepper J, et al. Acupuncture as a promising treatment for below-level central neuropathic pain: a retrospective study. J Spinal Cord Med 2003;26(1):21–6.

[128] Wong AM, Leong CP, Su TY, et al. Clinical trial of acupuncture for patients with spinal cord injuries. Am J Phys Med rehabil 2003;82(1):21–7.

[129] Alexander DN, Cen S, Sullivan KJ, et al. Effects of acupuncture treatment on poststroke motor recovery and physical function: a pilot study. Neurorehabil Neural Repair 2004;18(4):259–67.

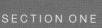
[130] Wayne PM, Krebs DE, Macklin EA, et al. Acupuncture for upper-extremity rehabilitation in chronic stroke: a randomized sham-controlled study. Arch Phys Med Rehabil 2005;86(12):2248–55.

[131] Yu YH, Wang HC, Wang ZJ. The effect of acupuncture on spinal motor neuron excitability in stroke patients. Zhonghua Yi Xue Za Zhi (Taipei) 1995;56 (4):258–63.

[132] Fink M, Rollnik JD, Bijak M, et al. Needle acupuncture in chronic poststroke leg spasticity. Arch Phys Med Rehabil 2004;85 (4):667–72.

[133] Mukherjee M, McPeak LK, Redford JB, et al. The effect of electro-acupuncture on spasticity of the wrist joint in chronic stroke survivors. Arch Phys Med Rehabil 2007;88(2):159–66.

[134] Zhao JG, Cao CH, Liu CZ, et al. Effect of acupuncture treatment on spastic states of stroke patients. J Neurol Sci 2009;276 (1–2):143–7.

[135] Cheng PT, Wong MK, Chang PL. A therapeutic trial of acupuncture in neurogenic bladder of spinal cord injured patients – a preliminary report. Spinal Cord 1998;36(7):476–80.

[136] Honjo H, Naya Y, Ukimura O, et al. Acupuncture on clinical symptoms and urodynamic measurements in spinal-cord-injured patients with detrusor hyperreflexia. Urol Int 2000;65(4):190–5.

[137] Keppel Hesselink JM, Kopsky DJ. Acupuncture for bladder dysfunctions in multiple sclerosis. Medical Acupuncture 2005;17(1):38–9.

[138] Klauser AG, Rubach A, Bertsche O, et al. Body acupuncture: effect on colonic function in chronic constipation. Z Gastroenterol 1993;31(10):605–8.

[139] Deluze C, Bosia L, Zirbs A, et al. Electroacupuncture in fibromyalgia: results of a controlled trial. BMJ 1992;305 (6864):1249–52.

[140] Vickers AJ, Straus DJ, Fearon B, et al. Acupuncture for postchemotherapy fatigue: a phase II study. J Clin Oncol 2004;22(9):1731–5.

[141] Martin DP, Sletten CD, Williams BA, et al. Improvement in fibromyalgia symptoms with acupuncture: results of a randomized controlled trial. Mayo Clin Proc 2006;81(6):749–57.

[142] Luo HC, Jia YK, Li Z. Electro-acupuncture vs. amitriptyline in the treatment of depressive states. J Tradit Chin Med 1985;5(1):3–8.

[143] Röschke J, Wolf C, Muller MJ, et al. The benefit from whole body acupuncture in major depression. J Affect Disord 2000;57(1–3):73–81.

[144] Allen JJ, Schnyer RN, Chambers AS, et al. Acupuncture for depression: a randomized controlled trial. J Clin Psychiatry 2006;67(11):1665–73.

[145] Wang SM, Peloquin C, Kain ZN. The use of auricular acupuncture to reduce preoperative anxiety. Anesth Analg 2001;93 (5):1178–80, table.

[146] Karst M, Winterhalter M, Munte S, et al. Auricular acupuncture for dental anxiety: a randomized controlled trial. Anesth Analg 2007;104 (2):295–300.

[147] MacGowan DJ, Janal MN, Clark WC, et al. Central poststroke pain and Wallenberg's lateral medullary infarction: frequency, character, and determinants in 63 patients. Neurology 1997;49(1):120–5.

[148] Moulin DE, Hagen N, Feasby TE, et al. Pain in Guillain–Barré syndrome. Neurology 1997;48 (2):328–31.

[149] Weimar C, Kloke M, Schlott M, et al. Central poststroke pain in a consecutive cohort of stroke patients. Cerebrovasc Dis 2002;14(3–4):261–3.

[150] Siddall PJ, McClelland JM, Rutkowski SB, et al. A longitudinal study of the prevalence and characteristics of pain in the first 5 years following spinal cord injury. Pain 2003;103(3):249–57.

[151] Jahnsen R, Villien L, Aamodt G, et al. Musculoskeletal pain in adults with cerebral palsy compared with the general population. J Rehabil Med 2004;36(2):78–84.

[152] Kogos Jr SC, Richards JS, Banos JH, et al. Visceral pain and life quality in persons with spinal cord Injury: a brief report. J Spinal Cord Med 2005;28 (4):333–7.

[153] Nampiaparampil DE. Prevalence of chronic pain after traumatic brain injury: a systematic review. JAMA 2008;300(6):711–9.

[154] Ruts L, Rico R, van KR, et al. Pain accompanies pure motor Guillain–Barré syndrome. J Peripher Nerv Syst 2008;13(4):305–6.

[155] Beiske AG, Loge JH, Ronningen A, et al. Pain in Parkinson's disease: Prevalence and characteristics. Pain 2009;141(1–2):173–7.

[156] Dyson-Hudson TA, Kadar P, LaFountaine M, et al. Acupuncture for chronic shoulder pain in persons with spinal cord injury: a small-scale clinical trial. Arch Phys Med Rehabil 2007;88 (10):1276–83.

[157] Hibbard MR, Uysal S, Kepler K, et al. Axis I psychopathology in individuals with traumatic brain injury. J Head Trauma Rehabil 1998;13(4):24–39.

[158] Kreutzer JS, Seel RT, Gourley E. The prevalence and symptom rates of depression after traumatic brain injury: a comprehensive examination. Brain Inj 2001;15(7): 563–76.

[159] De Wit L, Putman K, Baert I, et al. Anxiety and depression in the first six months after stroke. A longitudinal multicentre study. Disabil Rehabil 2008;30 (24):1858–66.

[160] Brown RF, Valpiani EM, Tennant CC. Longitudinal assessment of anxiety, depression, and fatigue in people with multiple sclerosis. Psychol Psychother 2009;82:41–56.

[161] Migliorini CE, New PW, Tonge BJ. Comparison of depression, anxiety and stress in persons with traumatic and non-traumatic post-acute spinal cord injury. Spinal Cord 2009;47 (11):783–8.

[162] Pontone GM, Williams JR, Anderson KE, et al. Prevalence of anxiety disorders and anxiety subtypes in patients with Parkinson's disease. Mov Disord 2009;24(9):1333–8.

Practical application of Western medical acupuncture in neurological conditions

5

CHAPTER CONTENTS

KEY POINTS

- Acupuncture can be very valuable for a wide range of symptoms in neurological conditions.
- Dividing symptoms into broad categories of sensory, motor, visceral and generalized dysfunction simplifies the clinical reasoning process.
- The lack of large randomized controlled trials does not mean that acupuncture may not be beneficial.
- Acupuncture clinical reasoning is a logical process and requires consideration of aspects such as level of stimulation and duration of treatment.

Introduction

Research has indicated possible applications for acupuncture in neurological conditions. However there are many cases when the evidence base is inadequate to guide practice. Clinicians regularly meet patients who might benefit from acupuncture. The development of a coherent clinical reasoning framework allows practitioners to devise treatment schedules for any patient who may present to the clinic, drawing insights from Western scientific literature.

Clinical reasoning framework

A clinical reasoning framework can be based around the major problems that people with neurological conditions may complain of, namely sensory, motor, visceral and generalized disorders (Table 5.1). The literature regarding these presentations has been explored in Chapter 4.

There follows a series of practical cases which aim to illustrate a range of possible approaches to treatment. Each case provides information regarding the 'dose' of treatment such as choice of points, level of stimulation, duration of treatment and course of treatment.

Part 1: Sensory function

Case study 5.1: level 1: Nociceptive pain in multiple sclerosis

A 53-year-old woman with multiple sclerosis fell and fractured her right calcaneum. She was unable to put any weight through her heel due to pain.

Table 5.1 Clinical reasoning framework in neurological conditions

Key issue	Examples	Acupuncture options
Sensory problems	Impaired sensation Pain Hypersensitivity Unpleasant provoked or spontaneous sensations such as tingling or burning	Needle locally in area of sensory loss or pain Needle extrasegmentally for generalized pain-relieving effects Consider use of EA for strong stimulation, e.g. to influence impaired sensation or chronic pain presentations Consider scalp acupuncture over sensory line
Motor problems	Weakness or inactivity Spasticity or rigidity	Needle into muscle of interest Consider trigger point acupuncture to gain muscle relaxation and reduction in pain Consider EA to gain contraction of muscle and to encourage increased activity Consider EA to gain muscle contraction as a prelude to muscle relaxation where excess muscle activity is present Consider scalp acupuncture over motor line
Visceral problems	Bladder or bowel dysfunction	Consider the autonomic supply to the organ and needle segmentally Also needle extrasegmentally for generalized effects on the organ
Generalized problems	Insomnia Fatigue and reduced energy levels Depression Anxiety or agitation	Use important points, particularly those on the front of the body or those in the back over the sympathetic outflow between T1 and L2 Consider points on the head to influence the trigeminal system Consider ear acupuncture to gain general calming effects, e.g. via vagus nerve

EA, electroacupuncture.

Consequently, she walked with a marked limp and had to lean on her husband for support. Pain on weight-bearing was 6–7/10. She was only able to walk 100 metres with difficulty and with assistance and was at risk of falling again. Her timed 10-metre walk took 31 seconds and she scored 42/56 on a Berg Balance Scale.

Treatment

She received a course of six acupuncture treatments over 3 weeks, each treatment lasting 25 minutes. The needles were stimulated initially for Deqi and then again at 5-minute intervals.

Points

Right ST 36, SP 5; bilateral LI 4, LR 3.

Outcome

Pain reduced to 0–1/10. This allowed her to put weight through her heel, and to participate actively in rehabilitation to improve balance, strength and mobility. After treatment she was able to walk up to 200 metres independently with elbow crutches. Her balance and safety were improved. Timed 10-metre walk took 12 seconds and Berg Balance Score was 47/56.

Comment

Local points combined with generalized points resulted in an excellent result for this patient. The calcaneus is innervated by the medial calcaneal nerve and the first branch of the lateral plantar nerve. Both nerves arise from the tibial nerve (L4–S3). Selection of local points in the muscles sharing a common innervation with the calcaneus allowed modulation of pain on a segmental basis. This case illustrates how useful acupuncture can be within a physiotherapist's range of skills.

Case study 5.2: level 1: Pain from active trigger point in Brown-Séquard syndrome

A 34-year-old man presented with a 1-month history of right shoulder pain. He had developed right-sided C5 Brown-Séquard syndrome 7 months previously. This had affected the right side of his spinal cord, leaving him with impaired movement below C7 on the right and impaired sensation below T10 on the left. The patient was able to walk independently indoors but needed to use one crutch outdoors. The patient's social worker had contacted the patient's physiotherapist to enquire whether an increase in funding for additional carers was required due to the patient's increasing difficulty in managing daily activities.

On assessment the patient reported constant pain in the right shoulder, rating this as 8/10. He had poor dexterity in his hands and the addition of shoulder pain made it difficult for him to dress independently. There was no history of recent shoulder injury. Examination indicated weakness throughout the upper limb, including the shoulder region, and a local increase in muscle tone in right upper trapezius. This region was locally tender and palpation reproduced the patient's pain.

Treatment

The patient received one acupuncture treatment to deactivate trigger points in upper fibres of trapezius. LI 4 was added bilaterally for 15 minutes for generalized pain relief. In addition he was provided with activities to improve stability and strength of the right shoulder. He received one follow-up session 6 months later, providing advice on sleeping position.

Points

Trigger points in upper fibres of trapezius, LI 4 bilaterally.

Outcome

Pain reduced immediately to 3/10 and in the next few days reduced further to 0/10. There was no recurrence until 6 months later. At this time advice on supported sleeping position was provided. There were no further reports of pain. No increase in funding for carers was required.

Comment

This is a good example of one treatment having a major impact. Impaired upper-limb function following the development of Brown-Séquard syndrome meant that this patient's ability to function independently was more vulnerable to minor change. The presence of shoulder pain raised the possibility of an increase in care package to support him. The application of acupuncture avoided this necessity and represents an invaluable treatment option.

Case study 5.3: level 1: Paraesthesia and dysaesthesia in transverse myelitis

A 32-year-old woman presented with unpleasant sensations in her legs since the onset 6 weeks previously of transverse myelitis at T12/L1. She reported problematic pins and needles and feelings of 'tightness' in her legs, particularly in the thighs. Assessment revealed low tone, weakness and quadriceps spasticity as well as sensory and proprioceptive impairment in the lower limbs. In addition she was incontinent of urine.

Functional ability

She was unable to stand unassisted and used a sliding board for moving from bed to wheelchair. She was independently mobile in a wheelchair. She needed the assistance of one person for activities of daily living.

Treatment

The patient received 12 acupuncture treatments lasting 30–40 minutes over 3 weeks. The needles were not stimulated at any point. She also received ongoing physiotherapy to improve her ability to stand and walk.

Points

Local needling was carried out into the area of unpleasant sensations using bilateral ST 31, ST 34, GB 31 and GB 34.

Outcome

This patient reported significant improvement as a result of the acupuncture treatment and stated that it had 'kickstarted everything else'. During the treatments the patient reported a pleasant tingling sensation in both legs and a feeling of deep relaxation. Following treatments she noticed a reduction in unpleasant sensations, improved sensation in the soles of the feet and a 'better sense of her legs being there'. In addition she noted increased muscle activity in her left foot and improved right quadriceps control in gait directly after treatment.

Comment

Needling into the area of discomfort with long treatment times and no stimulation reduced dysaesthesia. The treatments were provided intensively in an attempt to make a sustained difference and to allow the patient to progress. This amount of treatment time looks substantial. However these treatments may easily be provided within the context of a busy neurorehabilitation gym. Needle insertion takes just a few minutes. The patient can then be distantly monitored whilst other patients are being treated. In fact this can be a very efficient treatment option.

Case study 5.4: level 2: Back and hip pain in choreoathetoid cerebral palsy

A 42-year-old woman presented with a 2-year history of low-back and left hip pain. Pain had recently become more severe and she rated both pains as 8/10. The pain affected her ability to concentrate at university and she was becoming low in mood. She reported that the back pain was worse when standing or transferring into her wheelchair. These were positions which caused lumbar extensor spasm. Hip pain was worse when standing or lying on the left side at night.

Examination indicated severe choreoathetoid movements affecting all four limbs and trunk. Hyperextension of lumbar spine was evident on standing with bilateral spasm of paraspinals. In addition malalignment was evident in her legs with severe hyperextension of the knees and dystonic foot posture. Palpation revealed local tenderness over both L5/S1 facet joints, acute tenderness over the left greater trochanter and active trigger points in right and left gluteus medius and minimus. Assessment suggested facet joint problem at L5/S1 due to severe and repeated hyperextension of the lumbar spine, combined with gluteal enthesopathy.

Functional ability

The patient was able to transfer in and out of her wheelchair independently. She used an electric wheelchair for mobility. She received daily assistance with washing and dressing from carers.

Treatment

A range of different options were trialled, including acupuncture and transcutaneous electrical nerve stimulation (TENS). She received a course of eight acupuncture treatments over 5 weeks. Early treatments involved the deactivation of trigger points in gluteus medius and gluteus minimus at the beginning of the session. This was often followed by the insertion of 5–6 needles around and over the left greater trochanter combined with bilateral ST 36. Needles were gently stimulated initially for Deqi and then left in situ for 20–25 minutes. Acupuncture was trialled for treatment of the back pain but was difficult, carried safety risks due to the patient's involuntary movements and was of limited benefit. TENS at 110 Hz over the lumbar spine was therefore trialled with greater success. In addition she received physiotherapy to try and improve selective control at the trunk as well as providing stretches into flexion for lumbar spine.

Points

Gluteus medium and minimus trigger points; Huatojiaji points bilaterally at L4 and L5 (trialled twice). Six points immediately around and over greater trochanter; ST 36 bilaterally.

Outcome

The patient experienced good short-term relief of hip and buttock pain with pain reducing to 2/10. There was no sustained change in back pain secondary to needling but good pain relief was obtained by using TENS on the lumbar spine overnight. This patient required ongoing monitoring and was later referred on for review by the pain team.

Comment

Acupuncture provided substantial relief of hip pain for 3 months. However it was difficult to sustain pain relief due to the extreme stresses placed upon the patient's joints due to the choreoathetoid movements. Treatment of back pain in the presence of involuntary paraspinal spasms was very difficult and issues of safety raised by Watson [1] are relevant in this situation. Trial of TENS was more successful and provided a simple option that she could use whenever the back pain was problematic. In complex presentations it is important to remember the limitations of any one technique and involve other professionals as necessary.

Case study 5.5: level 1: Impaired sensation affecting dexterity in stroke

A 61-year-old man presented with marked sensory impairment in his right upper limb, 2 months after a stroke. He had impaired awareness of light touch, deep touch, thermal sensation and proprioception. Assessment indicated good motor ability. However, his sensory impairment hampered his ability to complete functional activities requiring fine dexterity; for example, he was unable to do up buttons. He was able to walk independently and was independent in daily activities but slow due to poor manual dexterity. He had been unable to work since his stroke.

Treatment

The patient received eight acupuncture treatments over 8 weeks. Each treatment lasted for 30 minutes. Needles were stimulated initially for Deqi and then restimulated at 5-minute intervals. No other interventions were provided during this time.

Points

Right LI 4, LI 5, LI 10, LI 11 and SI 3.

Outcome

The patient experienced substantial improvement in sensation and proprioception which resulted in improved manual dexterity and improved function; for example he was able to do up buttons. This improved dexterity allowed him to return to his job working in a bar.

Comment

Studies have demonstrated improved motor dexterity following somatosensory stimulation in stroke [2]. These studies usually provide stimulation over a peripheral nerve such as the median nerve and aim for the patient to feel strong paraesthesia. This physiotherapist used points throughout the upper limb local to the area of sensory deficit, provided strong stimulation and gained improvements in sensation and motor function. In planning such treatments it would be useful to consider the peripheral nerves supplying the target areas and select points to stimulate these nerves.

Part 2: Motor function

Case study 5.6: level 1: Inability to move fingers following spinal stroke

A 54-year-old woman presented with difficulty with finger movement following a spinal stroke 6 months previously. The stroke had affected the anterior portion of the spinal cord extending from C5 to T1. On assessment she had severe limitation of movement in both hands. On the left she had no finger flexor activity and this could not be stimulated by the use of electrical nerve stimulation.

Functional ability

The patient had lived with her daughter since the stroke. She was able to walk independently. She was able to wash independently but needed help with fine finger tasks such as tying her shoe laces.

Treatment

She received five electroacupuncture treatments over 2 weeks. Needles were inserted into the target muscle and stimulated at 2 Hz for 25 minutes. Visible finger flexion was obtained on each occasion during treatment. In addition she completed upper-limb active exercise, stretches and functional tasks for hand muscles.

Points

Needles were inserted into either flexor digitorum superficialis or flexor digitorum profoundus. Usually only two needles were inserted, with one at either end of the muscle belly.

Outcome

After two treatments this patient was able actively to flex her fingers through a few degrees. After four treatments she began using her finger flexors as part of basic functional tasks such as picking up a plastic beaker. In addition attempts to stimulate the muscles using electrical stimulation transcutaneously were now successful in obtaining finger flexion.

Comment

This case highlights the possibility of stimulating muscle activity more easily and more specifically when needles are inserted directly into the muscle. This may be of benefit to some individuals at early stages of their rehabilitation and for muscles which are located more deeply. In addition, the intensity required for electroacupuncture is much lower than that required for transcutaneous stimulation since the high electrical impedance of the skin has been overcome. Electroacupuncture is therefore more

comfortable for many patients and provides a therapeutic option for those who are unable to tolerate transcutaneous electrical stimulation.

Case study 5.7: level 2: Inability to move arm or leg poststroke

A 57-year-old man presented with dense right hemiplegia and sensory impairment 6 weeks after a middle cerebral artery infarction. On assessment he had severe low tone throughout the right side except for clonus in right plantarflexors. He had no active movement in his arm or leg, grade 0/5, after 6 weeks of intensive inpatient rehabilitation on a specialist stroke unit using a wide range of modalities. Motor Assessment Scale score was 9/48.

Functional ability

He was able to stand but his right leg was inactive. He was unable to walk and was dependent on a wheelchair for mobility. He needed help with daily activities.

Treatment

The patient received eight scalp electroacupuncture treatments at 100 Hz for 25 minutes over 4 weeks. First treatment was given to the motor line over the lesioned (left) hemisphere. All subsequent treatments needled the motor line over intact hemisphere. Intensity was turned up until the patient could feel a gentle buzzing sensation of the scalp. Active assisted movement of right arm and leg was carried out during acupuncture treatment. His inpatient rehabilitation programme continued.

Points

Four needles were inserted along the length of the motor line. Electroacupuncture was attached to needles at either end of this line of needles.

Outcome

There was no change after treatment 1. During treatment 2 there was the sudden development of active movement in the right arm and leg after

10 minutes of stimulation as follows: grade 1+ in finger flexors, shoulder flexors and abductors; grade 2– in elbow flexors (through 45°), and knee extensors (60°); grade 3– in hip flexors (30°). By the end of eight treatments there had been continued improvement in movement as follows: grade 2– in finger flexors (20°), hip extensors (20°), knee flexors (30°); grade 3– in elbow flexors (60°), shoulder flexion (40°), shoulder extension (30°), hip flexion (70°); grade 4– at knee extension. The patient had developed basic arm movement but was unable to use this functionally. He was able to stand with more activity in his right leg and was able to walk 10–15 metres with the assistance of one person. Motor Assessment Scale score was 17/48.

Comment

The physiotherapist was trying to understand how scalp acupuncture might influence motor ability. Papers reporting inhibition of lesioned hemisphere by the intact hemisphere seemed relevant, as well as those reporting the application of transcranial magnetic stimulation over the intact hemisphere to reduce this transcallosal inhibition and improve motor ability in stroke [3, 4]. Therefore during treatment 2 she provided electroacupuncture stimulation over the intact hemisphere. During this treatment she elicited the first active movement in 6 weeks. This sudden development of movement resembles improvements reported in Chinese texts on scalp acupuncture. We cannot be sure what mechanisms are at work in this case. However the outcome was improved motor ability so that the patient could use his right leg and begin to walk. Scalp acupuncture has received very little attention in the scientific literature despite repeated reports of benefit for cerebral conditions from China. Research seems long overdue.

Case study 5.8: level 1: Spasticity in legs affecting walking in multiple sclerosis

A 48-year-old woman developed increased spasticity in her left hamstrings. She had been diagnosed with multiple sclerosis 12 years previously. She had been able to walk short distances with a frame until she was recently admitted to hospital with

pneumonia. Assessment revealed bilateral spasticity, particularly of the hamstrings, with flexor spasms affecting the left leg more than the right. She had substantial muscle weakness of legs and trunk. She was unable to put weight through her left leg and was unable to walk. Physiotherapy over the previous 4 weeks had tried a wide range of treatments to improve her mobility. The physiotherapist had therefore discussed with the patient and her family the real possibility that she might not regain the ability to walk.

Treatment

The patient received four acupuncture treatments over 3 days in prone lying. Trigger points in up to seven different areas in the left hamstrings were located and deactivated using fanning technique. High-intensity, low-frequency electroacupuncture at 2 Hz eliciting strong muscle twitches of the left hamstrings was then applied for 10 minutes. Physiotherapy to assist her to stand followed immediately after acupuncture.

Points

Trigger points in hamstrings. Electroacupuncture points were selected at either end of the medial and lateral hamstrings within the muscle belly and connected up along the length of the muscle.

Outcome

Immediately after the first treatment she was able to stand and take weight through her left leg for the first time since her recent illness. Further acupuncture treatments before physiotherapy gained a similar outcome. She regained the ability to walk independently with a frame 8 weeks later. At this point her timed 10-metre walk took 56 seconds. She has continued to maintain this level of independent walking ability over subsequent years.

Comment

In this case the physiotherapist had tried every option to help the patient to walk. Focal weakening of the hamstrings with botulinum toxin was considered. This option may have reduced the flexor spasm but was unlikely to have helped her regain the ability to stand. Acupuncture was very much the last attempt to help this patient. The immediate improvement after the first treatment was unexpected but allowed physiotherapy to build on this ability and eventually help the patient to regain independent mobility. This treatment would not work for all patients. Indeed in some patients electroacupuncture applied to the leg muscles might exacerbate the flexor spasms. However it is an option worth trying.

Case study 5.9: level 1: Dyskinesia and 'off' symptoms in Parkinson's disease

A 64-year-old man presented with increasing motor symptoms of dyskinesia, 'off' periods and freezing. He also reported neck pain of 8/10. The patient had been diagnosed with Parkinson's disease 7 years previously and attended a specialist Parkinson's clinic for regular monitoring. He was able to walk independently with one stick but reported frequent falls.

Treatment

This man received eight acupuncture treatments over 4 weeks. Each treatment lasted 25 minutes. Needles were initially stimulated for Deqi. No further stimulation was provided. The presence of involuntary dyskinesia during treatment required the use of a substantial number of pillows to ensure he was well supported and comfortable. He was monitored closely throughout treatment.

Points

Left GB 21, LI 14, bilateral LI 4, SI 3. During later treatments GV 20, bilateral GB 20 and LR 3 were added.

Outcome

The patient experienced a rapid reduction of neck pain to 0/10. Dyskinesias were reduced with fewer 'off' periods and fewer falls. He was also able to reduce his parkinsonian medications.

Comment

The physiotherapist treating this patient had hoped to gain a reduction in the patient's neck pain. However after a number of treatments it was obvious that his motor symptoms were also improving. This is an intriguing finding in view of the possibility that pain and dyskinesia share some common pathophysiological mechanisms [5].

Part 3: Visceral dysfunction

Case study 5.10: level 1: Overactive bladder in multiple sclerosis

A 23-year-old woman with multiple sclerosis presented with frequency, urgency, urge incontinence and nocturia. This had become worse over the last few months since a recent relapse of multiple sclerosis. Physiotherapy treatment sessions of 45 minutes were regularly interrupted 2–3 times every day due to frequency, i.e. approximately 10–15 times per week. Incontinence Impact Questionnaire (IIQ-7) score was 19/21. Bladder scan following micturition indicated effective bladder emptying. Urinalysis was normal. This patient's symptoms suggested overactive bladder syndrome with detrusor hyperreflexia.

Functional ability

The patient was able to walk up to 5 metres with a frame but was very unsteady due to trunk and lower-limb ataxia and weakness as well as mild plantarflexor spasticity. She needed help from one person for activities of daily living.

Treatment

She received eight acupuncture treatments over 4 weeks, each treatment lasting 25 minutes. Electroacupuncture at 20 Hz [6] was trialled on the first treatment but this caused flexor spasms. Therefore all treatments involved manual acupuncture with no stimulation.

Points

SP 6, SP 4 bilaterally for first treatment. SP 6, LR 3 bilaterally for all subsequent treatments.

Outcome

Frequency, urgency and nocturia were reduced. The patient also reported improved sleep and improved daytime energy levels. Her physiotherapy sessions were less disrupted. On average she needed to go to the toilet only once or twice during physiotherapy sessions over the entire week. This allowed her to concentrate on work to improve balance and mobility. Her IIQ-7 score was 14/21.

Comment

Parasympathetic outflow to the detrusor emerges at spinal levels S2–4 (see Chapter 4). SP 6 in flexor digitorum longus (S1–2) and LR 3 in the first dorsal interosseous muscle (S2–3) ensured that afferent information would arrive at relevant levels of the sacral spinal cord, with the aim that this would modulate bladder function.

Case study 5.11: level 2: Constipation in multiple sclerosis

A 52-year-old woman with multiple sclerosis presented with a range of symptoms including low mood, irritability, anger and tearfulness, headaches most days, infrequent bowel activity, opening bowels once each week with difficulty, poor sleep, waking frequently, daytime fatigue and numb left arm. In addition she had poor condition of skin below her knees which was dry, red and in places cracked. She could transfer with help from one person but was unable to walk.

Treatment

She received 10 treatments over 5 weeks. Each treatment lasted 25 minutes. Needles were stimulated initially for Deqi. No further stimulation was given. During the early treatments the condition of the skin on her legs prevented the use of any points below the knee. However by treatment 6 the skin condition had improved so much that ST 36 could be needled.

Points

Bilateral LI 11, LI 4 and Yintang in treatments 1–5. Bilateral ST 36 added in subsequent treatments.

Outcome

Early treatments resulted in decreased irritability, reduction in headaches, increased energy levels, increased sensation in left arm and improved skin condition of legs from broken skin to healed skin. The improved skin condition permitted the safe addition of ST 36 bilaterally. Needling this point resulted in an immediate impact on bowel function with sensations in the abdomen after treatment and bowels opened later that day. Following subsequent treatments bowel activity increased to bowels open on alternate days. She reported feeling better for having more regular bowel activity.

Comment

ST 36 is highlighted as an important point to influence bowel activity and this was relevant in her case. The needle at this point is inserted into tibialis anterior, which is innervated by the deep peroneal nerve (L4–5). Skin overlying this point is supplied by the lateral cutaneous nerve of calf (L4–5, S1). Innervation of the bowel emerges from L1–2 and S2–4. Needling of ST 36 therefore does not enter the same spinal segments as those controlling bowel activity, although there will be links between adjacent segments via interneurones. Part of acupuncture's influence on the bowel is through generalized effects of stimulating the limb rather than purely segmental mechanisms.

Part 4: Generalized symptoms

Case study 5.12: level 1: Insomnia in cervical myelopathy

A 61-year-old woman presented with insomnia. She had recently had cervical spine decompression for cervical myelopathy and exhibited mild bilateral lower-limb spasticity and generalized weakness.

She was able to stand but was unable to walk. She was dependent on a wheelchair for mobility and on carers for assistance to wash and dress. A persistent lack of sleep was interfering with her ability to participate actively in rehabilitation.

Treatment

The patient received four acupuncture treatments of 25 minutes over 2 weeks. Needles were stimulated for Deqi initially but no further stimulation was given.

Points

Yintang, bilateral HT 7, ST 36, SP6.

Outcome

There was marked improvement in sleep allowing her to participate more effectively in rehabilitation, with a reduction in daytime sleepiness. After the second treatment the patient reported: 'I cannot remember the last time I slept that well'.

Comment

Improvement of sleep is one of the commonest reports following acupuncture for any reason in patients with neurological conditions.

Case study 5.13: level 1: Fatigue affecting daily activities in multiple sclerosis

A 38-year-old woman presented with fatigue limiting her ability to carry out daily activities, including looking after her children, particularly later in the day when her fatigue was more pronounced. She had been diagnosed with multiple sclerosis 5 years previously. She was able to walk with one stick. The fatigue had become worse recently since she had started Tysabri. Modified Fatigue Impact Scale (MFIS) was 54/84.

Treatment

The patient received eight acupuncture treatments, of 25 minutes over 6 weeks. Needles were stimulated for Deqi at the beginning of the treatment and once more halfway through treatment.

Points

CV 6, bilateral LI 4, LR 3, SP 6, ST 36.

Outcome

The patient experienced reduced fatigue, improved sleep pattern and increased energy levels. She reported that she was able to look her after children more easily. She also reported fewer side-effects from Tysabri. MFIS reduced to 33/84.

Comment

Fatigue is common and problematic in neurological conditions. A relatively short course of acupuncture resulted in substantial benefits for this patient as well as for her family. It also helped to reduce medication side-effects.

Case study 5.14: level 2: Depression in multiple sclerosis

A 42-year-old woman presented with depression, uncertainty about the future, muzzy head and generalized fatigue. She was on antidepressant medications. She was able to walk unsteadily with elbow crutches. On assessment truncal ataxia and mild lower-limb spasticity were evident. She had recently retired from work due to ill health.

Treatment

The patient received eight treatments of 25 minutes over 4 weeks. Needles were stimulated initially for Deqi. There was no further stimulation.

Points

Points included a selection from bilateral ST 36, SP 10, SP 6, SP 3, LR 3, KI 3 as well as right LI 11, left HT 7, GV 20, Yintang, bilateral Huatojiaji at T 3, 4, 7, BL 20, ST 44 and ST 40. On average eight needles were used for each treatment.

Outcome

The patient was calm and relaxed during and after treatment. She reported that her head felt clearer, her mood was lighter and she felt more optimistic and more self-confident. She also said that she felt less stressed and 'more like her old self back again'. She felt she could tackle things more easily. She also noted an improvement of circulation in her hands and feet.

Comment

Key features of depression include feelings of low self-confidence and little optimism about the future. This patient's impairments and functional ability changed very little but the provision of acupuncture provided a substantial effect on her outlook. She felt she was in a position to look to the future and move forward with her life. In turn this allowed her to make best use of the rehabilitation services that she was accessing at that time.

Case study 5.15: level 2: Acute anxiety following traumatic brain injury

A 48-year-old man presented with acute anxiety. He had sustained a traumatic brain injury 2 months previously. He was functionally very able but presented with cognitive impairment and acute anxiety. He was withdrawn and finding it difficult to participate in cognitive-behavioural therapy sessions which he was receiving to help manage his anxiety. General Health Questionnaire-12 (GHQ-12) score was 27/36. He was previously fit and active, worked fulltime and enjoyed a healthy social life.

Treatment

The patient received 14 treatments over 6 weeks with initial treatments provided on alternate days. There was no stimulation of needles on the first two treatments. In subsequent treatments the needles were stimulated at 10-minute intervals. Early sessions lasted 25 minutes. Sessions gradually increased to 35–40 minutes.

Points

Yintang, bilateral LI 4, ST 36, KI 6. In later treatments some points were substituted with HT 7, LR 3, GB 34 and back Shu points.

Outcome

The patient experienced a reduction in anxiety, was able to participate effectively in cognitive-behavioural therapy sessions and spontaneously began socializing with other patients on the unit after the second treatment. GHQ-12 score was 9/36.

Comment

Acupuncture resulted in a general calming of this man who had recently undergone a very stressful traumatic accident. This allowed him to engage more effectively in therapies to assist him to move forwards in his life. After the first couple of treatments he started becoming more sociable on the unit, coming out of his room and talking with other patients. The physiotherapist had noticed this effect with other patients she had treated with acupuncture after traumatic brain injury.

Case study 5.16: level 2: Agitation secondary to pain in stroke

A 59-year-old man presented with agitation due to severe central neuropathic pain throughout the left side of his body. He had sustained a stroke 5 weeks previously causing dense left hemiplegia, moderate spasticity in upper and lower limb, left hemisensory impairment and inattention to left side of space. He exhibited severe agitation and called out on any attempts to move his left side. Medications had limited effect. He was completely unable to participate in rehabilitation due to pain.

Functional ability

He was unable to use his left arm, stand or walk. He was dependent on a hoist and on two people to move him from bed to wheelchair. He required the assistance of one to two people to assist him with all daily activities.

Treatment

The patient received 16 acupuncture treatments over 5 weeks with initial treatments closer together. Each treatment lasted 20–25 minutes according to how long the patient was able to lie still. There was no stimulation of needles. The physiotherapist sat immediately by the patient's right side throughout treatment and limited movement of his right arm on the occasions when he attempted to move it.

Points

Bilateral LI 4, LR 3.

Outcome

The patient experienced a substantial reduction in agitation. He became very relaxed by the end of each treatment, allowing effective therapy immediately after acupuncture. Pain gradually reduced over the course of treatment and he was therefore able to participate in rehabilitation. He eventually developed the ability to stand and take a few steps.

Comment

This may not be the case to attempt when you are fresh from your first acupuncture course. However with close and careful monitoring such patients may gain substantially from treatment. Body acupuncture was selected in this case. Ear acupuncture might have been another good option to consider, perhaps in combination with body needling on the left side, which he was unable to move. This would have eliminated the risk posed by the man moving his right arm restlessly.

Summary of clinical reasoning in neurological conditions

Selection of points

To gain specific effect in local tissues, select points in those tissues; to gain a generalized effect, needle 'big' points on arms and legs, e.g. LI 4, LR 3, ST 36.

Depth of needling

To gain a specific segmental effect consider whether the needle needs to be in the dermatome, myotome or sclerotome. Trigger point acupuncture or electrical stimulation of muscles will require needles to be in the muscles. Otherwise needle to the usual recommended depth.

Stimulation

This will depend on both the state of the patient and the desired outcome. If the patient is agitated, anxious or in substantial pain minimal or no stimulation would generally be more helpful. In situations which are chronic, difficult to change or where you are aiming to influence sensory or motor inactivity, select stronger stimulation which might include electroacupuncture. In spasticity you may select minimal or no stimulation or you may select strong electroacupuncture stimulation according to the effects you are aiming for and the response of the individual patient.

Course of treatment

This will depend on the response of the patient. Some patients may need just a few treatments, often backed up by other options such as physiotherapy. Some may need a longer course of treatment. The possibility of follow-up would be useful for some patients.

References

[1] Watson P. Modulation of involuntary movements in cerebral palsy with acupuncture. Acupunct Med 2009;27(2):76–8.

[2] Conforto AB, Cohen LG, dos Santos RL, et al. Effects of somatosensory stimulation on motor function in chronic cortico-
subcortical strokes. J Neurol 2007;254(3):333–9.

[3] Boggio PS, Alonso-Alonso M, Mansur CG, et al. Hand function improvement with low-frequency repetitive transcranial magnetic stimulation of the unaffected hemisphere in a severe case of
stroke. Am J Phys Med Rehabil 2006;85(11):927–30.

[4] Murase N, Duque J, Mazzocchio R, et al. Influence of interhemispheric interactions on motor function in chronic stroke. Ann Neurol 2004;55(3):400–9.

[5] Lim SY, Farrell MJ, Gibson SJ, et al. Do dyskinesia and pain share common pathophysiological mechanisms in Parkinson's disease? Mov Disord 2008;23(12):1689–95.

[6] Kabay SC, Yucel M, Kabay S. Acute effect of posterior tibial nerve stimulation on neurogenic detrusor overactivity in patients with multiple sclerosis: urodynamic study. Urology 2008;71(4):641–5.

Section 2

Clinical conditions

Acquired brain injury: stroke, cerebral palsy and traumatic brain injury

6

CHAPTER CONTENTS

KEY POINTS

- Stroke is commonly treated in physiotherapy departments and the rehabilitation process is frequently long and complex.
- Some manifestations of the brain injury will respond to acupuncture.
- There is a high risk of a second stroke so preventive acupuncture may be appropriate.
- Some of the side-effects produced by drug therapy will also respond to acupuncture.
- Treatment will be a mixture of traditional Chinese medicine (TCM) and Western theory.
- In TCM terms stroke is associated with both Wei and Feng syndromes.
- Cerebral palsy is considered separately, but the acupuncture treatment does not differ greatly from that in stroke rehabilitation.
- Traumatic brain injury manifests in similar damage and will require similar treatment.

Part 1: Stroke

Definition

A stroke is defined as a syndrome of rapidly developing clinical signs of focal (or global) disturbance of cerebral function, with symptoms lasting 24 hours or longer, or leading to death, with no apparent cause other than that of vascular origin [1]. The damage to the brain tissue is caused by thrombosis, embolus or haemorrhage. This leads to hemiplegia or some form of hemiparesis. The description of the stroke or cerebrovascular accident (CVA) as 'right' or 'left'

can be misleading as the resulting paralysis is usually on the side opposite to the brain lesion. This also assumes, incorrectly, that all the adverse effects will be unilateral.

This definition includes subarachnoid haemorrhage but excludes transient ischaemic attack (TIA), subdural haematoma and haemorrhage or infarction caused by infection or tumour. TIA is defined as a neurological deficit due to cerebrovascular disease that lasts less than 24 hours. Hemiplegia is defined as the paralysis of muscles on the side of the body opposite to the area of cerebral damage.

Incidence

An estimated 150 000 people have a stroke in the UK each year, with over 67 000 deaths due to stroke, making stroke the most common cause of death in England and Wales after heart disease and cancer [2].

Stroke has a greater disability impact than any other disease, with many thousands of people living with moderate to severe disabilities as a result [3].

The direct cost of stroke to the NHS is estimated to be £2.8 billion and the cost to the wider economy is £1.8 billion. The informal care cost is around £2.4 billion, with the total costs of stroke predicted to rise in real terms by 30% between 1991 and 2010. Stroke patients occupy around 20% of all acute hospital beds and 25% of long-term beds [4].

It is thought that there has been an overall reduction in the numbers of strokes in the UK. Work undertaken in the Oxford region has shown that, as a result of the use of preventive medicines, including drugs that lower blood pressure and cholesterol and those that thin the blood, together with the reduction in heavy smoking, the incidence of stroke has dropped by 40% [5]. The current decline in incidence and case fatality may also be due to dietary changes and the emphasis on the treatment of hypertension [6]. There is a possibility that the predisposition to stroke runs in families, although this is likely to be linked to hypertension as the risk factor [7].

Mortality

Stroke is a devastating condition for both patients and carers, with a high mortality rate throughout the first year after the lesion: 30% at 3 weeks, 40% at 6 months and 50% at 1 year [8]. Morbidity is high, with 12% estimated to be in long-term care 1 year after the event [9]. The risk of recurrence is also high: 7% for at least 5 years after the initial stroke and 15 times the stroke risk for the general population [10]. The figures suggest that each health district can expect 550 patients to present with stroke each year and each general practitioner can expect to see four or five new cases a year and be caring for 12 survivors, of whom seven or eight will be disabled [11]. Stroke is therefore a major financial burden to the NHS and consumes more than 4% of total NHS expenditure and more than 7% of community health and social care resources [12].

Risk factors

There are many health factors which appear to predispose a patient to stroke. Age is the most important factor [13], but in general raised blood pressure [14], smoking [15] and alcohol consumption [16] are associated with a greater risk of occlusive and haemorrhagic stroke. Diabetes mellitus is associated only with occlusive stroke. Other factors that may be important are obesity, poor diet, febrile illness, oral contraception, taking hormone replacement therapy and, in some cases, wide seasonal variation in temperature, although this can be either extreme cold or heat [17]. It has also been suggested that the seasonal availability of vitamin C may be a factor [18], although with the wide variety of non-seasonal foods now available this may not be an issue in industrial nations.

Diagnosis

Differentiation from other diseases

Transient ischaemic attack

TIA is defined as a 'clinical syndrome characterized by acute loss of cerebral or monocular function with symptoms lasting less than 24 hours'. These patients are often unaware of what has happened to them and unlikely to present for treatment; however they do retain a heightened risk of stroke and if discovered should be seen by a primary care doctor for preventive treatment [19]. TIA is not described as a true stroke.

(Acupuncture may have some thing to offer at this stage; see the syndrome 'Rising Liver Fire',

linked to Kidney Yin Xu, in Chapter 1. Treatment is aimed at prophylaxis, including the lowering of blood pressure.)

Clinical stroke syndromes

It is relatively easy to distinguish vascular strokes – those caused by emboli, haemorrhages and infarcts – from non-vascular pathology. However, up to 13% of patients thought initially to have had a vascular stroke turn out to be suffering from other pathology [20, 21]. Stroke is most commonly confused with epilepsy, delirium and loss of consciousness, tumours, depression and dementia syndromes.

Dementia manifests as a global impairment of higher mental function, without loss of consciousness. Multiple cerebral infarcts are the predominant pathology in 10–30% of patients and as many again have mixed pathology with vascular signs. The site of the infarction may generally be more important than the absolute volume of brain tissue lost. Cardiac embolism is likely to be an important factor but is of unknown incidence and difficult to diagnose with certainty [6].

Stroke can be divided into four subgroups with distinctive clinical characteristics. The following definitions are taken from *Stroke: Epidemiology, Evidence and Clinical Practice* [6, 22].

Total anterior circulation infarct (TACI)

TACIs have a combination of:

1. new higher cerebral dysfunction (dysphasia, dyspraxia, dyscalculia, visuospatial disorders)
2. homonymous hemianopia (one-sided visual field defect)
3. unilateral motor and/or sensory deficits in at least two of the face, arm and leg.

Impaired consciousness rendering testing impossible is interpreted as a deficit. These symptoms are consistent with occlusion of the proximal middle cerebral artery, in isolation or associated with internal carotid artery occlusion. Two-thirds of these infarcts are embolic; the rest are thrombotic.

This group has a poor chance of good functional outcome and mortality is high.

Partial anterior circulation infarcts (PACIs)

PACIs comprise two of the three elements of a TACI, higher cerebral dysfunction alone or a motor/sensory deficit more limited than that defining a TACI (i.e. one limb alone or hand and face but not the whole arm). These are presumed to be due to embolic occlusion of one of the two divisions of the middle cerebral artery or a smaller branch.

This group of patients is more likely to have a second stroke in the first year.

Lacunar infarcts (LACIs)

LACIs present with pure motor or sensory stroke, sensorimotor stroke, ataxic hemiparesis (cerebellar-type ataxia with ipsilateral pyramidal signs), dysarthria, 'clumsy hand' syndrome or acute focal movement disorders. Motor/sensory signs must involve at least two of the face, arm and leg. These represent thrombotic occlusion of the deep perforating branches of the middle cerebral artery, supplying the internal capsule or pons.

Despite the relatively small area of infarct many of these patients remain substantially handicapped.

Posterior circulation infarcts (POCIs)

A POCI presents with ipsilateral cranial nerve palsy, plus contralateral motor/sensory deficit, disorder of conjugate eye movement, isolated cerebellar dysfunction or isolated homonymous hemianopia. These infarcts are in the vertebrobasilar arterial territory: only one fifth are embolic, the rest are thrombotic.

This group of patients is more likely to have a second stroke within the first year, but has the best chance of a good functional outcome.

Silent infarcts

A silent infarct is one diagnosed on computed tomography (CT) or magnetic resonance imaging (MRI) scanning without corresponding signs or symptoms. It may be silent because of a relatively benign location or because the symptoms are either only transient or are simply not reported by the patient.

Prevalence of silent infarction increases with age and the risk factors are no different from those for symptomatic stroke. The increased likelihood of cognitive impairment among subjects reporting stroke symptoms in the absence of a diagnosed stroke or TIA suggests that such symptoms are not benign and may warrant clinical evaluation that includes cognitive assessment [23].

CT and MRI scans

It is important to be exact in the early diagnosis of stroke because this has a bearing on the relative safety of the subsequent treatment in the acute phase. A CT scan should be performed to ensure that there is no sign of continuing haemorrhage or any other abnormality before a thrombolytic agent can be used. MRI is a newer imaging modality and offers better pictures. However it is less comfortable for the patient, being more claustrophobic and, in the case of stroke, serves the same function as a CT scan in ruling out the presence of a continuing bleed. The techniques can also be used in the subacute phase to confirm the establishment of collateral circulation to the cerebral hemispheres.

Medical treatment

Acute

Most patients with stroke are admitted to hospital, although some, those with generally less severe symptoms, remain at home for their nursing and subsequent rehabilitation. In practice it is difficult to be certain how many people are not admitted to hospital because they are not routinely recorded.

A welcome innovation has been a widespread advertising campaign to alert the public to the first signs of stroke [24], emphasizing that stroke should be recognized as a medical emergency requiring fast admission and specialist management. Patients who have suffered a stroke remain at increased risk of a further incident: therefore secondary prevention is part of treatment.

Measurement of the underlying structural changes within the brain has only recently become routine. Now the idea of cell death or apoptosis is better understood, it is becoming clear that there are two types of damage. Firstly, the focus of the stroke, where the cells are deprived of oxygen, for whatever reason, and subsequently die, and, secondly, the so-called penumbra or area surrounding the focal point, where the cells are damaged by pressure from temporarily swollen tissues but may not necessarily be destroyed. Since the penumbra has the potential to be reperfused there is a limited time period for interventions to be effective before the cells die. It would be desirable to increase the blood supply to the penumbra without increasing the haemorrhage.

Considerable research has been undertaken to investigate drug treatment in the immediate aftermath of stroke. Drugs such as aspirin and heparin seem to have some purpose in preventing further damage immediately after the stroke but two recent major studies have not entirely supported their use.

The International Stroke Trial investigated 19 435 patients within 48 hours of acute stroke and randomized them between two different doses of heparin or placebo [25]. The design also randomized patients to receive daily aspirin or no aspirin. The researchers used a 2×2 factorial design with patients randomized to one of four possible groups: heparin and aspirin, aspirin or heparin alone or no treatment. Treatment lasted 14 days or until discharge, if sooner.

The results from the International Stroke Trial study showed that there was no overall benefit in mortality or limitation of brain damage from the use of heparin; indeed, there was a slightly higher – 9 per 1000 – rate of haemorrhagic strokes and more deaths within 14 days. Neither heparin regimen gave any clinical advantage at 6 months. There was no interaction between heparin and aspirin in the main outcomes.

The other major study, the Chinese Acute Stroke Trial [26], randomized 20 000 patients to daily low-dose aspirin or a placebo, also within 48 hours of the stroke. Treatment lasted 4 weeks. The Chinese Acute Stroke Trial study showed that aspirin started in the acute stage was associated with small benefits. The difference in death rates between the aspirin and control groups was only 0.5%. Combining the data from these two very large trials detects a small treatment effect for aspirin, thus supporting the early prescribing of aspirin, as long as continuing haemorrhage has been excluded. As aspirin is prescribed in any case for long-term prevention it becomes imperative that CT scans take place routinely very soon after stroke.

Thrombolytic drugs have also been investigated, particularly tissue plasminogen activator (tPA, alteplase) given within just 3 hours of an acute ischaemic stroke. The most recent Cochrane review [27] balances the increase in deaths within the first to seventh days and deaths at final follow-up with the reduction in disability in the survivors. It suggests that intravenous recombinant tPA may be the best method of delivery but is cautious about recommending general use.

However the current advice given to physicians [28] is that thrombolytics may be given but haemorrhage must definitely be excluded and that the patient should be in a specialist centre with appropriate experience and expertise.

Subacute

The most important first step is an assessment of disability. Swallowing, management of dysphagia and nutrition will be checked, along with bowel and bladder function. Immediate complications will be prevented by careful monitoring of temperature, dehydration and risk of pressure sores. Possible areas of impairment and also social context need to be assessed before full rehabilitation is started.

Spasticity is a motor disorder characterized by a velocity-dependent increase in tonic stretch reflexes. It commonly leads to muscle shortening and joint contractures. Signs of change in muscle tone are observable within a few days of the initial brain damage. A relatively new drug used to combat spasticity is botulinum toxin (BTX or BoNT). A number of trials among stroke patients have shown a significant decrease in muscle tone. The effects of the BTX were shown to decrease after 3 months, but if the patients were regaining control of their muscles, that could be seen as an advantage. Several studies have shown a good effect in stroke rehabilitation situations [29–31]. The trial by Lai et al. [31] shows that an increased effect is gained by serial splinting to maintain the increase in range of movement gained by the relaxing muscle spasm. It would be interesting to compare that with the muscle-relaxing effect of acupuncture, either in place of, or used with, BTX.

Management and rehabilitation

Input is necessary from a range of health professionals in addition to the medical team. Physiotherapists, speech and language therapists and occupational therapists are all important members of the team and need to understand what each can contribute. Social services and community health staff will also join the team to enable the ultimate easy discharge of the patient into the community.

Correct positioning of stroke patients is a widely advocated strategy to prevent the development of abnormal muscle tone, contractures, pain, skin breakdown and respiratory complications. Since this and the other supportive treatments require a constant team effort, it has been demonstrated that patients in specialist stroke units are likely to do better [32].

Rehabilitation should be a long-term process with a seamless transition from acute to community services. Training in the skills of independent living may be necessary for up to a year after the stroke, but is rarely available in the straitened circumstances prevailing throughout the NHS.

Prognosis

Body structure and function, activity and participation

The effect of stroke, or indeed any neurological condition, is described in varying ways. The *International Classification of Functioning, Disability and Health* (ICF) suggests that an individual's disability and resultant function is a result of the interactions between his or her health condition and contextual factors such as the physical environment or social attitudes [33]. A full description is included in this chapter, although it applies equally to the others.

ICF highlights the relationship between problems with body structure and function and the individual's level of activity and participation (Table 6.1).

ICF goes on to identify three levels of functioning of the human: at the body level, at the whole-person level and within society in general.

Disability involves functional difficulties in one or more of these levels and may include the following:

● Impairment refers to problems in body function or structure resulting from the health condition; in the example of stroke, impairments might include paralysis, sensory loss, visual disturbance, pain, cognitive impairment, speech problems or impairment of consciousness.

● Activity limitations are difficulties an individual may have in carrying out activities and might include an inability to walk to the toilet or the inability to drive.

● Participation restrictions refer to problems the individual may have when involved in day-to-day life situations.

Contextual factors also contribute to the overall disability. External environmental factors might include steps into the person's home limiting access or uneven footpaths en route to the local shops posing a risk of tripping. Personal factors might include the individual's personal coping style and past experience as well as educational and social background.

Disability is often measured in terms of the ability to carry out activities of daily living (ADL) using scales such as the Barthel ADL Index. The main emphasis in stroke research has been on the domains of physical activity and self-care but it is useful to remember that the World Health Organization definition of disability is much broader than this.

The relationships between impairments and activity or participation restriction are not fixed. Individuals with very severe impairment may participate fully within their local community with an appropriate level of support. Another individual with relatively mild impairment may be severely restricted in activity and participation, possibly due to substantial impact of contextual factors. This highlights the complexity of carrying out research in the stroke population.

Effects of stroke

The primary effect of stroke is impairment of muscle function caused by motor and/or sensory deficits commonly affecting the face, arm and leg on the contralateral side. This will result in the characteristic hemiparesis or hemiplegia leading to physical disability of a temporary or permanent nature.

Unfortunately there are many other possible effects, depending on the site of the brain lesion and the quality of the poststroke care. Among them are:

● dysphagia or dysphasia
● incontinence
● infections, urine or respiratory
● cognitive impairment

Table 6.1 Definitions of major International Classification of Functioning, Disability and Health categories

Category	World Health Organization definition (33)
Body structure	Anatomical parts of the body such as organs, limbs and their components
Body function	Physiological functions of body systems, including psychological functions
Activity	The execution of a task or action by an individual
Participation	Involvement in a life situation

- mood changes
- pressure sores
- deep-vein thrombosis
- pulmonary embolus
- pain, particularly in the shoulder
- falls and fractures.

Depending on the site of the lesion there may be varying degrees of speech loss or swallowing difficulties and there is a real danger of food aspiration in the acute stage of stroke. Most patients with moderate to severe stroke are incontinent at admission, and many are discharged still incontinent. Both urinary and faecal incontinence are common in the early stages and need urgent management in order to prevent these problems delaying the patients' eventual rehabilitation. Urinary incontinence directly after stroke is an indicator of poor prognosis for both survival and functional recovery [34]. Care must be taken to prevent infection.

Anxiety is an equally common problem accompanied by feelings of fear and apprehension with physical symptoms such as breathlessness, palpitations and trembling. The specific causes of anxiety after stroke are not known; it may simply be a product of the sudden physical disability or may more closely resemble an anxiety disorder and require antidepressive drug treatment. Anxiety after stroke has certainly been shown to be associated with increased severity of depressive symptoms and greater functional impairment [35].

Long periods of inactivity produce a danger of skin breakdown and the possibility of pressure sores is increased if the patient is also incontinent. The lack of voluntary movement also increases the risk of deep-vein thrombosis and pulmonary embolus. Early mobilization after stroke has been shown both to cut rates of poststroke depression by 50% and also to be cost-effective [36, 37]. This has implications for early acupuncture treatment of this condition. The link between exercise and general feeling of well-being and mood elevation is well documented in healthy subjects [38], and the chemical action of acupuncture has often been compared to that of exercise [39].

A further complication of recovery is spastic hypertonia associated with exaggerated deep tendon reflexes. This is often associated with central nervous system disorders due to lesions in the brain that affect descending tracts normally inhibiting spinal reflex pathways. The resulting excessive muscle tone can cause many problems, including loss of free

movement, difficulties performing daily activities and pain [40]. It may also cause the limb to become 'frozen' or fixed in an uncomfortable position.

Pain is most common in the affected shoulder. It is to be hoped that it is less often present now that much emphasis is placed on correct positioning of the paralysed limbs [41]. Unfortunately the initial loss of muscle tone in the hemiplegic arm often results in damage to the capsule with subsequent pain. Use of functional electrical stimulation can help prevent this unpleasant complication [42].

Falls are not uncommon in elderly patients even if they have not suffered a stroke. Paretic limbs become osteopenic or less dense and since the stroke patient is likely to fall to the affected side, poststroke fractures are a frequent complication in the process of rehabilitation. Fear of falling can be damaging too, leading to reduction in possible mobility and social withdrawal.

Patterns of recovery

The aim of all treatment should be independence in self-care within a year after the stroke. This is achieved in a range between 60% [43] and 83% [44] of surviving patients, both measured at 1 year after stroke. However the same data suggest that between 16 and 31% may be institutionalized by the end of the year.

Recovery of rolling, sitting balance, transfers and walking among patients referred for rehabilitation seems to follow a relatively predictable pattern over the first 8 weeks [45]. The majority of muscle recovery occurs within the first 3 months after the stroke with subsequent recovery taking place at a slower pace [46]. Some useful recovery still occurs between the sixth and twelfth months. In the hemiplegic hand it is thought that if there is no active hand grip after 3 weeks there is unlikely to be much improvement [47].

The accepted wisdom within the physiotherapy profession is that there is little to be gained from the rehabilitation process as late as 2 years after the stroke, but there may be unused potential for physical improvement in the period before this cut-off, depending on previous access to treatment. Overall recovery is thought to be adversely affected by the patients' age [48]. This assumes that there may be co-pathology, including mobility problems such as osteoarthritis.

Recurrence

One in five strokes is a recurrent stroke and a patient who has had one stroke is at 10-fold increased risk of another [49]. Despite similar neurological impairments, patients with recurrence on the opposite side to their original episode tend to have markedly more severe functional disability after completed rehabilitation than patients with an ipsilateral recurrence, implying that functional ability to compensate is decreased. These figures serve to underline the importance of a prophylactic dose of aspirin or even acupuncture.

Stroke and physiotherapy

Current physiotherapy

Physiotherapists are an important part of the hospital rehabilitation team and, working alongside the occupational therapists, are particularly concerned with regaining functional movement in the paralysed limbs. In order to achieve this many of the primary movement patterns need to be relearned by the patient. Progress is often hindered by the state of the muscle tissue, which may exhibit weakness, spasticity or no tone at all, remaining flaccid. Progress can also be inhibited by the development of contractures and resulting pain produced by poor postural positioning in the bed and chair. This will also be made worse by early, incorrect attempts at movement.

The modalities used by the physiotherapist are many and varied, based essentially on the retraining of physical movement and incorporating forms of biofeedback to retrain balance and proprioception [50], functional electrical stimulation [51], gait retraining and treadmill training [52]. Transcutaneous electrical nerve stimulation (TENS) has also been used successfully [53], usually utilizing acupuncture points. Approaches to treatment vary but may also include techniques drawn from the Bobath approach, movement science and, on occasion, proprioceptive neuromuscular facilitation. Research has failed to identify substantial differences between the different approaches but a clear finding is the need for intensive training [54]. More research on the individual components of rehabilitation is still required.

Spontaneous neurological recovery is considered by many to be responsible for most of the functional recovery after stroke but in a critical review Kwakkel et al. suggested that simple biological variability may encourage rehabilitation-induced effects and that comprehensive functional therapy incorporating elements of intensive and task-specific strategies may ultimately produce the best effects [55].

Application of acupuncture

Physiotherapists working in neurological rehabilitation units are in close daily contact with their patients and, as acupuncture appears to be an effective intervention in the stroke recovery process, are ideally placed to use it.

Prevention of stroke by traditional Chinese medicine (TCM) acupuncture depends on meticulous TCM diagnosis and is both complicated and unproven, but the type of acupuncture applied after stroke to combat the paralysis is not complex and is well within the capacity of any physiotherapist with basic acupuncture training. The state of current research is confused but indicates possible applications [56].

Neurological basis

The specific neurological changes that could benefit a stroke patient are described in detail in Chapter 4. However the demonstrable physiological effects of acupuncture in stroke are as follows.

Changes in cerebral circulation

Given the pathology of stroke, it is clear that an acupuncture intervention that could maintain peripheral circulation to the cerebral hemispheres when the central supply is compromised would be useful acute therapy [57].

Of course, since the same conditions would apply as with aspirin or thrombolytic drugs, it must be ascertained that there is no continuing haemorrhage.

Changes in blood composition, velocity and general circulation

Changes in blood flow and velocity, noted by Yuan et al. [57] and Litscher et al. [58], could be helpful in preventing further emboli and aiding with reperfusion of temporarily damaged brain tissue. Indeed, these changes may mirror the actions of tPA or aspirin and could be considered as an alternative if the acupuncture could be administered quickly enough.

Effects on muscle tissue

A general increase in blood flow could be beneficial to recovering muscle tissue, particularly that which has been damaged by long-term disuse. One of the main perceived problems with rehabilitation is the increase in muscle tone and acupuncture has been shown to have a potentially useful decreasing effect [55, 59, 60]. In a good-quality trial, but with small numbers, clinically relevant changes in spasticity were observed to be comparable to those produced by botulinum toxin injections [61].

More work is needed on this aspect of acupuncture and stroke. A more general effect on muscle tissue, leading to an increase in muscle strength in healthy subjects, has been demonstrated, although only in small studies [62, 63]. In a larger study carried out in the UK, the Motricity Index was used to measure muscle strength recovery in stroke patients and the researchers found that acupuncture appeared to produce a boost for this in the early stages of recovery [64].

The use of electroacupuncture raises a further set of questions for the researcher but does seem to be effective in some situations, for example in post-stroke shoulder subluxation, where electroacupuncture has been shown to have a useful effect if applied in the early stages [65] (Figure 6.1).

Using electroacupuncture, Shen et al. [66] showed that the combination of electroacupuncture and exercise therapy improved limb function in the hemiplegic patient, and, additionally, that the therapeutic effect of exercise was increased if it was given after the acupuncture.

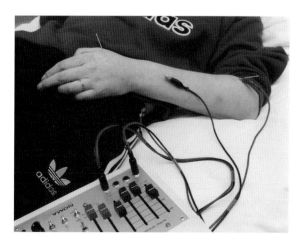

Figure 6.1 • Electroacupuncture applied in stroke (TE 5 and LI 10).

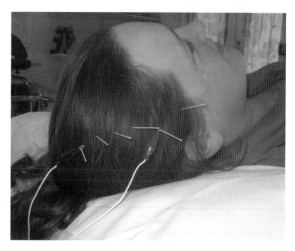

Figure 6.2 • Scalp acupuncture in stroke, motor line.

A paper in Chinese suggests that scalp acupuncture, a form of electroacupuncture, (see Chapter 12: Figure 6.2), works better if used in combination with exercise therapy in stroke rehabilitation [67].

Effects on mood

Acupuncture is associated with improvements in mood and energy, due in part to the observed increase in serotonin and endorphins. This evidence has been around for some time [68] but the positive psychological effects are coming under closer scrutiny now [69]. Since it has been suggested that depression and anxiety after stroke are associated with increased severity of depressive symptoms and greater functional impairment [35], this alternative to drug therapy may be very acceptable and will assist with patient compliance with taxing exercise programmes [70].

Effects on energy levels

There is a lot of anecdotal evidence linking acupuncture with an increase in energy level but little hard research, particularly in the field of neurology. However, an interesting study by Molassiotis et al., working with oncology patients, showed a significant decrease in fatigue after the application of acupuncture [71]. Given the known effect of the acupuncture stimulus on the limbic system it is not unreasonable to assume that this would be the case. A similar effect was detected in the Hopwood trial of acupuncture in stroke patients with just subsignificant results on the Nottingham Health Profile scale for emotional reaction and energy levels, in favour of the acupuncture group at 24 weeks after their stroke [64].

A Canadian project to create guidelines for 13 types of physical rehabilitation interventions used in the management of adult patients (>18 years of age) presenting with hemiplegia or hemiparesis following a single clinically identifiable ischaemic or haemorrhagic CVA was developed in 2006 [72]. This group identified and synthesized evidence from comparative controlled trials. The group then formed an expert panel which developed a set of criteria for grading the strength of the evidence and the recommendation. Patient-important outcomes were determined through consensus, provided that these outcomes were assessed with a valid and reliable outcome scale.

The Ottawa Panel developed 147 positive recommendations of clinical benefit concerning the use of different types of physical rehabilitation interventions involved after stroke. Among those listed were therapeutic exercise, task-oriented training, biofeedback, gait training, balance training, treatment of shoulder subluxation, electrical stimulation, TENS, therapeutic ultrasound and acupuncture [72].

Table 6.2 offers a summary of the symptoms that are likely to be present to a greater or lesser degree in most stroke patients. Obviously one of the characteristics is the unilateral nature of the impairment but otherwise these symptoms are common throughout this group of neurological conditions.

Table 6.2 Symptom picture for stroke

Symptom	Characteristic presentation	Stroke
Decreased mobility	Hemiparesis or hemiplegia	○ ○
Fatigue	Lack of energy	○
Respiratory problems	Weak cough	X
Muscle spasm	Increased tone	○ ○
Contractures	Stiffness and rigidity leading to deformity	○
Autonomic changes	Slowing circulation	○
Cognition/ mood	Emotional lability, poststroke depression	○
Communication	Sometimes hampered by facial palsy (loss of speech with right cerebrovascular accident)	○ ○
Bladder problems	Occasional	X
Visual problems	Hemianopia, single-sided visual neglect	○

X, usually absent; ○, common, ○○, very frequent.

Links to TCM

TCM recognized the effects of stroke and categorized the symptoms over 2000 years ago (Table 6.3). Before the Tang and Song dynasties, the pathomechanism of stroke was seen as the result of some internal deficiency followed by a Pathogenic attack. Later the condition was considered to be primarily a result of internal Wind. Contemporary Chinese TCM doctors now view this disease as deficiency of upright Qi leading to an internal stirring of Liver Wind. Onset is also related to disorders involving the Yin and Yang of the Heart and Liver, Spleen and Kidney, in their Zang Fu sense.

The risk factors of diet, obesity, high blood pressure and a sedentary occupation have been acknowledged in the sizeable literature dealing with stroke treatment using both herbs and acupuncture [73–75]. The very fact that this type of treatment has been reported as clinically successful for so long underlines the need for more rigorous research in this field.

TCM treatment depends on the perceived cause of the stroke. A lot of treatment may be undertaken to prevent stroke ever happening, with the deficiency of Yin in both Liver and Kidney being tackled along with support for the Spleen and advice on diet and lifestyle.

Physiotherapists are rarely in a position to prevent this kind of neurological catastrophe but are very much concerned with the treatment and rehabilitation of the patient after it has occurred. The consensus of opinion in TCM terms seems to be that an energetic policy, stimulating the points of the Yang meridians, is most successful. The aim is to move the stagnation of Qi and Blood. Electroacupuncture is often added, as is scalp acupuncture. It is useful to stimulate both Spleen and Stomach in order to aid and regulate digestion and points for Kidney and Liver are sometimes added to prevent recurrence.

Table 6.3 Traditional Chinese medicine (TCM) effects of stroke

Structures affected in TCM terms

Collaterals	Channels	Yang organs	Yin organs	Sequelae
External Wind	Internal Wind	Internal Wind	Internal Wind	Qi Xu
Weak Wei Qi	Liver and Kidney Yin deficiency			Blood stasis
Numbness in extremities, minimal motor impairment Mild facial paralysis	Hemiplegia Facial paralysis Stiff tongue	Coma Hemiplegia Constipation Retention of urine	Coma Hemiplegia Cold limbs Double incontinence	Conscious Hemiplegia/hemiparesis Facial paralysis Speech problems

Simple acupuncture formula for windstroke sequelae

Upper-limb points

GB 20 Fengchi, LI 15 Jianyu, LI 11 Quchi, LI 10 Shousanli, LI 4 Hegu, TE 5 Waiguan.

Lower-limb points

GB 31 Fengshi, ST 31 Biguan, ST 36 Zusanli, SP 10 Xuehai, GB 39 Xuanzhong, GB 43 Xiaxi, LR 3 Taichong.

The resulting paralysis may not affect both limbs, so the points used to free the channels should only be used where necessary. The points selected to support the major Zang Fu organs should be used in all cases.

Some authorities recommend the use of points on the unaffected limb, some use them bilaterally but there seems to be no clear guide as to which is better. From the point of view of a stimulus to the nervous system to prevent stroke-side neglect, it seems logical to treat only the affected side. It also seems logical to add electroacupuncture using a current of 2 Hz in order to produce a muscle twitch. However bilateral treatment makes sense too; stimulation of both dorsal horns will maximize the effect. TCM sometimes advises starting with the unaffected side and progressing to both sides [76].

The TCM approach to the physical sequelae of stroke is to mobilize the Qi in the affected limbs but in modern texts the selection of points, although still based on syndrome differentiation, follows a more segmental pattern, recognizable to Western medical acupuncture practitioners.

The TCM differentiation of stroke offers four patterns, similar to those in the West:

1. a mild stroke involving only the superficial channels and collaterals (Zhong Luo)
2. a more serious incident involving the channels themselves and resulting in recognizable hemiplegia (Zhong Jing)
3. stroke involving the bowels or 'tense' stroke (Zhong Fu). The patient loses consciousness and on regaining it may show hemiplegia and changes in continence or constipation
4. a severe form of stroke is that involving the viscera (Zhong Zang), where the patient is unconscious and comatose with open mouth, and loose lips failing to contain the saliva.

It is the Zhong Jing type that is most likely to be treated by physiotherapists and, if the Zhong Fu and Zhong Zang survive they will show the same one-sided paralysis of the limbs and sometimes the face [77].

The fundamental causative factors are thought to be linked to the Wei and Feng syndromes (see Chapter 1).

Syndromes identified in stroke

As with most neurological conditions the state or balance of all the body system is seen to be disturbed and the following syndromes are often found within the umbrella classification of 'poststroke'. Table 6.4 offers collections of acupoints which can be used if the symptoms fit.

The energy that is present in the body is all that is available so this treatment can sometimes be very slow and should not be undertaken if the patient is very weak or if the results of the brain lesion are severe.

Table 6.4 Common syndromes in stroke

Syndrome	Main points	Comments
Attack on the channels with external Pathogens still retained in the body	LI 4 Hegu TE 5 Waiguan ST 8 Touwei GB 20 Fengchi	Early treatment, first 10 days only
Deficiency of Yin with an excess of Yang, Liver/GallBladder fire flaring upward	GV 20 Baihui LR 3 Taichong GB 43 Xiaxi KI 3 Taixi	Cooling points
Liver/Kidney Yin Xu together with generalized Yin and Yang Xu	BL 23 Shenshu KI 3 Taixi GV 4 Mingmen SP 6 Sanyinjiao	Supporting Kidney energy
Spleen/Kidney Yang Xu with Phlegm and stasis in the channels	CV 12 Zhongwan ST 40 Fenglong ST 36 Zusanli SP 6 Sanyinjiao	Kid 3 could be added
Qi and Blood Xu with malnourishment of the sinews and vessels	ST 36 Zusanli SP 6 Sanyinjiao GB 34 Yanglingquan BL 20 Pishu	Plus local points where weakness is marked
Underlying Blood stasis	LR 2 Xingjian LR 3 Taichong SP 6 Sanyinjiao SP 6 Diji LU 1 Zhongfu LU 11 Shaoshang PE 6 and UB 60	More general, powerful moving points

Acupuncture is rarely used in isolation in TCM. Specific Chinese herbal medicine will also be prescribed to invigorate blood and transform stasis. Table 6.5 offers a more eclectic selection of points, mostly chosen on the basis of myotomes and muscle innervation or useful Yang meridians.

Summary

Stroke is a major health problem in the UK and treatment and rehabilitation of stroke patients are considerable expenses to the NHS. Modern diagnostic techniques make it possible to identify which areas of the brain are damaged. However, at present there are no completely effective treatments available in the acute phase and very few therapies that have been proven to change the rate of improvement after the initial swelling in the brain tissue has resolved.

A form of therapy which could decrease the resulting disabilities is certainly worth investigating. Physiotherapists, as part of the rehabilitation team, are able to use acupuncture at appropriate times in the process but should also be able to refer to specialist clinics outside the NHS if more long-term treatment is required.

Relatively weak but cumulative evidence from the recent research literature indicates that investigation of the effect of acupuncture on both motor power and spasticity is not yet complete [56, 61, 64, 78–80]. Although the evidence for acupuncture in acute stroke remains equivocal, the borderline trends

Table 6.5 Acupuncture points used in stroke

Problem	Acupoints	Comments
Paralysis of the extensor groups of the Upper Limb (Yang aspect)	GB 21 Jianjing LI 15 Jianyu LI 11 Quchi TE 5 Waiguan Baxie (Extras) GB 10 Fubai	Chinese texts also suggest LI 17 Tianding but this is awkward to needle and most relevant with loss of voice
Paralysis of the flexor groups of the Upper Limb (Yin aspect)	LU 10 Yuji PE 8 Laogong HR 8 Shaofu Baxie (Extras)	PE 8 is not easy to needle, but suggested for 'trembling' of the hand Although not strictly Yin in aspect, the Baxie points are useful in hemiplegia
Paralysis of the Lower Limb (Yang aspect)	GB 30 Huantiao ST 31 Biguan GB 34 Yanglingquan BL 36 Chengfu Bafeng (Extras)	GB 31 also useful
Paralysis of the Lower Limb (Yin aspect)	SP 10 Xuehai SP 6 Sanyinjiao LR 2 Xingjian KI 3 Taixi Bafeng (Extras)	SP 9 if oedema present
Shoulder pain	Eyes of the Shoulder SI 11 Tianzhong LI 11 Quchi SJ 9 Sidu Baxie (Extras)	Support subluxation
Facial paralysis, deviation of the mouth	Qianzheng (Extra) ST 2 Sibai ST 4 Dicang CV 24 Chengjiang	Also used in Bell's palsy
Deviation of the tongue and aphasia	Ear Shenmen CV 24 Chengjiang GV 15 Yamen	Speech generally HT 5 Tongli
General trunk weakness and asymmetry	GB 20 Fengchi Bailao (Extra) BL 23 Shenshu BL 25 Dachangshu	Could also open Du meridian with SI3 Houxi and BL 62 Shenmai
Internal problems including loss of appetite, constipation difficulties with urination	CV 12 Zhongwan CV 4 Guanyuan ST 25 Tianshu ST 36 Zusanli	Sp 6 Sanyinjiao also helpful
To eliminate pathogenic Wind	GB 20 Fengchi TE 17 Yifeng GB 12 Wangu	GV 20 Baihui and GV 16 Fengfu may also be used

in the Cochrane review [81] indicate further work on two aspects, motor recovery and overall morbidity, with perhaps more accurate distinction between haemorrhagic and non-haemorrhagic stroke.

Since stroke is the most common cause of neurological damage affecting the elderly we should consider any modality that may help with the rehabilitation process. Patients may receive 2–3 months of physiotherapy after which they will be managing their own recovery. Lack of additional formal therapy has the potential to slow rehabilitation especially in the presence of substantial muscle weakness, atrophy, spasticity and reduced physical fitness. This may further lead to decreased activity impacting on independence and quality of life, thus becoming a major socioeconomic problem.

Case studies

Case study 6.1: level 1 case study

A 52-year-old male had a stroke 8 weeks previously. He was left with mild right-sided weakness with the leg worse than the arm. He complained of sensory changes in the arm, feeling 'heavy' with pain around the shoulder. There was no loss of range of movement in the arm but the patient was very anxious about what he perceived as a lack of dexterity and the change in sensation.

Initially the visual analogue scale (VAS) was measured for feeling of 'heaviness' 8/10 and the outcome measure Nine-Hole Peg Test was also used (for finger dexterity); time taken was 49 seconds.

Treatment

Treatment lasted only 10 minutes and only LI 15 and TE 14 (Eyes of the Shoulder) were needled to address general shoulder pain on the first occasion. Deqi achieved without manipulating needles.

Once the patient was used to the feeling of the needles, the 'Four Gates' (LI 4 and LR 3 bilaterally) were added for relaxation and global pain. Then, progressively, the following points were added over the first three treatments:

- LI 14 Binao for neuralgia and paresis of the upper extremity
- LI 10 Shousanli and LI 11 Quchi for motor impairments and pain in the upper limb
- GB 21 Jianjing for pain in the shoulder girdle and referred pain into the arm

- Yintang for relaxation and calming the mind
- Baxie points for changes in superficial sensation.

The sessions were gradually increased in length to 30 minutes and 12 treatments were given in total over a period of 4 weeks. Manipulation of needles was used to achieve Deqi if possible.

Results

The acupuncture treatment regime had a very positive effect on this patient. His VAS for the 'heaviness' he felt went from 8/10 to 3/10. The time taken to perform the Nine-Hole Peg Test improved from 49 to 23 seconds.

Part of this improvement could be attributed to natural recovery and the desensitization work carried out in additional physiotherapy sessions and in the patient's own time, but both the patient and the therapist felt that the acupuncture had a definite beneficial effect on his arm sensation and this directly improved his dexterity.

Case study 6.2: level 2 case study

The patient was a 59-year-old woman with a left CVA thrombosis 5 years previously. She had been discharged after a period of inpatient rehabilitation.

Main complaint

There was no hand activity present. The patient was being taught weight transfer techniques. Previous treatment during the year after the stroke by a professional acupuncturist was unsuccessful. Now she was being treated by the community physiotherapist every 2 weeks, working on increased central control and mobilizing the right hand and forearm.

Aim of physiotherapy

The aim of physiotherapy was to decrease high tone in pronators and flexors and increase potential extensor ability. Acupuncture was introduced twice weekly to attempt this.

Acupuncture treatment

Points: first treatment: LI 11, LI 10, LI 4 and Baxie 15 minutes. Deqi was felt at all points.

Passive/active activity with supination, pronation and wrist and finger extensors was carried out. Nine further treatments followed and the points were not changed.

Results

After the first session there was a flicker of activity with facilitation in wrist extensors. Nothing was noted in the fingers. Some activity was seen in triceps with shoulder protraction. Subjectively, the patient reported a 'buzzing' feeling in her arm for 2 hours afterwards and the friend who carried out the daily stretching exercises said it was looser the following morning.

The patient continued to get a strong 'buzzing' response afterwards. The physiotherapist reported more potential for movement but no functional changes and further commented, 'The improvements noted: right scapular stabilization, some mid-range shoulder medial and lateral rotation, mid-range elbow extension, supination and pronation, wrist extension and flickers of finger extension were remarkable as they had not been observed in the 4 years since her stroke despite continuous good-quality neurophysiotherapy input.'

Case study 6.3: level 3 case study

A 62-year-old French-speaking male was admitted via A&E after collapsing and losing consciousness at home. He was doubly incontinent at the time of collapse and had subsequent left-sided weakness on gaining consciousness. Since his admission he reported blurred vision, dizziness with nausea, severe headache, fatigue, reduced sensation on the left side but high levels of perceived pain throughout the left side. He quickly regained full continence. CT scan confirmed right-sided LACI and evidence of small-vessel disease.

Prior to his admission, he had been fully independent. He had just arrived in the UK from abroad the day before his collapse. Whilst abroad, he had been subjected to a 6-month period of significant physical abuse whilst in a political prison. Although he reported not having any lasting significant physical injuries as a result of this, he described feeling traumatized by it. He had some history of hypertension which was well controlled since his admission. He was a controlled diabetic, had persistent sinusitis for which he was under the care of the Ear, Nose and Throat team, and was diagnosed with hepatitis C since his admission.

At the time of assessment he described generalized, constant pain on the left side of his body with a VAS of 9/10. This pain was unchanging irrespective of position or time of day. He also described experiencing 'intense burning'-type sensations, different to his constant pain, when touched on that side. This was considered to be allodynia since it was elicited by a normally non-painful stimulus. He was unable actively to move the left side due to pain. His other predominant symptom was constant dizziness and nausea (vertigo), worsened by all head movements and change of position. He was sitting out of bed daily and transferring through standing with the assistance of two people. He was only tolerating standing with the support of one person for a few minutes at a time and was refraining from weight-bearing through his left side due to pain.

Treatment

Acupuncture was suggested as his pain and vertigo were preventing him from attending other therapy sessions (Table 6.6).

Comment

Nociceptive pain is always located in the periphery, i.e. in the nociceptors; neuropathic pain may be peripheral (involving the peripheral nervous system) or central (involving the central nervous system, as in stroke).

Pain is another common symptom following stroke, and can be either central or peripheral in origin. Peripheral nociceptive pain is caused by the stimulation of body nociceptors. Often it can be attributed to postural dysfunction exacerbated by limited mobility often following stroke, or the disrupted biomechanical alignment of joints due to the weak and/or altered tonicity of the affected muscles. Poststroke shoulder pain associated with subluxation of the joint has been reported as one of the most common sources of pain, occurring in up to 80% of survivors.

Centrally generated or central neuropathic pain results from damage to the central nervous system. Central poststroke pain (CPSP) is estimated to occur in up to 8% of patients following a stroke and can begin up to a month after the event [82]. It is thought that damage to the spinothalamic pathways is responsible for this pain. The most common treatment for CPSP is the use of amitriptyline, which is also commonly used as an antidepressant. This was prescribed early on in the patient's management. However, it seemed to be of no benefit. Gabapentin, another neuropathic painkiller, was subsequently prescribed but made the patient very drowsy and he chose to cease taking it.

Table 6.6 Summary of acupuncture treatment in level 3 case study

Day	Pretreatment	Treatment	Posttreatment
1	Vertigo+++, unable to move head Pain, generalized left side, VAS 9/10	Right HT 7, PE 6, LI 11, LR 3 25 minutes	Less vertigo – able to extend neck with minimal symptoms
2	Vertigo returned on rising this morning Pain ISQ	As above and LI 4 30 minutes	Reduced vertigo – as yesterday
3	Much less vertigo, no symptoms from LTS, some on head movement	As day 2 and Sp 6 30 minutes	No vertigo
4	No vertigo Slight decrease in pain 9/10 Decreased allodynia, tolerating light touch upper limb	Bilateral LI 4 and LR 3 – Four Gates 30 minutes	Decreased pain 8/10 AROM right GH flexion 45°
7	Mild vertigo returned last night Less generalized pain	Four Gates and right HT 7 30 minutes	Vertigo gone Pain only in joints
8	Mild vertigo Pain IM, VAS 7/10	Four Gates and bilateral PE 6 30 minutes	Vertigo gone, full neck ROM
9	No vertigo Moving arm, pain 5–6/10 and IM Tolerating firm touch	As day 8	AA ROM 160° Pain 5/10
14	Pain 5/10, joints only UL and LL Constipated for 2 days	Four Gates and TE 5 30 minutes	UL power grade 4/5 LL power 3/5 Pain 5/10
15	Full AROM UL with minimal pain 2/10 LL pain persists, including with WB 5–8/10	Four Gates and bilateral St 36 30 minutes	Independent STS Mobile 5 metres with ZF LL pain 5/10
16	Pain LL 5/10, PNs on WB UL joint pain 4/10	Left LR 3, LR 7, SP 6, LI 4 and LI 11 30 minutes	Pain UL and LL 3/10 PNs persist
17	Mobile 10 metres with ZF Pain 3/10	As day 16	ISQ
28	Independently mobile, no aid UL joint pain 3/10 GH stiffness, AROM 150° LL pain 1/10 and mild PNs on WB	LI 4, LI 11, LI 14, LI 15, TE 14 and ST 38 30 minutes	UL pain 1/10 Full GH movement
29	UL joint pain 3/10 GH AROM 170°	As day 28	UL and LL pain 1/10 Strength UL and LL Grade 4+/5 Discharged home

VAS, Visual Analogue Scale; ISQ, in status quo; LTS, lying to sitting; AROM, active range of movement; GH, glenohumeral; IM, intermittent; AA, active assisted; ROM, range of movement; UL, upper limb; LL, lower limb; WB, weight-bearing; STS, sit to stand; ZF, zimmer frame; PNs, pins and needles

Rationale for treatment

The decision to try acupuncture for this patient was mainly driven by the fact that he was not able to comply with his rehabilitation sessions with either physiotherapy or occupational therapy, nor had he responded to the prescribed analgesia. He was becoming despondent and frustrated with his limitations. The clinical presentation of his painful symptoms associated with weakness and sensory disturbance associated with the stroke meets the diagnostic criteria of CPSP.

Initial treatment was administered to his non-stroke side due to the allodynic symptoms he was experiencing on the left. It was hoped to impact the pain of the other side via diffuse noxious inhibitory control, stimulation of the descending inhibition pathways and deactivation of the limbic system. LI 4, which is considered the most powerful analgesic point, was not chosen initially for precisely this reason. If he proved to be a strong responder, the experience might have been too overwhelming. LI 11 was chosen initially as it is indicated in the treatment of pain and hemiplegia of the arm, and is considered a tonification point. LR 3 and especially PE 6 were predominantly chosen for their indication in cases of dizziness and nausea, with SP 6 added on day 3 to accentuate this effect. As well as HT 7, both LR 3 and PE 6 are also useful in calming the mind. The addition of LI 4 was indicated on the second session as the patient had experienced no adverse effects from the first treatment. He was also suffering from nasal congestion, for which LI 4 can also be effective.

The patient was very pleased with the results of his first three sessions, with significant improvement in his vertiginous symptoms and reduced allodynia, allowing him to move more freely. His generalized pain however remained essentially unchanged so direct treatment to the left side was deemed appropriate to include. Siguan; the 'Four Gates' were chosen as this is thought to be useful in the treatment of more global pain. HT 7 and PE 6 were added to this combination on separate occasions to try to eradicate the vertigo which was now intermittent, yet mild. TE 5 was combined with the 'Four Gates' due to onset of constipation, but then replaced with ST 36. This point is a homeostatic point, restoring balance to the system, and is implicated in sinusitic Phlegm stagnation. ST 36 is also a useful point for lower-limb pain, which was now more dominant than the upper limb.

Treatment progressed well, with elimination of the vertigo, improved allodynia allowing firm touch, much-reduced upper-limb pain limited to the joints, moderately reduced lower-limb pain and improved range of movement and strength in both limbs. All of these contributed towards markedly improved function, allowing him to mobilize short distances with a walking frame and participate in his therapy sessions. Focus was then changed to treat only the left side at days 16 and 17, after which he was given a 10-day break from acupuncture treatment to focus on his mobility and functional therapies. In this time, he gained independence in his mobility unaided and his leg pain improved. However, some pain persisted in the shoulder with some self-reported stiffness and reduced range of motion. He was treated on two consecutive days with the 'Eyes of the Shoulder' (LI 15 and TE 14), LI 11, LI 4 and ST 38. ST 38 is commonly used to release shoulder stiffness. The following day he was discharged from hospital with full mobility, full active range of motion in the arm and leg, and with only mild strength impairment. He was still aware of some mild pain, rated as 1/10 on VAS, but his allodynia was mostly gone. Pins and needles on the sole of his left foot were still experienced on weight-bearing. Unfortunately we have not been able to follow this patient up after discharge.

It is interesting that, throughout acupuncture treatment, this patient often felt the scratch of the needle penetrating the skin, but described none of the sensations associated with Deqi after insertion. These include numbness, heaviness, aching or tingling. Some authors have suggested that the perception of Deqi is necessary for acupuncture to be effective and that the lack of this feeling in acupuncture might negate its effects. The sensations associated with Deqi are thought to be transmitted via the type II and III muscle afferents via the spinothalamic tract. Damage to the spinothalamic tract is implicated in the pathophysiology of CPSP and this might explain the lack of Deqi felt by this patient.

Conclusion

Although CPSP is one of the less common sequelae of stroke, it can be incredibly debilitating for those who experience it and is notoriously difficult to manage. Pharmaceutical management is often inadequate and can be associated with unpleasant side-effects. The outcome of this case study supports that of Yen and Chen [83], that the use of acupuncture alongside standard Western rehabilitation can be effective in the management of CPSP. Further investigation into the use of acupuncture for the management of this kind of neuropathic pain would be of great interest.

Part 2: Cerebral palsy

Introduction

Cerebral palsy is included in this section of the book because it is an acquired brain injury, although in most cases this injury occurs before or during birth.

The condition is caused by abnormalities in the parts of the brain that control muscle movements. This means that, while cerebral palsy seriously affects movement and posture, it often does not become apparent until the child reaches an age where independent movement is the norm. The majority of children with cerebral palsy are born with it, although it may not be detected for several years. A minority of children may have cerebral palsy as a result of brain damage in the first few months or years of life. Causes can be as varied as bacterial meningitis, viral encephalitis, head injury from child abuse or a road traffic accident.

Symptoms

The most common signs are difficulty when performing voluntary movements, a lack of muscle coordination, which may result from ataxia or athetosis, spasticity and exaggerated reflexes causing stiff or tight muscles or, conversely, muscle tone that is too floppy. An unusual walking pattern, walking on the toes or tending to crouch or with one foot or leg dragging is often an early sign. Speech problems may be apparent, often as a result of muscle weakness affecting respiratory control or laryngeal and soft-palate function. The articulation of the jaw may also be affected. The seriousness of this problem depends on the general degree of muscle weakness. Other communication disorders (e.g. hearing loss, language delay or disorder) may also be associated with cerebral palsy.

Prognosis

Cerebral palsy does not always cause profound disabilities. While one child with severe cerebral palsy might be unable to achieve independent mobility and need extensive, lifelong care, another with mild cerebral palsy might be only slightly awkward and require no special assistance. Supportive treatments, medications and surgery can help many individuals improve their motor skills and ability to communicate with the world.

Treatment

It is not possible to cure cerebral palsy, but treatment will often improve a child's capabilities. Many children go on to enjoy near-normal adult lives if their disabilities are properly managed. In general, the earlier treatment begins, the better chance children have of overcoming developmental disabilities or learning new ways to accomplish the tasks that challenge them. Treatment may include physical and occupational therapy, speech therapy, drugs to control seizures, relax muscle spasms and alleviate pain; surgery to correct anatomical abnormalities or release tight muscles; braces and other orthotic devices; wheelchairs and rolling walkers; and communication aids such as computers with attached voice synthesizers.

Cerebral palsy and physiotherapy

A physiotherapist will concentrate on improving the development of the large muscles of the body, in the arms, legs and abdomen, and those concerned with posture and locomotion, the gross motor skills. Children are taught better ways to move and balance. Help will be given with the use of wheelchairs, independent standing and the safe use of stairs. Work is also done on the fun skills such as running, kicking and throwing or learning to ride a bike. Therapy usually begins in the first few years of life or soon after the diagnosis is made, and may continue for many years.

In the UK physiotherapy is likely to include Bobath techniques for correcting posture and guiding functional movement. The aim is to help children change the abnormal posture that they are forced into by weakened or shortened muscles. Therapists can help parents to understand their child's needs. Parents are shown the most appropriate ways of positioning in order to help their child to move and how to incorporate these into the child's daily life.

The Voita method is also used to a certain extent. This aims to release inner, innate movement reflexes by constant repetition.

Children with cerebral palsy also grow and develop, but their patterns of growth and development are delayed or arrested at a certain stage. The brain controls all movements, so that when some part of the brain is damaged, as in cerebral palsy, the control is disordered, resulting in movement problems. Each case is different and each child has to be treated according to individual need. One child may be able to move his lower limbs more easily than his upper limbs, or the other way round. This will interfere with his development. Sometimes many stages of movement development are missing altogether. If, for example, a child cannot lie on her tummy, lift her head up or support herself with her arms she will not learn to use the muscles of her neck and her back which she needs for sitting up straight or standing up. This may also interfere with the control of breathing and speech.

Physiotherapists use specific sets of exercises to work toward the prevention of musculoskeletal complications. An example of this is preventing the weakening or deterioration of muscles that can result from lack of use. Also, physiotherapy can help avoid contractures, in which muscles become fixed in a rigid, abnormal position. The focus of treatment is on enabling the child to grow and develop as normally as possible, ideally in mainstream education.

Acupuncture

The focus of acupuncture treatment will be very similar to that for stroke.

The emphasis lies mainly on the use of Yang meridians, as in the sequelae of stroke. Body points such as LI 4, LI 11, GB 34, GB 39, SP 6, TE 5 and PE 6 to open the channels, and scalp acupuncture for the upper- and lower-limb motor regions can also be used.

There has been some useful Chinese research in this field but much of it has failed to spark enthusiasm in the West due to a large number of the available trials being uncontrolled. Imposing a controlled protocol and an inert placebo intervention on a child could be seen as unethical in China, or indeed anywhere, so better protocols are needed. The following are good examples of the work undertaken but lacking rigorous controls or outcome measures.

Researchers at the Children's Hospital, Zhejiang Medical University, in China spent over a year researching the effects of acupuncture and acupressure treatment on children suffering from infantile cerebral palsy. Seventy-five children took part in the study which involved comprehensive meridian therapy, including scalp and body acupuncture supplemented with acupressure and massage. The number of treatments each child received ranged from a minimum of 10 to a maximum of 120, the exact number being assessed according to the child's needs.

The effect of the treatment was measured by evaluating the children's performance of physical exercise, social adaptability and their intelligence quotient (IQ) both before and after the treatment period. The results revealed 'a very positive improvement in the children's physical capability and an increase of their intelligence' [84].

A clinical study of acupuncture looking at both the Bobath approach, commonly used by physiotherapists, and acupuncture was undertaken in 2005 [85]. This involved the treatment of 90 cases of spasmodic cerebral palsy patients aged from 1 to 10 years. The patients were randomly divided into three groups, with 30 members in each group: group A (acupuncture group), group B (rehabilitation training group) and group C (acupuncture and rehabilitation training group).

Group A was treated by both scalp and body acupuncture; group B received physical therapy following the Bobath and Voita methods; and group C was treated by acupuncture and received physical therapy at the same time. All three groups took 90 days as one course of treatment. The results showed that the total effective rate of groups A and C were significantly higher than group B; the developmental quotient of both groups A and C were higher than that of group B after treatment. It appears that acupuncture can add something to the quality of life of cerebral palsy patients.

In a similar study, again with a mixture of exercise, Bobath techniques and acupuncture, Mu et al. [86] suggest that the combination of techniques can be effective. More recently a single case study [87] seemed to indicate that in the child studied a simple acupuncture intervention, regular needling of GB 34 and St 36, resulted in temporary cessation of involuntary extension contractions of the erector spinae muscle. This was not maintained between treatments. Although of limited value evidentially this case indicates that there may be a response worth full investigation in the future.

Acupressure as a single intervention has been recommended for cerebral palsy but this has little evidence base and seems to need to be undertaken regularly over a very long period [87]. Many of the acupressure points offered as useful for general mobilization of the soft tissues in cerebral palsy patients correspond clearly with trigger points known to Western medical acupuncture [88]. A form of light massage given regularly to areas of muscle with perceived physiological changes can be helpful in decreasing muscle tone; this type of massage is sometimes termed Tuina.

Successful and early prevention and/or control of contracture may prevent the need for later corrective surgery, so this often takes precedence in any physiotherapy programme. It is important to work with both the parents and the school to maximize the independence of the child and when the neurophysiology of acupuncture is better understood we may find it has a useful place in the treatment regime. At present it seems to do no harm.

Case study 6.4: level 1 case study: back pain and abnormal posture

A 54-year-old woman presented with chronic low-back pain of 7/10, radiating down the lateral aspect of her right leg as far as the knee. She reported long-standing abnormal standing posture and movement difficulties when walking secondary to cerebral palsy. She complained of poor-quality sleep which was disturbed by involuntary 'jumping' of her legs. She was independent in daily activities.

Treatment

This patient was referred for physiotherapy to address her posture and movement difficulties as well as her back pain. Following detailed assessment it was clear that the patient needed to complete a range of activities to improve activation of core stability muscles, to improve strength and endurance of abdominal muscles and to mobilize the lumbar spine. However the presence of pain meant

that completing these activities was impossible. Therefore acupuncture was used to reduce pain to allow subsequent muscle re-education.

Pain was localized to particular points, and palpation reproduced the patient's pain. Points which were tender on palpation were needled. This included BL 27 bilaterally as well as BL 54, GB 30, GB 31 and GB 34 on the right side. The patient responded strongly during treatment and during these early sessions some needles had to be removed after a few minutes due to localized pain, for example, GB 34. Gradually the points became less tender and other points were palpated and selected. General points for pain relief were also chosen. Points needled included extra point Shiqizhuixia (M-BW-25), LR 3, BL 60, Yintang, GV 4 and GV 20. A course of 10 acupuncture treatments was provided over a period of 6 weeks. Needles were stimulated initially for Deqi and then every 10 minutes during the 30-minute treatment.

Outcome

At the end of individual treatment sessions the patient appeared calm and less anxious. By the end of the course of treatment the back and leg pain had reduced to 0/10 and there was a marked improvement in her posture and functional ability. The patient was able to stand with a more upright posture and was able to walk greater distances. Both the patient and the physiotherapist were surprised and delighted by the degree of improvement, especially in view of the long-standing nature of the condition. In addition the patient reported a range of general benefits, including a reduction of involuntary movements of the legs, improved sleep quality, improved mood, reduced anxiety, improved self-confidence and an overall sense of enhanced well-being.

Part 3: Traumatic brain injury

Introduction

Traumatic brain injury is a form of acquired brain injury resulting from sudden trauma to the brain. This injury is commonly caused by road traffic accidents, but may also result from falls, assault, gunshot wounds and sporting injuries [89]. The brain may be damaged by accelerating, decelerating and impacting on the inside of the skull leading to bleeding, bruising and damage to nerve cells and fibres. The skull may remain intact or may be fractured [90]. Traumatic brain injury is a leading cause of death and disability worldwide, causing up to 1.5 million deaths annually. It causes severe disability for 150–200 people per million each year and is the leading cause of disability for those aged under 40 years [91]. Injuries are more common in people aged 15–24 or over 75 years [92].

Symptoms

Presenting symptoms depend upon the initial severity of injury but may include motor difficulties including paralysis, spasticity and ataxia, visual difficulties, sensory impairment, aphasia as well as difficulties with attention, perception, memory, problem-solving and judgement. Mood swings, irritability and aggression, disinhibited sexual behaviour, poor initiation and apathy may also be evident. Recognised sequelae of traumatic brain injury include the development of seizures, chronic pain, particularly headache, and disturbed function of the hypothalamopituitary axis.

Prognosis

Outcome following traumatic brain injury depends on the severity of initial damage. Improvement in acute management means that some of those with severe injuries will now survive. These individuals are likely to develop substantial disability and require long-term support. Those with less severe injuries may be left with minor or moderate residual symptoms. However some of those with apparently minor injuries may experience long-lasting difficulties which have a substantial impact on their functional ability and participation within the wider community [92].

Treatment

Initial treatment focuses on saving life and minimizing further damage to the brain. Many patients will require artificial ventilation to ensure adequate oxygenation of the brain. Other injuries, such as fractures and soft-tissue injuries, will be assessed and managed appropriately. Particular care will be taken to screen for spinal fractures. Neurosurgical

intervention may be required to evacuate significant haematomas or to remove any debris resulting from penetrating injuries to the skull. After the acute phase, treatment will aim to improve the functional ability of the patient and support the patient and family to adjust to any residual difficulties. Input will be provided by a multidisciplinary team.

Traumatic brain injury and physiotherapy

Physiotherapy will begin in the acute stage and involve respiratory care. Management of the musculoskeletal system will begin from the acute stage and continue throughout the rehabilitation process. Interventions will aim to maintain range of movement, promote motor control and balance as well as to restore functional abilities. The physiotherapist will work closely alongside other members of the specialist neurorehabilitation team as well as actively involving the patient's family.

Traumatic brain injury and acupuncture

The focus of acupuncture shares similarities with the approach to stroke and includes the use of Yang meridians in the upper and lower limbs. However, the sudden and traumatic onset of injury may result in areas of local Qi or Blood stagnation as well as the effect of shock on the Heart and Kidney, causing depletion [75]. Common TCM patterns noted in traumatic brain injury include blood stasis, hyperactivity of Liver Yang, obstruction of Phlegm, deficiency of Kidney Essence and deficiency of Qi and Blood [93].

Very little research has been conducted in this condition. A Chinese study by He et al. [94] reported the use of acupuncture in 30 cases of post-traumatic coma. Patients in the treatment group (n = 15) received acupuncture and point injection in addition to standard care. This study reported that patients in the acupuncture group showed 'obvious' improvement in symptoms such as aphasia, hemiplegia, facial weakness and eye movement in comparison to the control group. These are interesting results but studies with more rigorous design and outcome measurements are required. A number of case reports have noted benefits from acupuncture in traumatic brain injury. Chen used needling of Shendao (GV 11) complemented by Guanyuan (CV 4) to improve circulation through the Governor and Conception Vessels [93]. He reported greater benefits from this option for relief of spasticity than from body, scalp or ear acupuncture. Donnellan reported benefits from body acupuncture for the relief of central neuropathic pain and mood disturbance in a patient with severe traumatic brain injury and multiple fractures [95].

Case study 6.5: level 1 case study

A 58-year-old man presented with left upper-limb pain and sensory disturbance following traumatic brain injury 2 months previously. The pain was disturbing him throughout the day and affecting his participation in therapy sessions. He reported anxieties about the future, including whether he would be able to return to work. Examination indicated central neuropathic pain with extreme sensitivity and agitation in response to touch of his arm. Pain numerical rating scale = 9/10. He had mild weakness in the arm but function was limited by pain and sensory impairment rather than motor ability. He was able to walk but required supervision for safety.

Treatment

In the first few treatments, points throughout the left upper limb were needled, including TE 14, LI 15 and LI 10 as well as the use of LI 4 bilaterally for its generalized effect on pain. In sessions 3 and 4 lower-limb points were used, including GB 34 for its generalized effect on sinews and joints and GB 39 for its influence on 'the Marrow'. The patient received a total of nine treatments over a period of 4 weeks.

Treatments lasted 25 minutes initially but were increased to 40 minutes. Needles were stimulated initially for Deqi but received no further stimulation.

Results

Acupuncture resulted in substantial benefits for this patient. The degree of pain and distress had prevented his participation in rehabilitation at a relatively early stage of his recovery. Pain medications had provided limited effect on the pain. The provision of acupuncture resulted in a reduction of pain to 4/10 on numerical rating scale and a general calming effect on the patient. Subsequently he was able to participate fully in his physiotherapy and occupational therapy sessions.

References

[1] World Health Organization WHO. Cerebrovascular Disorders. Geneva: Offset publications; 1978.

[2] Peterson S, Peto V, Scarborough P, et al. Coronary Heart Disease Statistics. London: British Heart Foundation; 2005.

[3] Adamson J, Beswick A, Ebrahim S. Is stroke the most common cause of disability? J Stroke Cerebrovasc Dis 2004;13(4):171–7.

[4] National Audit Office U. Reducing brain damage: faster access to better stroke care. London: The Stationery Office; 2005.

[5] Goldacre MJ, Duncan M, Griffith M, et al. Mortality rates for stroke in England from 1979 to 2004: trends, diagnostic precision, and artifacts. Stroke 2008;39 (8):2197–203.

[6] Ebrahim S, Harwood R. Stroke: Epidemiology, evidence and clinical practice. 2nd ed Oxford: Oxford University Press; 1999.

[7] Wannamethee SG, Shaper AG, Ebrahim S. History of parental death from stroke or heart trouble and the risk of stroke in middle-aged men. Stroke 1996;27:1492–8.

[8] Wade DT. Stroke (acute cerebrovascular disease). In: Stevens ARJ, editor. Health care needs assessment: the epidemiologically based needs assessment reviews. Oxford: Radcliffe Medical Press; 1994. p. 111–255.

[9] Legh-Smith J, Wade DT, Langton-Hewer R. Services for stroke patients one year after stroke. J Epidemiol Community Health 1986;40:161–5.

[10] Burn J, Dennis M, Bamford J. Long-term risk of recurrent sstroke after a first- ever stroke. Stroke 1994;25:333–7.

[11] Wade DT, Langton Hewer R. Epidemiology of some neurological diseases with special reference to work load on the NHS. Int Rehabil Med 1987;8(3):129–37.

[12] Department of Health. Saving Lives: Our Healthier Nation. London: Stationery Office; 1999.

[13] Balarajan R. Ethnic differences in mortality from ischaemic heart disease and cerebrovascular disease in England and Wales. BMJ 1991;302:560–4.

[14] Juvela S, Hillbom M, Palomaki H. Risk factors for spontaneous intracerebral haemorrhage. Stroke 1995;26:1558–64.

[15] Robbins AS, Manson JE, Lee IM, et al. Cigarette smoking and stroke in a cohort of US male physicians. Ann Intern Med 1994;120:458–62.

[16] Gill JS, Zezulka AV, Shipley MJ, et al. Stroke and alcohol consumption. N Engl J Med. 1986;315:1041–6.

[17] Christie D. Stroke in Melbourne, Australia: an epidemiological study. Stroke 1981;12:467.

[18] Bulpitt CJ. Vitamin C and vascular disease. Br Med J 1995;310:1548–9.

[19] Kirshner HS. Prevention of secondary stroke and transient ischaemic attack with antiplatelet therapy: the role of the primary care physician. Int J Clin Pract 2007;61(10):1739–48.

[20] Norris JW, Hachinski VC. Misdiagnosis of stroke. Lancet 1982;i:328–31.

[21] Libman RB, Wirkowski E, Alvir J, et al. Conditions that mimic stroke in the emergency department: implications for acute stroke trials. Arch Neurol 1995;52:1119–22.

[22] Bamford J, Sandercock P, Dennis M, et al. Classification and natural history of clinically identifiable subtypes of cerebral infarction. Lancet 1991;337 (8756):1521–6.

[23] Wadley VG, McClure LA, Howard VJ, et al. Cognitive status, stroke symptom reports, and modifiable risk factors among individuals with no diagnosis of stroke or transient ischemic attack in the REasons for Geographic and Racial Differences in Stroke (REGARDS) Study. Stroke 2007;38(4):1143–7.

[24] The Stroke Association. Stroke is a Medical Emergency. UK. Northampton: The Stroke Association; 2008.

[25] IST. The International Stroke Trial (IST): a randomised trial of aspirin, subcutaneous heparin, both, or neither among 19435 patients with acute ischemic stroke. Lancet 1997;349:1569–81.

[26] Chinese Acute Stroke Trial. CAST: randomised placebo-controlled trial of early aspirin use in 20 000 patients with acute ischemic stroke. Chinese Acute Stroke Collaborative Group. Lancet 1997;349(9066):1641–9.

[27] Wardlaw JM, del Zoppo G, Yamaguchi T. Thrombolysis for acyute ischaemic stroke (Cochrane review). The Cochrane Library 2002;(3).

[28] Intercollegiate Working Party. Care after Stroke or Transient Ischaemic attack. London: Royal College of Physicians; 2008. Clinical Standards.

[29] Ashford S, Turner-Stokes L. Management of shoulder and proximal upper limb spasticity using botulinum toxin and concurrent therapy interventions: A preliminary analysis of goals and outcomes. Disability & Rehabilitation 2009;31(3):220–6.

[30] Elovic EP, Brashear A, Kaelin D, et al. Repeated treatments with botulinum toxin type a produce sustained decreases in the limitations associated with focal upper-limb poststroke spasticity for caregivers and patients. Arch Phys Med Rehabil 2008;89 (5):799–806.

[31] Lai JM, Francisco GE, Willis FB. Dynamic splinting after treatment with botulinum toxin type-A: A randomized controlled pilot study. Adv Ther 2009;26(2):241–8.

[32] Ottenbacher KJ, Jannell S. The results of clinical trials in stroke rehabilitation research. Arch Neurol 1993;50:37.

[33] World Health Organization. Towards a common language for functioning, disability and health: International Classification of Functioning, Disability and Health. Geneva: World Health Organization; 2002.

[34] Patel M, Coshall C, Lawrence E, et al. Recovery from poststroke urinary incontinence: associated factors and impact on outcome. J Am Geriatr Soc 2001;49 (9):1229–34.

[35] Schultz S, Castillo C, Kosner J, et al. Generalised anxiety and depression: assessment over 2 years after stroke. Am J Geriatr Psychiatry 1997;5:229–37.

[36] Bernhardt J, Dewey H, Thrift A, et al. A very early rehabilitation trial for stroke (AVERT): phase II safety and feasibility. Stroke 2008;39(2):390–6.

[37] Tay-Teo K, Moodie M, Bernhardt J, et al. Economic evaluation alongside a phase II, multi-centre, randomised controlled trial of very early rehabilitation after stroke (AVERT). Cerebrovasc Dis 2008;26(5):475–81.

[38] Jones M, O'Beney C. Promoting mental health through physical activity: examples from practice. Journal of Mental Health Promotion 2004;3(1):39–47.

[39] Andersson S. Physiological mechanisms in acupuncture. In: Hopwood V, Lovesey M, Mokone S, editors. Acupuncture and Related Techniques in Physiotherapy. London: Churchill Livingstone; 1997. p. 19–39.

[40] Bakheit AMO, Thilmann AF, Ward AB, et al. A randomized, double-blind, placebo-controlled, dose-ranging study to compare the efficacy and safety of three doses of botulinum toxin type A (Dysport) with placebo in upper limb spasticity after stroke. Stroke 2000;31(10):2402–6.

[41] Braus DF, Kraus JK, Strobel J. The shoulder–hand syndrome after stroke: a prospective clinical trial. Ann Neurol 1994;36:728–33.

[42] Chantraine A, Baribeault A, Uebelhart D, et al. Shoulder pain and dysfunction in hemiplegia: effects of functional electricaal stimulation. Arch Phys Med Rehabil 1999;3:328–31.

[43] Aho K, Harmsen P, Hatano S, et al. Cerebrovascular disease in the community: results of a WHO collaborative study. Bull World Health Organ 1980;58(1):113–30.

[44] Skilbeck CE, Wade DT, Hewer RL, et al. Recovery after stroke. J. Neurol. Neurosurg. Psychiatry 1983;46:5–8.

[45] Partridge CJ, Johnston M, Edwards S. Recovery from physical disability after stroke: normal patterns as a basis for evaluation. Lancet 1987;i:373–5.

[46] Wade DT, Langton Hewer R. Functional abilities after stroke: measurement, natural history and prognosis. J Neurol Neurosurg Psychiatry 1987;52:1267–72.

[47] Humphrey P. Stroke and transient ischaemic attacks. J Neurol Neurosurg Psychiatry 1994;57:534–43.

[48] Barer DH, Mitchell JR. Predicting the outcome of acute stroke: do multivariate models help? Quarterly Journal of Medicine 1989;70:27–39.

[49] Jorgensen HS, Nakayama H, Reith J, et al. Stroke recurrence: predictors, severity, and prognosis. The Copenhagen Stroke Study. Neurology 1997;48:891–6.

[50] Dursun E, Hamamci N, Donmez S. Angular biofeedback device for sitting balance of stroke. Stroke 1996;26:1354–7.

[51] Glanz M, Klawansky S, Stason W, et al. Functional electrostimulation in post-stroke rehabilitation: a meta-analysis of the randomised, controlled trials. Arch Phys Med Rehabil 1996;77:549–53.

[52] Visintin M, Barbeau H, Korner-Bitensky N, et al. A new approach to retrain gait in stroke patients through body weight support and treadmill stimulation. Stroke 1998;29:1122–8.

[53] Tekeoolu Y, Adak B, Goksoy T. Effect of transcutaneous electrical nerve stimulation (TENS) on Barthel Activities of Daily Living (ADL) index score following stroke. Clin Rehabil 1998;12:277–80.

[54] Kwakkel G. Impact of intensity of practice after stroke: Issues for consideration. Disabil Rehabil 2006;28(13/14):823–30.

[55] Kwakkel G, Wagenaar C, Twisk J, et al. Intensity of leg and arm training after primary middle cerebral artery stroke: a randomised trial. Lancet 1999;354:191–6.

[56] Mukherjee M, McPeak LK, Redford JB, et al. The effect of electro-acupuncture on spasticity of the wrist joint in chronic stroke survivors. Arch Phys Med Rehabil 2007;88(2):159–66.

[57] Yuan X, Hao X, Lai Z, et al. Effects of acupuncture at Fengchi point (GB 20) on cerebral blood flow. J. Tradit. Chin Med 1998;18 (2):102–5.

[58] Litscher G, Schwarz G, Sandner-Kiesling A, et al. Effects of acupuncture on the oxygenation of cerebral tissue. Neurol Res 1998;20(Suppl. 1):528–32.

[59] Yu Y, Wang H, Wang Z. The effect of acupuncture on spinal motor neuron excitability in stroke patients. Chin Med J (Taipei) 1995;56:258–63.

[60] Zhao ZQ. Neural mechanisms underlying acupuncture analgesia. Prog Neurobiol 2008;85:335–75.

[61] Wayne PM, Krebs DE, Macklin EA, et al. Acupuncture for upper-extremity rehabilitation in chronic stroke: a randomised sham-controlled study. Arch Phys Med Rehabil 2005;86 (12):2248–55.

[62] Ludwig M. Influence of acupuncture on the performance of the quadriceps muscle. Deutsche Zeitschrift fur Akupunktur 2000;43(2):104–7.

[63] Huang L, Zhou S, Lu Z, et al. Bilateral effect of unilateral electroacupuncture on muscle strength. J Altern Complement Med 2007;13(5):539–46.

[64] Hopwood V, Lewith G, Prescott P, et al. Evaluating the efficacy of acupuncture in defined aspects of stroke recovery: a randomised, placebo controlled single blind study. J Neurol 2008;255(6):858–66.

[65] Ada L, Foongchomcheay A. Efficacy of electrical stimulation in preventing or reducing subluxation of the shoulder after stroke: a meta-analysis. Aust J Physiother 2002;48(4):257–67.

[66] Shen FF, Wu Q, Lin ZR, et al. Effects of different interference orders of electroacupuncture and exercise therapy on the therapeutic effect of hemiplegia after stroke [in Chinese]. Zhongguo Zhen Jiu 2008;28 (10):711–3.

[67] Ouyang Q, Zhou W, Zhang CM. The key of increasing the therapeutic effect of scalp acupuncture on hemiplegia due to stroke. Zhongguo Zhen Jiu 2007;27(10):773–6.

[68] Han JS. Electroacupuncture: an alternative to antidepressents for treating affective diseases? Int J Neurosci 1986;29:79–92.

[69] Sawazaki K, Mukaino Y, Kinoshita F, et al. Acupuncture can reduce perceived pain, mood disturbances and medical expenses related to low back pain among factory employees. Ind Health 2008;46(4):336–40.

[70] He J, Shen PF. Clinical study on the therapeutic effect of acupuncture in the treatment of post-stroke depression. Zhen Ci Yan Jiu 2007;32(1):58–61.

[71] Molassiotis A, Sylt P, Diggins H. The management of cancer-related fatigue after chemotherapy with acupuncture and acupressure: A randomised controlled trial. Complement Ther Med 2007;15 (4):228–37.

[72] Khadilkar A, Phillips K, Jean N, et al. Ottawa panel evidence-based clinical practice guidelines for post-stroke rehabilitation. Top Stroke Rehabil 2006;13(2):1–269.

[73] Huang P, Liu M. Stroke and Parkinson's Disease. Beijing: Peoples' Medical Publishing House; 2007.

[74] Maclean W, Lyttleton J, Windstroke . Clinical Handbook of Internal Medicine. Sydney: University of Western Sydney Macarthur; 1998. p. 624–54.

[75] Maciocia G. The Foundations of Chinese Medicine. New York: Churchill Livingstone; 1989.

[76] Beijing College. Essentials of Chinese Acupuncture. Beijing: Foreign Languages Press; 1980.

[77] Chan HPY. Clinical trials of the treatment of stroke using various traditional acupuncture methods. Acupuncture for Stroke Rehabilitation. Boulder: Blue Poppy Press; 2006. p. 27–32.

[78] Alexander DN, Cen S, Sullivan KJ, et al. Effects of acupuncture treatment on poststroke motor recovery and physical function: a pilot study. American Society of Neurorehabilitation and Neural Repair 2004;18(4):259–67.

[79] Fink M, Rollnik J, Bijak M, et al. Needle acupuncture in chronic poststroke leg spasticity. Arch Phys Med Rehabil 2004;85 (4):667–72.

[80] Park J, White AR, James MA, et al. Acupuncture for subacute stroke rehabilitation. Arch Intern Med 2005;165:2026–31.

[81] Zhang ZH, Liu M, Asplund K, Li L. Acupuncture for acute stroke. Cochrane Database Syst Rev 2005;CD00317(2):1–22.

[82] Bowsher D. Central post-stroke ('thalamic syndrome') and other

central pains. Am J Hosp Palliat Care 1999;16(4):593–7.

[83] Yen HL, Chen W. An east–west approach to the management of central post-stroke pain. Cerebrovasc Dis 2003;(16):27–30.

[84] Zhou XJ, Chen T, Chen JT. 75 infantile palsy children treated with acupuncture, acupressure and functional training. Chung Kuo Chung Hsi I Chieh Ho Tsa Chih 1993;13(4):220–2.

[85] Wu Q, Chen H. The effect of acupuncture on improving the quality of life of cerebral palsy patients. International Journal of Clinical Acupuncture 2005;14 (4):251.

[86] Mu R, Chen L, Liu L, et al. Combined acupuncture and functional exercises for infantile cerebral palsy in 45 cases. Journal of Acupuncture and Tuina Science 2003;1(6):13–4.

[87] Watson P. Modulation of involuntary movements in cerebral palsy with acupuncture. Acupuncture Med 2009;76–7.

[88] Dorsher PT, Fleckenstein J. Trigger points and classical acupuncture points: part 3: relationships of myofascial referred pain patterns to acupuncture meridians. Deutsche Zeitschrift fur Akupunktur 2009;52(1):9–14.

[89] Dobkin BH. Traumatic brain injury. The clinical science of neurologic rehabilitation. Oxford: Oxford University Press; 2003. p. 497–546.

[90] Campbell M. Acquired brain injury: trauma and pathology. In: Stokes M, editor. Physical management in neurological rehabilitation. Edinburgh: Elsevier; 2004. p. 103–24.

[91] De Silva MJ, Roberts I, Perel P, et al. Patient outcome after traumatic brain injury in high-,

middle- and low-income countries: analysis of data on 8927 patients in 46 countries. Int J Epidemiol 2009;38(2):452–8.

[92] RCP and BRSM. Rehabilitation following acquired brain injury: national clinical guidelines. Royal College of Physicians; 2003.

[93] Chen YX. Puncturing Shendao in treating hemiplegia following head injury. International Journal of Clinical Acupuncture 1997;8 (3):293–4.

[94] He J, Wu B, Zhang Y. Acupuncture treatment for 15 cases of post-traumatic coma. J Tradit Chin Med 2005;25 (3):171–3.

[95] Donnellan CP. Acupuncture for central pain affecting the ribcage following traumatic brain injury and rib fractures – a case report. Acupuncture In Medicine. Acupunct Med 2006;24 (3):129–33.

Parkinson's disease and related conditions

7

KEY POINTS

- Parkinson's disease (PD) is commonly treated in physiotherapy departments but success is not usually enduring.
- Some of the symptoms will respond to acupuncture.
- Some of the side-effects produced by drug therapy will also respond to acupuncture.
- Treatment will be a mixture of traditional Chinese medicine (TCM) and Western theory.
- In TCM terms PD is associated with Feng syndromes.

Introduction

Definition

Parkinson's disease (PD) is one of a group of conditions which are thought to be primarily due to the gradual loss of dopamine-producing brain cells, situated in the substantia nigra. It is considered to be a chronic disorder of the motor system primarily causing mobility problems. Postural problems are associated with later stages of the disease.

Incidence

It is unusual to find PD diagnosed before the age of 50 but the prevalence increases with age, becoming as high as 4% in older age groups, particularly in more industrialized countries. The incidence of PD in the UK is 18 per 100 000 population per year, amounting to approximately 10 000 new cases each year [1]. Sex distribution is approximately equal.

Mortality

PD is not generally considered to be a fatal disease. Major morbidity and mortality are less than 1%, having been reduced considerably by the modern drug regimes.

Risk factors

The root cause remains obscure but parkinsonism results from many different pathological processes, including ageing, environmental and genetic factors. Ageing is not thought to be a primary cause of PD, although the substantia nigra containing dopamine-producing neurons declines with age. It is possible that injury or infection in early life may predispose the patient to accelerated loss of this tissue. It has been suggested that PD can be a side-effect of certain psychotropic drugs [2]. Analytic studies generally reveal an inverse association between PD and ciga-rette smoking, although epidemiologic evidence does not support a direct protective effect of smoking [3].

It has also recently been suggested that gout can protect from PD. The value of the increased uric acid present in the system needs to be fully evalu-ated but first results are interesting [4]. The associ-ation between ischaemic stroke, vascular risk factors and PD has been addressed in several studies [5].

Shy–Drager syndrome is very similar to Parkinson's in symptomatology but differs in one major respect, respiratory problems. It is described as multiple-system atrophy with autonomic failure and is a pro-gressive disorder but is often first recognized by an increase in loud and strident snoring while the patient is sleeping.

This disorder is generally characterized by postural hypotension – an excessive drop in blood pressure which causes dizziness or momentary blackouts upon standing or sitting up. There are three types of Shy–Drager syndrome: (1) parkinsonian type, which may include symptoms of PD such as slow movement, stiff muscles and mild tremors; (2) cerebellar type, which may include problems such as loss of balance and the tendency to fall; and (3) combination type, which may include symptoms of both types.

There has been some argument over the years about other similar pathologies, known as vascular parkinsonism. The condition has been named and renamed several times, with terms such as arterio-sclerotic parkinsonism, arteriosclerotic pseudopar-kinsonism and lower-body parkinsonism. Despite the progress in our understanding of other parkinso-nian syndromes, such as progressive supranuclear palsy and multiple-system atrophy, and significant developments in neuroimaging techniques, the con-cept of vascular parkinsonism is still unclear and the clinical diagnosis is often difficult [5], but from a physiotherapy or acupuncture perspective it does not differ greatly from PD.

Diagnosis

Differential diagnosis

Early symptoms are subtle and make their appear-ance gradually, with those closest to the patient often unaware of what the diminished energy and depression may foreshadow. Normal voluntary and spontaneous movements are lacking. In some people the disease progresses more quickly than in others, leading to a rapid decrease in the ability to perform daily activities due to the shaking or tremor.

The definitive symptoms of PD are tremor at rest; involuntary trembling in the hands, arms, legs or jaw; rigidity or stiffness of the limbs and trunk; a general slowness of movement (bradykinesia); and impaired balance and coordination, often involving postural instability. 'Dropped-head' syndrome is charac-terized by severe neck flexion but minor thoracic or lumbar curvature. It results from neck extensor weakness or increased tone of the flexor muscles. This symptom is usually reported in neuromuscular diseases such as amyotrophic lateral sclerosis, myas-thenia gravis and polymyositis or in extrapyramidal disorders, but does also occur in PD [6].

Patients may also have difficulty in walking or talking and completing small motor tasks becomes problematic.

In addition to these motor changes, there may be other symptoms, including depression and other emotional changes; difficulty in swallowing, chewing and speaking; urinary problems or constipation; skin problems; and sleep disruptions. There is noticeably decreased facial expression, apathy, fatigue and sometimes pain. This fatigue, combined with worsening functional status, can be a significant contributor to poor quality of life [7].

Some cognitive changes can be suspected early in the disease, particularly frontal lobe executive dysfunction. Parkinsonians find it difficult to turn thought into action. A slowing-down of mental processes is sometimes mistaken for dementia, but as a rule of thumb, if you give a Parkinson's patient time to answer a question, he or she will answer. A patient suffering from Alzheimer's will tend to forget the question. As the disease develops psychiatric problems can dominate the clinical picture. Depression is the most common of these, with about a third of patients suffering from depression at some stage in their disease [1].

Tests

The differential diagnosis is based on both medical history and a neurological examination. Early signs of value include infrequent blinking, the lack of arm swinging, and cogwheel or plastic rigidity accentuated when the opposite side is stressed. The disease can be difficult to diagnose accurately in the early stages so doctors may sometimes request brain scans or laboratory tests in order to rule out other diseases.

Medical treatment

Pharmacology

Various pharmacologic and surgical therapies have been developed to deal with the dysfunction caused by this disease. A variety of drugs provide some relief from the symptoms. Usually, patients are given levodopa combined with carbidopa. Carbidopa delays the conversion of levodopa into dopamine until it reaches the brain. Nerve cells can use levodopa to make dopamine and replenish the brain's dwindling supply. Although levodopa helps at least three-quarters of parkinsonian cases, not all symptoms respond equally to the drug. Bradykinesia and rigidity respond best, while tremor may be only marginally reduced.

Problems with balance and other symptoms may not be improved at all. Anticholinergics may be used to help control tremor and rigidity. Other drugs, such as bromocriptine, pramipexole and ropinirole, mimic the role of dopamine in the brain, causing the neurons to react as they would to dopamine. An antiviral drug, amantadine, also appears to reduce symptoms. A relatively new drug, rasagiline (Agilect), can also now be used along with levodopa for patients with advanced PD or as a single-drug treatment for early PD. Constipation is a common problem, often as a result of decreased intestinal peristalsis induced by anticholinergics.

Continuous levodopa treatment for PD patients is frequently associated with the development of motor complications such as dyskinesias and a tailing-off of effect towards the end of the dose. Medical management for this includes careful manipulation of the dose to establish the optimum treatment schedule and improve absorption, incorporating catechol-O-methyl transferase inhibition, monoamine oxidase-B (MAO-B) inhibition, dopaminergic agonists, amantadine and continuous dopaminergic infusions.

Surgery

Surgery was in vogue for PD before the 1970s but became less popular until recently. It may be appropriate if the disease fails to respond to drugs or the effect of the drugs diminishes. Transplanted fetal mesoencephalic cells, harvested from aborted fetuses, grown in cell culture and injected into the brain in a form of cell suspension, have been shown to replace the production of natural dopamine, producing some good results, although the technique itself remains controversial [8]. A technique called deep-brain stimulation uses electrodes implanted into the brain and connected to a small pulse generator which can be externally programmed. This can decrease the need for some of the drugs, reducing the unwanted side-effects, most often the increased involuntary movements associated with levodopa [9]. The deep-brain stimulation can also reduce the fluctuation of symptoms, allowing for greater freedom of movement generally. Early results have been good but the technique is not yet widely used.

Prognosis

Impact on patient

PD is similar to other neurological problems in that it varies widely from patient to patient. With some the tremor is the most limiting factor while others seem untroubled by that, but far more concerned by their lack of mobility or difficulty communicating by facial expression. Clinical experience suggests that there is, however, a great deal of unreported depression and often quite a lot of pain brought about by the rigidity and overall poverty of muscle movement [10].

When investigating the lifestyle impact of PD, Kuopio et al. found that women scored significantly lower on five of the eight dimensions of the SF-36 outcome measure. This study found depression to be more common among women than men [11]. They concluded that, to improve the quality of life in PD patients, it is necessary to recognize and treat the depression. Parkinsonian symptoms and symptoms of autonomic dysfunction such as constipation and sexual impotence in males predominate early in the course of the disease and certainly have an effect on mood. Constipation may be unrelenting and hard to manage in some patients.

Shy–Drager syndrome may be difficult to diagnose in the early stages; however, within a year of onset most patients develop postural hypotension. For the majority of patients, blood pressure is unstable – often fluctuating up and down and may cause severe headaches. Other symptoms may also develop, such as generalized weakness, double vision and/or other vision disturbances, impairment of speech, sensory changes, difficulties with breathing and swallowing, often causing pronounced snoring; dysphagia is a late symptom and affects both solids and liquids. This difficulty arises either from an inability to force the food down the throat or rigidity of the voluntary muscles of the throat and leads to complaints of food getting stuck in the throat. Ingestion of only small portions of food and careful chewing, one morsel being swallowed before the next is taken, may help. The problem is important because of the risk of aspiration. Other symptoms may include irregularities in heart beat, inability to sweat and diarrhoea.

Parkinson's disease and physiotherapy

Exercise has long been a popular form of treatment with physiotherapists, although the effects seem to be best in the short term. A recent study by Morris et al. [12] confirms this. For the exercise group, quality of life improved significantly during inpatient hospitalization and this improvement was retained at follow-up. Inpatient rehabilitation produced short-term reductions in disability and improvements in quality of life in people with PD. Exercise training has also been found to decrease significantly the number of falls experienced by these patients [13]. Other techniques, including auditory cues [14] or the use of treadmills, have been tried with some success [15], but all the studies were relatively small and none appear to hold the key. As a novel way of combining both forward and backward walking in a pleasurable environment, tango lessons have been investigated, with some success [16].

The Royal College of Physicians guidelines have recommended the following:

'Physiotherapy should be available for people with PD. Particular consideration should be given to:

- Gait re-education, improvement of balance and flexibility
- Enhancement of aerobic capacity
- Improvement of movement initiation
- Improvement of functional independence, including mobility and activities of daily living
- Provision of advice regarding safety in the home environment' [17].

All of the above will be tackled in a course of physiotherapy treatment at any stage of the disease but the addition of acupuncture may be of considerable benefit. There have been several studies investigating the effect of acupuncture on the symptoms of PD and a recent systematic analysis summed the situation up well, concluding that 'there is evidence indicating the potential effectiveness of acupuncture for treating idiopathic PD'. The review found that, out of the 10 trials selected, nine claimed a statistically positive effect from the use of acupuncture [18].

The outcome measures most used were the Unified Parkinson's Disease Rating Scale (UPDRS) and the outdated Webster scales. The Motor Dysfunction Rating Scale for Parkinson's Disease (MDRSPD) was only used in one of the studies. The results were limited by the methodological flaws, unknowns in concealment of allocation, number of dropouts and blinding methods in the studies, but as acupuncture has been used clinically to treat the symptoms of PD for hundreds of years, the picture is encouraging for further research.

Acupuncture in Parkinson's disease

Acupuncture remains a popular treatment for PD in far-Eastern countries.

Occidental medicine has a given definition for PD and knowledge of PD pathophysiology has led to development of therapeutic management. PD, even if not named, is likely to have always existed in different parts of the world. Description and management of this neurodegenerative condition are found in ancient medical systems. The following section attempts to introduce the philosophical concepts of traditional Chinese medicine (TCM) and the description, classification and understanding of parkinsonian symptoms in TCM.

There has been a serious attempt to re-evaluate the traditional treatments in the light of modern knowledge, in particular the herbal remedies [19], but a scientific review of all TCM therapies in this context is now needed.

In a non-blinded pilot study, 85% of patients reported subjective improvement of individual symptoms, including tremor, walking, handwriting, slowness, pain, sleep, depression and anxiety [20]. There were no adverse effects; however there were only 20 patients in this study.

Electroacupuncture may be a refinement that will be more effective in treating PD. It is used on body needles and also on those inserted into the scalp (see section on scalp acupuncture, below).

Some interesting work has been done by a Chinese research group, where electroacupuncture was applied at a frequency of 100 Hz at the points GV 20 and GV 14 to MFB transected parkinsonian rats who had rotenone (3 µg) administered bilaterally and stereotaxically into the medial forebrain bundle (MFB) to produce parkinsonian symptoms [21]. An extension of this work to human patients might produce significant results.

Nonetheless, the following sections will offer a selection of acupuncture points and techniques with varying rationales. The reason for point selection may ultimately be less important than the point itself. Table 7.1 gives a summary of expected symptoms.

Body acupuncture

Acupuncture points, mainly on Yang meridians, can be used, as in all neurological diseases, to tackle the superficial musculoskeletal symptoms. Both pain

Table 7.1 Symptom picture for Parkinson's disease (including multiple-systems atrophy)

Symptom	Characteristic presentation	Parkinson's disease
Decreased mobility	Rigidity	o
Fatigue	Lack of energy	o
Respiratory problems	Snoring	X Shy–Drager syndrome only
Muscle spasm	Tremor	o
Contractures	Stiffness and rigidity	o
Autonomic changes	Slowing circulation	o o
Cognition/mood	Apathy Depression	o
Communication	Facial rigidity Unwilling to engage	o o
Bladder and bowel problems	Usually drug-induced	o
Visual problems	Rare	X

X, usually absent; o, common; o o, very frequent.

and movement problems can be addressed. The points can be selected according to symptoms and Table 7.2 gives some of the alternatives. Many problems are directly caused by the medical interventions and these have also been listed. Electroacupuncture may be used at some of the points; the recommended frequency for body points is 2 Hz, while that for scalp points is 100 Hz.

There is a danger of the list of acupoints becoming endless, so only the most specific points are given. These are selected for completeness from both Western medicine approaches and those more traditionally Chinese. Those that relate directly to the following TCM syndromes are also mixed in.

Scalp acupuncture

Perhaps surprisingly, scalp acupuncture is a technique frequently recommended for PD, in both Western and modern Chinese texts. This is a relatively modern idea and the technique claims to

Table 7.2 Parkinson's disease – useful points

Symptoms	Points	Rationale	Comments
Postural changes Dropped-head syndrome	GV 22 Xinhui BL 6 Chengguang GB 17 Zhengyang GB 10 Fubai	Extrapyramidal effect	Hard to influence
Stooping posture	GV 20 Baihui Moxa to GV 4 Mingmen KI 3 Taixi	GV meridian empty	Postural hypotension
Bradykinesia Slow and limited movement or difficulty initiating movement	ST 36 Zusanli SP 6 Sanyinjiao KI 3 Taixi GB 10 Fubai	Qi and Blood deficiency, Kidney Yang deficiency	Used both as a tonic and as a Qi boost
Uncoordinated movement	Du 20 Baihui Du 14 Dazhui	Regulation of central nervous system	Add Sishencong
Depression	Four Gates HT 7 Shenmen Ear Shenmen Sishencong Yintang	To lift the spirits and generally soothe and calm the psyche	Liver/Heart/GV influence
Cold and painful upper limbs	TE 6 Waiguan	Local point	Treats poor circulation
Cold and painful lower limbs	SP 10 Xuehai ST 31 Biguan	Circulation points	Treats poor circulation
Slow general circulation	Moxa to BL 17 Geshu	For general circulation	CV 6, Qihai, can be used to support body Qi
Mask-like face	HT 5 Tongli HT 7 Shenmen	Expression of emotion	Stimulates Spirit
Dull monotonous speech	HT 5 Tongli	Associated with speech	
Involuntary tremor	LR 3 Taichong SI 3 Houxi GV 16 Fengfu	Cogwheel rigidity	GV 16 expels Wind
Palpitation	HT 7 Shenmen PE 6 Neiguan CV 17 Shanzhong	Cardiac arrhythmia	
Irregular bowels	CV 4 Guanyuan ST 25 Tianshu LI 11 Quchi TE 5 Waiguan TE 6 Zhigou	Effect on Jin Ye circulation	Sometimes a drug side-effect
Drooling	HT 6 Yinxi HT 7 Shenmen		For excess of uncontrolled saliva
Dry mouth	CV 24 Chenjiang		Drug side-effect

| Table 7.2 Parkinson's disease – useful points—cont'd ||||
Symptoms	Points	Rationale	Comments
Incontinence or urinary retention	ST 36 Zusanli SP 6 Sanyinjiao BL 23 Shenshu KI 3 Taixi		
Fatigue	Any of the stimulating points Possible use of extra meridians	General acupuncture effects	Use in moderation; little surplus energy available

stimulate the surface of the brain, most particularly the sensory and motor cortices (see Chapter 12).

Points are located by identifying the anteroposterior median line as a reference (Figure 7.1).

In PD both motor and sensory lines should be treated with the addition of the chorea or tremor area (Figure 7.2).

The treatment can be used on either the unaffected side or bilaterally. The usual frequency should be between 100 and 200 Hz.

Some studies [22] have used scalp and body acupuncture together as an addition to the drug regime and there has been some attempt to analyse what may be happening in the brain during scalp acupuncture in a Parkinson's patient, particularly as regards dopamine production; however more work needs to be done [23].

Some authorities claim that scalp acupuncture used early enough can alleviate tremor without any additional drug treatment, but if the disease has

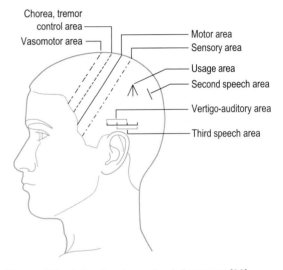

Figure 7.2 • Lateral surface stimulation areas [29].

been present for more than 2 years the improvement will only be temporary [24]. Once the patient has been taking regular drug medication for many years it would be unwise to try to replace this with acupuncture treatment.

TCM approach

Which TCM syndromes may be involved? According to Maciocia, the most likely syndromes will be Qi and Blood deficiency, Phlegm Heat agitating Wind or Liver and Kidney Yin deficiency [25].

In practical terms this means that the symptoms of these syndromes, described in detail below, have a chance of including those known to be common to PD patients.

Due to the usual lack of homogeneity among patients suffering from any type of neurological disease, there may of course be wide variation.

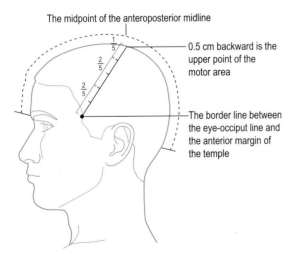

Figure 7.1 • Location of motor area [29].

There are other techniques for dealing with the broad spectrum of symptoms, including a use of abdominal acupuncture only in addition to the normal drug regime. This has some logic; many of the side-effects of the drugs – fatigue, constipation, for example – could be lessened this way, but little work has been published so far and there are many flaws in the methodology of the best published study [26].

Qi and Blood deficiency

Poor or absent circulation of Qi and Blood is seen in TCM as the cause of both pain and poor movement ability. The blockage may in fact be caused by early manifestations of Phlegm Heat (see below). Local points on the most affected limbs will also be useful.

Common symptoms include chronic tremor of a limb or limbs, sallow complexion, reluctant speech and lack of facial expression. Also found are stiff neck, cold painful limbs, general poverty of movement, unsteady gait with difficulty in taking the first step, dizziness and blurred vision.

Treatment

Tonify Qi, nourish Blood, energize the meridians and dispel Wind.

- ST 36 Zusanli tonifies Qi and Blood.
- SP 6 Sanyinjiao tonifies Qi and Blood.
- LR 8 Ququan nourishes Liver Blood.
- CV 4 Guanyuan nourishes Blood generally.
- SP 10 Xuehai improves Blood circulation in the lower limb.

Phlegm Heat agitating Wind (affecting Liver)

There are three different syndromes associated with the stirring of Liver Wind. They can be caused by:

1. internal Heat, caused by penetration of an exogenous Pathogen to the interior. This is characterized by serious febrile diseases in children, e.g. measles or meningitis
2. inability of the deficient Liver Yin to control the Liver Yang with subsequent internal Wind symptoms (this is more associated with PD)
3. deficiency of Liver Blood [25].

Treatment for all three causes will aim to subdue the Liver Wind, which can be very dangerous, frequently leading to Wind Stroke or cerebrovascular accident. Otherwise the Liver energies need controlling or tonifying according to whether the underlying symptoms exhibit excess or deficiency. The prevention of stroke depends on getting this balance correct but it will not really affect or prevent the onset of PD.

This syndrome is often associated with hypertension, stroke, epilepsy and trigeminal neuralgia. It may be exacerbated by prolonged frustration or anger, both of which are said to damage the liver. It is also linked to obesity and a lack of physical exercise.

The symptoms are likely to include vertigo, tremor, convulsion and spasms. Stiff neck, facial paralysis, tinnitus, apoplexy and hemiplegia may also occur.

Treatment

Calm Liver. Disperse Wind.

- LR 2 Xingjian Fire point disperses Fire in the Liver.
- LR 3 Taichong Liver source point balances Liver, moves Qi.
- GB 20 Fengchi expels Wind.
- BL 18 Ganshu Back Shu point for the Liver.
- LI 4 Hegu expels Wind and is used for face and neck.
- GV 20 Baihui is used to calm the Liver and expel Wind.
- KI 3 Taixi tonifies Kidney Yin and Yang.
- KI 7 Fuliu tonifies both Kidney and Liver.
- BL 23 Shenshu Back Shu point for the Kidneys.

Liver and Kidney Yin deficiency

This situation is often the precursor to Liver Yang rising. If the cooling Yin of the Liver is depleted the Yang becomes hyperactive and rises upwards, producing the symptoms of headache, dry eyes and tinnitus. The Heat also causes irritability and anger, emotions damaging to the Liver. This syndrome is a combination of both excess and deficiency, although the excess symptoms seem more obvious.

Liver Yang rising is a fairly common pattern and will be mentioned again in this book as it is closely associated with neurological damage. Stress, frustration, anger and resentment build up over a long period of time, obstructing the free flow of Liver Qi. This produces Heat, which dries up Yin. Yin thus cannot control Yang, which rises to the head. In contrast, the person could be relatively cool in the lower part of the body.

Symptoms include general frailty, dizziness, tinnitus, insomnia, headache, night sweats, low-back pain, stiff neck, back and knees and mental restlessness. Often also present will be lack of facial expression, poor memory and general physical clumsiness.

Treatment

Nourish Yin, dispel Wind, energize the meridians.

- CV 4 Guanyuan supports Kidney Yin.
- BL 23 Shenshu Back Shu point for the Kidneys.
- KI 3 Taixi nourishes Kidney Yin.
- SP 6 Sanyinjiao nourishes Kidney Yin.
- BL 18 Ganshu Back Shu point for the Liver.
- LR 8 Ququan nourishes Liver Yin.
- LR 3 Taichong Liver source point balances Liver and moves Qi.

In summary, in TCM terms PD provides a long and complicated list of symptoms, all of which combine to make up a picture that is not unlike the TCM idea of old age, a slow decline of supporting Kidney energy. It is not suggested that PD can be cured by acupuncture but it is reasonable to suppose that the known physiological effects may help with symptom control.

It is important to remember that these patients are characterized by a slowing-down of body processes and a general lack of energy. Acupuncture can be a draining type of therapy and should be used with caution. However, it can be seen that, with a basic understanding of TCM, a useful prescription can be drawn up for a patient manifesting with a clear neurological disease process [27]. Then it would be sensible to select specific points for symptoms, ensuring that some of the powerful end points are also used. One good argument for using acupuncture for the management of PD might be that it causes fewer adverse effects than drug treatment, particularly levodopa, and often addresses some of the associated problems [28].

However, it is always best to combine acupuncture with the type of physical retraining treatment described in the physiotherapy section of this chapter. PD has been described as a depression with physical symptoms. One of the well-documented side-effects of acupuncture is the improvement in mood. Parkinson's patients are hard to motivate and it is often difficult to perceive whether there is a response.

Teaching ways to initiate the first step, increasing control over simple tasks like walking or sit to stand will help immeasurably with daily life, while a feeling that all is not lost will help to maintain whatever progress is possible and motivate the patient further.

Case study 7.1: level 1 case study: PD immobility

General lack of movement

- Male PD patient, diagnosed over 4 years previously
- Community physiotherapist visiting
- Coping at home, living with his wife.

Presenting symptoms

- Very immobile facial features, blank staring face, slow to smile
- Hard to initiate walking, stiff gait, constant dull ache in legs
- On examination: poor circulation in lower limbs, blue and cold to the touch
- TCM impression: Qi and Blood deficiency.

Treatment

Treatment entailed acupuncture with ongoing physiotherapy to improve mobility. Six acupuncture treatments were provided over 4 weeks.

Points used bilaterally: SP 10 for lower-limb circulation, SP 6, ST 36 boost to system, ST 44 for leg pain. Manual acupuncture was given for 30 minutes. DeQi was obtained at most needle sites.

Outcome

- Within three treatments the patient's legs were noticeably pinker and warmer to touch and the patient stated that walking was subjectively 'easier' and that his legs 'belonged to him again'.
- Pain had diminished and sleeping had improved.

- This patient was only treated six times (twice in the first week) and not referred again but had a short-term relief from some of his symptoms.

Case study 7.2: level 3 case study

This patient was a 62-year-old man who had had PD for 8 years, and who was being managed by specialist PD services. He lives with his wife. He has a history of hypertension.

Main complaint

The patient's main complaint was worsening cervical pain associated with 'dropped-head' syndrome. He was taking paracetamol 1 gram 6-hourly and diclofenac 50–100 mg tds with limited effect.

Physical presentation

Walks independently; impaired standing balance; flexed posture; bradykinesia; upper-limb resting tremor.

Examination of neck

The patient had restricted passive joint range and muscle extensibility in his cervical spine. His neck was in a posture of flexion and right-side flexion with muscle weakness in the cervical spine. Locally tender on palpation, no active trigger points, non-dermatomal distribution of pain in neck radiating to shoulders. X-ray showed cervical spine degeneration.

Diagnosis

The diagnosis was regional myofascial pain syndrome.

Treatment

- Muscle re-education to improve range, alignment and strength around neck region
- Soft-tissue massage of cervical/shoulder region
- Maitland's joint mobilizations in cervical spine
- Acupuncture.

Acupuncture treatment

Bilateral LI 4, LI 11, LI 14, TE 5, TE 14.

On occasions the therapist used right unilateral SI 10, SI 11, SI 12, BL 11, GB 21 plus right LI 4, LI 11, LI 14 and TE 5. Acupressure to BL 10 was also included.

Treatments lasted 30 minutes; needles were simulated for Deqi at 10-minute intervals. The patient had a strong warm sensation during treatment; he commonly fell asleep. The first course of treatment was 18 sessions over 6 months; then the patient had a 5-month break from acupuncture; this was followed by a further 13 sessions over 3 months.

The patient was advised to try self-treatment with four-pole transcutaneous electrical nerve stimulation over the lower cervical spine at home during his second course of treatment.

Outcome

Acupuncture reduced his neck pain from 7/10 to 3/10. This made neck exercises easier to perform, with resultant benefits of improved neck flexibility, posture and strength.

He experienced an improvement in his mood and well-being due to this pain reduction. He was able to increase his level of activity and managed some painting and decorating in the house.

References

[1] Jones D, Playfer J. Parkinson's disease. In: Stokes M, editor. Physical Management in Neurological Rehabilitation. Edinburgh: Elsevier Mosby; 2004. p. 203–19.

[2] Keus SH, Munneke M, Nijkrake MJ, et al. Physical therapy in Parkinson's disease: Evolution and future challenges. Mov Disord 2008;24:1–14.

[3] Schoenberg BS. Environmental risk factors for Parkinson's disease: the epidemiologic evidence. Can J Neurol Sci 1987; 14(3):407–13.

[4] De Vera M, Rahman MM, Rankin J, et al. Gout and the risk of parkinson's disease: A cohort study. Arthritis Rheum 2008; 59(11):1549–54.

[5] Benamer HTS, Grosset DG. Vascular parkinsonism: a clinical review. Eur Neurol 2008;61:11–5.

[6] Kashihara K, Ohno M, Tomito S. Dropped head syndrome in Parkinson's disease. Mov Disord 2006;21(8):1213–6.

[7] Havlikova E, Rosenberger J, Nagyova I, et al. Impact of fatigue on quality of life in patients with Parkinson's disease. Eur J Neurol 2008;15(5):475–80.

[8] Hauser RA, Freeman MD, Snow BJ, et al. Long-term evaluation of bilateral fetal nigral transplantation in Parkinson disease. Arch Neurol 1999;56(2):179–87.

[9] Liang GS, Chou KL, Baltuch GH, et al. Long-term outcomes of bilateral subthalamic nucleus stimulation in patients with advanced Parkinson's disease. Stereotact Funct Neurosurg 2006;84(5–6):221–7.

[10] Findley L, Peto V, Pugner K. The impact of Parkinson's disease on quality of life: results of a research survey in the UK. Mov Disord 2000;15(3):179.

[11] Kuopio AM, Marttila RJHH, Toivonen M, et al. The quality of life in Parkinson's disease. Mov Disord 2000;15(3):216–23.

[12] Morris ME, Iansek R, Kirkwood B. A randomized controlled trial of movement strategies compared with exercise for people with Parkinson's disease. Mov Disord 2008.

[13] Ashburn A, Fazakerley L, Ballinger C, et al. A randomised controlled trial of a home based exercise programme to reduce the risk of falling among people with Parkinson's disease. J Neurol Neurosurg Psychiatry 2007; 78(7):678–84.

[14] Nieuwboer A, Kwakkel G, Rochester L, et al. Cueing training in the home improves gait-related mobility in Parkinson's disease: the RESCUE trial. J Neurol Neurosurg Psychiatry 2007;78(2):134–40.

[15] Protas EJ, Mitchell K, Williams A, et al. Gait and step training to reduce falls in Parkinson's disease. NeuroRehabilitation 2005;20 (3):183–90.

[16] Hackney ME, Earhart MG. Short duration, intensive tango dancing for Parkinson disease: An uncontrolled pilot study. Complement Ther Med 2008;17:203–7.

[17] National Collaborating Centre for Chronic Conditions. Parkinson's disease: national clinical guideline for diagnosis and management in primary and secondary care. London: Royal College of Physicians; 2006.

[18] Lam YC, Kum WF, Durairajan SSK, et al. Efficacy and safety of acupuncture for idiopathic Parkinson's disease: a systematic review. J Altern Complement Med 2008;14(6):663–71.

[19] Li Q, Zhao D, Bezard E. Traditional Chinese medicine for Parkinson's disease: a review of Chinese literature. Behav Pharmacol 2006;17(5–6):403–10.

[20] Shulman LM, Wen X, Weiner WJ, et al. Acupuncture therapy for the symptoms of Parkinson's disease. Mov Disord 2002;17(4):799–802.

[21] Wang X, Liang XB, Li FQ, et al. Therapeutic strategies for Parkinson's disease: the ancient meets the future – traditional Chinese herbal medicine, electroacupuncture, gene therapy and stem cells. Neurochem Res 2008;33(10):1956–63.

[22] Jiang XM, Huang Y, Zhuo Y, et al. Therapeutic effect of scalp electroacupuncture on Parkinson disease. Nan Fang Yi Ke Da Xue Xue Bao 2006;26(1):114–6.

[23] Jiang XM, Huang Y, Li DJ, et al. Effect of electro-scalp acupuncture on cerebral dopamine transporter in the striatum area of the patient of Parkinson's disease by means of single photon emission computer tomography. Zhongguo Zhen Jiu = Chinese Acupuncture and Moxibustion 2006;26(6):427–30.

[24] Lu S. Handbook of acupuncture in the treatment of nervous system disorders, PD. London: Donica Publishing; 2002.

[25] Maciocia G. The Practice of Chinese Medicine. Churchill Livingstone: Edinburgh; 1994.

[26] Chen Xh, Li Y, Kui Y. Clinical observation on abdominal acupuncture plus Madopa for treatment of Parkinson's disease. Zhongguo Zhen Jiu = Chinese Acupuncture and Moxibustion 2007;27(8):562–4.

[27] Hopwood V. Acupuncture in Physiotherapy. Oxford: Butterworth Heinemann; 2004.

[28] Lee MS, Shin BC, Kong JC, et al. Effectiveness of acupuncture for Parkinson disease: a systematic review. Mov Disord 2008; 23(11):1505–15.

[29] Yau PS. Scalp-Needling Therapy. Beijing: Medicine and Health Publishing; 1990.

Multiple sclerosis

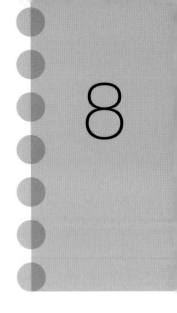

- Multiple sclerosis (MS) is commonly treated in physiotherapy departments but success is not always enduring.
- The symptoms of MS vary widely from patient to patient.
- Some of the symptoms will respond to acupuncture, as will some of the side-effects produced by drug therapy.
- Acupuncture appears to be able to aid with rehabilitation in early stages and to stabilize symptoms in middle or late stages.
- Treatment will be a mixture of traditional Chinese medicine (TCM) and Western theory.
- In TCM terms MS is associated with several major syndromes which relate to the various stages of the disease.
- Care must be taken not to overtreat and increase fatigue.

Introduction

Multiple sclerosis (MS) is the major cause of neurological disability in young adults. Around 85 000 people in the UK have MS. It is characterized by relapse and remission, making life very unpredictable for sufferers and their families. It is better known than some of the other neurological conditions partly because of the large number of sufferers and also partly because it is possible to have a version of the disease causing little disability.

Definition

MS is a chronic disease which occurs in the brain and spinal cord. It is the principal member of a group known as demyelinating diseases. It is the result of damage to the myelin sheath surrounding the axons of the nerve fibres in the central nervous system. The myelin is arranged in segments all along the nerve and the spaces between each myelin sheath are called the nodes of Ranvier. The myelin segment is called the internode. This arrangement allows for rapid and efficient axonal conduction by the process of saltatory conduction whereby the signal spreads rapidly and smoothly from one node of Ranvier to the next. If the myelin is lost or damaged, the insulation is damaged and the action potential is no longer conducted along the nerve, although the nerve itself is relatively undamaged.

It has been found that the central nervous system is able to overcome small areas of axon loss by finding ways to reroute messages around an area of damage through undamaged nerve cells. This ability to adapt in areas of damage is called plasticity. If the area of damage becomes too large, this rerouting process is no longer able to compensate and messages to or from that part of the central nervous system are permanently blocked, resulting in symptoms that do not improve. There seems to be a mixture of both grey and white matter affected by the demyelination process [1].

Incidences

MS has a peak incidence between 25 and 35 years and is twice as common in women as men.

Mortality

It appears that only about half the patients suffering from MS eventually die of causes related directly to it. Respiratory disease or cardiovascular complications, mainly brought about by demyelinating lesions, involving brain regions that regulate cardiorespiratory activity, could be considered as the immediate cause of death. But poverty of movement, trauma or even poor nursing care are also problems. The standardized mortality ratio in a recent study indicated that MS sufferers were almost three times as likely to die prematurely compared to the general population [2] but MS was not always given as cause on the death certificate.

Risk factors

It is now well established that there is a familial tendency to MS, although no clear pattern of inheritance has been found [3, 4]. Between 10% and 15% of patients with MS have an affected relative, a higher figure than could be predicted from population prevalence.

Diagnosis

Differential diagnosis

Early signs and symptoms will often include vague feeling of ill health for several years preceding diagnosis. Relatively minor discomforts, aches, pains and general lethargy, all easily dismissed by the patient as being trivial, can mount up steadily until a doctor is consulted. It is also important to remember that many people diagnosed with MS remain mobile and can live a near-normal life without the need to see a physiotherapist or an acupuncturist.

Probably the most common single symptom is an acute or subacute loss of vision in one eye, rarely both.

Tests

The diagnosis of MS is not an easy one to make and relies more on elimination of other causes than a direct confirmation.

1. A positive diagnosis requires at least two separate episodes of neurological symptoms, weakness or clumsiness, tingling or numbness, vision problems or balance problems, as confirmed by a neurologist. Each episode must have lasted at least 24 hours and occurred at different times at least 1 month apart.

2. In addition, a positive diagnosis requires symptoms that indicate injury to more than one part of the central nervous system, together with confirmatory magnetic resonance imaging (MRI) and laboratory tests with findings consistent with a diagnosis of MS.

MRI scans can be used to reveal lesions or plaques in the brain and a lumbar puncture may be done to evaluate the cerebrospinal fluid. MS sufferers tend to have a raised white blood cell count and abnormal levels of immunoglobulin.

Medical treatment

Pharmacology

Many MS patients do not require drug therapy; however, it is an incurable condition, and in order to manage acute episodes or specific symptoms some medication may be introduced.

Drugs to modify the disease are aimed at reducing the frequency and severity of relapses. Most commonly used are forms of interferon, given intrathecally, intramuscularly or subcutaneously.

Interferon has antiviral and immunomodulatory properties and is used because it is thought that MS may have a viral origin.

The mechanism of action of interferon-β1b in MS is not clearly understood, but is thought to involve immunoregulatory activities, including enhancing the suppressor activity of peripheral blood mononuclear cells. In a recent study looking at patients with a single clinical event suggestive of MS, the relative risk of clinically definite (CD) MS was reduced by 41% in those receiving interferon-β1b 250 μg every other day for 3 years (early-treatment group) compared with patients who were initially randomized to placebo then switched to interferon-β1b 250 μg every other day at the end of 2 years or at the onset of CD MS (delayed-treatment group) ($P < 0.01$). [5]. Thus there is some evidence that early doses of this particular type of interferon may be helpful in preventing further development of symptoms in some patients, but much more work is needed [6].

Surgery

Surgery is not commonly used in MS but in cases of very severe tremor deep-brain stimulation can be tried with implantation of a device within the brain, as in Parkinson's disease. In cases of disabling or painful spasticity a catheter or pump can be surgically placed in the lower spinal area to deliver a constant flow of medication, such as baclofen (Lioresal).

Prognosis

As has been discussed previously, there is a wide variation in symptoms and eventual outcome. Most people with MS will have a normal life expectancy but a small percentage may have infectious complications such as pneumonia, thus increasing the possibility of earlier death.

It has been suggested that those who experience few attacks after diagnosis with longer intervals between them, experiencing principally sensory damage, loss of vision and numbness, will tend to remain less disabled. This is referred to as the 'relapsing, remitting' form of the disease. Those patients with symptoms of tremor, poor coordination and difficulty walking, resolving only partially, within the first 5 years after diagnosis will not do so well.

There are some known triggers which can aggravate symptoms and these include fever, infection, high temperature and humidity and emotional trauma.

MS and physiotherapy

Physiotherapists are closely involved in the support and rehabilitation of MS patients, constantly seeking a way to reduce the disabling physical symptoms, treat pain and maximize mobility and independent living. In the last two aspects they work closely with occupational therapists. Physiotherapists usually work as part of a specialized team but will contribute their skills to tackling the following problems.

Fatigue

Contributing factors such as loss of sleep, poor diet or lack of aerobic exercise will be assessed.

Weakness and cardiorespiratory fitness

Patients are encouraged to undertake exercise targeted to their motor problems, allowing for any mobility problems.

Spasticity and spasms

Simple causative problems or aggravating factors such as pain or infection should be tackled. Passive stretching can be applied to the affected muscle groups and often families and carers are taught how to do this.

Contractures affecting joints

Specific positioning when at rest and gentle stretches should be continued to prevent contractures. Again, teaching the family is helpful.

If there is no response then splinting and serial casting may be tried.

Ataxia and tremor

Treatment techniques similar to those used in Parkinson's disease may be helpful. Pharmacological support may eventually be necessary.

Sensory losses, including visual problems

Where these affect mobility and daily activities, solutions will be sought, involving new ways of doing things.

Pain and other problems

Musculoskeletal pain

Primary musculoskeletal pain may occur in this group of patients as in any other population group. Exercises, passive movement, better seating or pain-relieving modalities such as heat, massage, transcutaneous electrical nerve stimulation or, indeed, acupuncture may be used.

Neuropathic pain

This is characterized by its sharp or shooting nature and may encompass allodynia or painful sensitivity to normal stimuli.

Cognitive loss

This may manifest as a difficulty in learning and remembering exercise routines and may mean patient compliance is a problem.

Depression, anxiety or emotionalism

These are not normally part of the physiotherapist's remit but are very important with regard to patient compliance. Treatment in specialist centres can be very helpful.

Swallowing or speech difficulties

These are usually dealt with by speech and language therapists but physiotherapists may help with secondary muscles or positioning for swallowing.

Pressure sores

These are the responsibility of the whole team and gentle movement, positioning, correct seating and prevention of contractures will all help to prevent this complication.

The above summaries are based on the suggestions by the National Collaborating Centre for Chronic Conditions in the National Institute for Health and Clinical Excellence guidelines.

Advice on complementary therapies is fairly unhelpful, suggesting that all patients try them out for themselves but recommending nothing in particular. An update is surely due [7].

Acupuncture research in MS

Acupuncture has been recommended as a safe alternative intervention for pain relief in MS [8]. However there remains a question as to whether muscle spasm is sometimes made briefly worse by deep needling [9].

There have been two systematic reviews of acupuncture in general neurology [10, 11]; both reports have concluded that the studies included showed no definitive data on the use of acupuncture for MS, although there might be a positive influence on the secondary symptoms. However, Hopwood & White [12] advise caution in reading systematic reviews, stating the review quality and conclusions depend on the research work included, mentioning in particular the difficulties facing researchers in adequately controlling acupuncture trials. Some qualitative work, including that by Pucci et al. [13], indicates that the use of acupuncture by MS patients is quite high and 61.5% of the patients interviewed in the Pucci study claimed that acupuncture was beneficial.

Acupuncture has been found to have a consistently beneficial effect on insomnia, although the quality of studies has been variable [14]. Auricular acupuncture for insomnia has also been investigated [15], offering moderately positive evidence for acupuncture. The auricular points used were mainly in the helix so could indeed have affected the parasympathetic nervous system and thus provided a calming effect. These were not investigations specific to MS but they are relevant.

A recent review of the use of complementary therapies in MS included acupuncture [16] and patients described it as generally relaxing but also a treatment which increased their energy and feelings of well-being. More specifically they said it reduced pain, increased flexibility, improved balance and reduced recovery time from relapses. The text does not offer information on the type of acupuncture given but it is likely to be of the traditional type as Western health professionals do not generally include acupuncture in the 'black box' of therapies for MS yet.

Acupuncture treatment for MS

Considering the symptoms in Table 8.1, it is clear that acupuncture may be able to affect most of them.

Body acupuncture

Body points can be selected according to local symptoms or according to the organ system that seems to be affected at the time. MS patients are subject to a considerable variation in severity of symptoms, and remissions and exacerbations are characteristic of the disease. A minimal selection of the appropriate points is necessary as overtreatment is very easy and patients can often be quite exhausted by their acupuncture treatment (Table 8.2). Needling is generally applied to the affected limbs.

Scalp acupuncture

This is occasionally used in MS but has no research evidence to support it. Logically, work on the motor or sensory cortical lines could be helpful when

Table 8.1 Symptom picture for multiple sclerosis

Symptom	Characteristic presentation	Multiple sclerosis
Decreased mobility	Rigidity	o
Fatigue	Lack of energy	o o
Pain		X
Muscle spasm	Tremor	o
Contractures	Stiffness and rigidity	o
Autonomic changes	Slowing circulation	o o
Cognition/ mood	Apathy Depression	o
Communication		o
Bladder problems		o
Constipation		o

X, usually absent; o, common; o o, very frequent.

Table 8.2 Multiple sclerosis – useful points

Symptoms	Points	Rationale	Comments
Postural changes Dropped-head syndrome	GV 22, BL 6, GB 17 GB 10	Extrapyramidal effect	Hard to influence
Cold, empty sensation in the back Poor posture	GV 20, Moxa to GV 4, KI 3 or BL 13, BL 20, BL 23, BL 24	Du meridian empty Local treatment	Postural hypotension Use for pain or fatigue in back
Trigeminal neuralgia	SI 18, SI 3	Local stimulus Can be used bilaterally	LI 4 could be used as an alternative distal point
Uncoordinated movement	GV 20	Regulation of central nervous system	Add Sishencong
Fatigue or paresis in upper limbs	LI 15, LI 11, LI 10, TE 5 and LI 4	Similar to treatment for CVA sequelae	Gentle low-frequency electroacupuncture with a perceptible muscle twitch may be helpful
Fatigue or paresis in lower limbs	ST 31, ST 32, SP 10, ST 36, GB 34, ST 40, GB 39, LR 3	Similar to treatment for CVA sequelae	
Muscle spasm	LR 3 and SI 3+ Distal points for pain	Same myotome or nerve distribution	Prevent contractures by careful positioning
Contractures	As above KI 1 can be used without needles	Minor Chakra. Used bilaterally for adduction flexion contractures of lower limb	Light finger pressure only
Depression	Four Gates HT 7 with KI 3 Ear Shenmen Sishencong Yintang	To lift the spirits and generally soothe and calm the psyche	Liver/Heart/Du influence
Night sweats	HT 6 and KI 7	Clears false Heat	
Insomnia	Ear Shenmen Insomnia points Extra points Anmian 1 and Anmian 2	Specific body points	Parasympathetic effects from the ear
Cold and painful upper limbs	TE 6	Local point	Treats poor circulation
Cold and painful lower limbs	SP 10, ST 31	Circulation points	Treats poor circulation
Slow general circulation	Moxa to BL 17 Geshu	For general circulation	Ren 6, Qihai, can be used to support body Qi
Emotional lability	PE 6, HT 7 ST 36, TE 5	Inappropriate expression of emotion	Calm Spirit Free the Jing Luo flow
Involuntary tremor	LR 3 and SI 3	Muscle tremor	Muscle weakness

Table 8.2 Multiple sclerosis – useful points—cont'd

Symptoms	Points	Rationale	Comments
Palpitation	HT 7, PE 6, CV 17	Cardiac arrhythmia	
Irregular bowels	CV 4, ST 25, LI 11 TE 5 TE 6	Effect on Jin Ye circulation	Sometimes a drug side-effect
Incontinence or urinary retention	ST 36, SP 6, SP 9 BL 23, BL 28, K 3, BL 40 CV 3	Activate Jin Ye circulation, decrease damp, support Kidney	Actual cause needs investigation Bladder or Zang Fu?
Fatigue	Any of the stimulating points Possible use of extra meridians	General acupuncture effects	Use in moderation, little surplus energy
Feeling of 'disconnection' between upper and lower halves of the body	GB 41 and TE 5	Dai Mai extra meridian (Girdle vessel)	Use with caution, low reserves of energy in multiple sclerosis

CVA, cerebrovascular accident.

treating changes in limb function. Jiao Shunfa has made anecdotal claims that scalp acupuncture can help with pain, paralysis and vertigo in MS [17].

TCM approach

Traditional Chinese medicine (TCM) offers an apparently complex approach to what is a complex disease process but when considered as separate and distinct stages the syndrome theories can be easily applied. The most commonly adopted TCM staging for MS was originated by British acupuncturists Blackwell and MacPherson [18] and offers a logical framework for treatment.

MS can be considered as four stages (Table 8.3): the first stage is remission, either before the disease process has really started or, far more likely, as an interval where symptoms recede and a near-normal state is regained.

The second stage is where the meridian symptoms predominate and the patient is aware of sensory or minor motor changes.

As the disease progresses, evidence of Zang Fu organ failure becomes apparent, with the patient now feeling fatigued and often ill. Chinese theory holds that MS is fundamentally an invasion of Damp Heat and this will begin to affect the Stomach,

Table 8.3 Staging of multiple sclerosis

Stage 1	Stage 2
Remission	Meridian problem Support Spleen and Stomach

Stage 3	Stage 4
Spleen Qi Xu Liver Blood Xu	Kidney Xu

Spleen and Liver, leading to a mixed picture of symptoms. Ultimately this internal state will affect Kidney energy and the final picture in the fourth stage is that of a serious Kidney energy deficit.

This is an infinitely variable process and, fortunately, many patients do not reach stage 4, perhaps not even stage 3. However the aim of acupuncture is to treat and support the evident problems in the current stage and return the patient to the stage preceding.

Stage 1: remission

For the sake of clarity, it is assumed that in a remission stage there are no active symptoms so the only therapy required will be preventive. Since the patient is undergoing a major disease process, support for the Stomach and Spleen will be useful, allowing the regenerative processes of the body full support from nutrition and digestion. Also in this stage it is useful to emphasize lifestyle advice, attention to diet generally, relaxation and rest when appropriate, and some form of recreational exercise.

Stage 2: external channel problem

Often there is a sudden onset, sometimes preceded by an emotional trauma. The symptoms are acute in nature and appear to be caused by Damp Phlegm or Damp Heat in the meridians, possibly originally caused by an invasion of Cold Damp.

The symptoms include weakness, heaviness, tingling and numbness in the extremities, cold limbs, and aching in the back or shoulders. Quite often patients complain of vertigo, blurred or double vision. The tongue has a greasy white coating, indicating Damp, and the pulse is slippery or empty.

Points to be used include: Zhongwan CV 12, Fenglong ST 40, Sanyinjiao SP 6, Yinlingquan SP 9, Pishu BL 20 and Zusanli ST 36. Blockages in the meridians causing local problems such as numbness in the feet should be dealt with by inclusion of local points such as Bafeng.

Stage 2: moving inwards (Damp Heat invades and obstructs channels)

This indicates a progression of the disease and the symptoms may now include numbness in the lower limbs with accompanying weakness, slackness of joints and gravitational oedema. The whole body feels heavy and the legs may feel cold, although the feet may feel hot. The joints are often painful. The patient does not react well to heat and may complain of tightness of the chest. Occasionally there is fever with frequent, urgent, dark yellow urine. The tongue is greasy with a yellow coat and the pulse is rapid and slippery.

Points to be used include Dazhui GV 4, Hegu LI 4, Yinlingquan SP 9 and Taibai SP 3. Plum blossom needling can be used to influence stagnation over the Huatuojiaji points, and other points for local, superficial symptoms should still be included.

(Plum blossom or seven star needling uses a flexible 6-inch (15-cm) hammer with a group of short

Table 8.4 Damp in the channels changing to Liver Blood Xu

Damp affecting the channels	Liver blood deficiency
Widespread numbness	Extremities numb and tingling
Heavy, aching limbs	Stiff limbs, increased muscle tone
Variable onset and progression	Slow gradual onset
Continuous symptoms	Symptoms much worse when the patient is tired
Emotions mostly unchanged, possible depression with generally low motivation	Either apathetic or anxious with tight, brittle emotions
Pulse full or normal	Pulse choppy or thready

needles on the head. The skin is lightly tapped in order to produce an erythema over the area.)

Blackwell and MacPherson [18] offer a helpful differentiation between stages 2 and 3 (Table 8.4).

Stage 3: Middle Jiao involvement

This tends to be the stage that is most often seen by physiotherapy services. All the preceding symptoms may be present, the resulting disability cannot be ignored and the patient seeks help. In TCM terms the production of Qi and Blood by the Spleen is now diminishing, resulting in deficiency. The retention of Damp in the system weakens the Spleen further, initiating a vicious circle.

The Zang Fu organs of the Middle Jiao will need support, starting with the Spleen but progressing to the Liver.

Stage 3.1: Spleen Qi Xu

The symptoms include tiredness, listlessness, flaccidity of muscles and a tendency to fatigue. The patient may have a poor appetite and a pale sallow complexion and suffer from bowel problems, in particular loose stools. The tongue will be swollen and tooth-marked and the pulse empty, thin and weak.

Points to be used include Zusanli ST 36, Taibai SP 3, Zhangmen LR 3, Weishu BL 21, Sanyinjiao SP 6, Zhongwan CV 12 and Pishu BL 20. As usual,

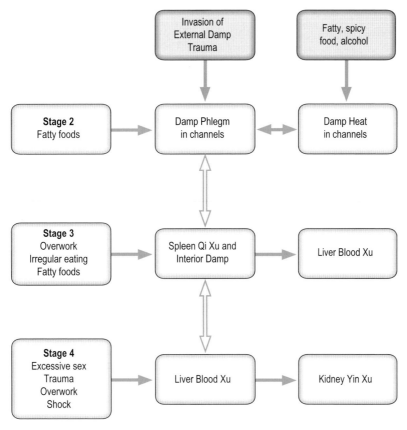

Figure 8.1 • Moving through the stages of multiple sclerosis in traditional Chinese medicine terms. After Blackwell and MacPherson [18].

add points to deal with superficial or channel problems as necessary. Figure 8.1 shows how the different syndromes which may be present are interlinked and interdependent.

Stage 3: Liver Blood Xu

The symptoms include blurred vision, always worse when tired, and a pale dull face. There may be muscle stiffness with cramps, spasticity and mild tremor.

The tongue will tend to be pale and dry and the pulse thin and choppy.

Points that can be used include Zusanli ST 36, Ququan LR 8, Geshu BL 17, Pishu BL 20, Sanyinjiao SP 6, Guanyuan CV 4 and Ganshu BL 18. As before, use local points for superficial symptoms.

Stage 4: Kidney Xu

In this stage the problem is predominantly one of Kidney deficiency and is characterized by weakness, fatigue and emaciation. Both Yin and Yang Kidney need tonification. The chronic Spleen Qi Xu depletes the Kidney Yang and the chronic Liver Blood Xu depletes both Kidney Jing and Kidney Yin.

Symptoms include severe weakness and fatigue. The patient often appears spiritless and there may be a pale complexion and premature ageing. Muscle weakness and atrophy are likely to be marked. Stiffness and muscle spasm are also common with severe tremor and ataxia. Low-back pain is often very distressing but it will be useful to check the wheelchair provision as well as using acupuncture. When a patient spends long periods of time in a chair it is essential to make sure the chair fits correctly. Other symptoms are urinary urgency, incontinence or retention. The tongue will be pale and wet and the pulse weak.

Points to use include Taixi KI 3, Shenshu BL 23, Xuanzhong GB 39, Guanyuan CV 4, Ciliao BL 32. Mingmen GV 4 is added for Kidney Yang Xu and Zhaohai KI 6 for Kidney Yin Xu (Figure 8.2).

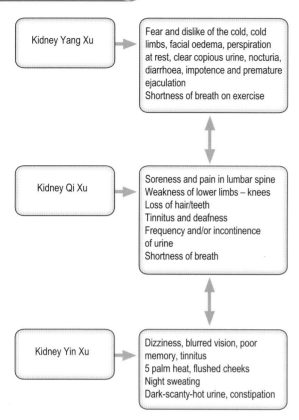

Figure 8.2 • Differentiation of kidney syndromes.

Summary

The use of acupuncture points in stages 1 and 2 will be indicated by the local symptoms but will tend to be distal. In stage 3, support is needed for the organs: ST36, SP 6, LR 3 plus back Shu points. In stage 4 use back Shu points and Kidney points, particularly KI 3.

Other syndromes which may occur in MS

Qi and blood deficiency

Poor or absent circulation of Qi and Blood is seen in TCM as the cause of both pain and also poor movement ability. The blockage may in fact be caused by early manifestations of Phlegm Heat (see below). Local points on the most affected limbs will also be useful.

Common symptoms are: chronic tremor of a limb or limbs, sallow complexion reluctant speech and lack of facial expression. Also found are stiff neck, cold painful limbs, general poverty of movement, unsteady gait with difficulty in taking the first step, dizziness and blurred vision.

Treatment

Tonify Qi, nourish Blood, energize the meridians and dispel Wind.

- ST 36 Zusanli tonifies Qi and Blood.
- SP 6 Sanyinjiao tonifies Qi and Blood.
- LR 8 Ququan nourishes Liver Blood.
- CV 4 Guanyuan nourishes Blood generally.
- SP 10 Xuehai improves Blood circulation in the lower limb.

Phlegm Heat agitating Wind (affecting Liver)

There are three different syndromes associated with the stirring of Liver Wind. They can be caused by:

1. internal heat, caused by penetration of an exogenous pathogen to the interior. This is characterized by serious febrile diseases in children, e.g. measles or meningitis.
2. inability of the deficient liver Yin to control the liver Yang with subsequent internal Wind symptoms (more associated with Parkinson's disease)
3. deficiency of Liver Blood [19].

Treatment for all three will aim to subdue the Liver Wind, which can be very dangerous, frequently leading to Wind Stroke or cerebrovascular accident. Otherwise the Liver energies need controlling or tonifying according to whether the underlying symptoms exhibit excess or deficiency. The prevention of stroke depends on getting this balance correct but it will not really affect or prevent the onset of Parkinson's disease or MS.

Liver Wind is often associated with hypertension, stroke, epilepsy and trigeminal neuralgia (often found in the later stages of MS). It may be exacerbated by prolonged frustration or anger, both of which are said to damage the Liver. It is also linked to obesity and a lack of physical exercise.

The symptoms include vertigo, tremor, convulsions, muscle spasms and stiff neck. Facial paralysis, tinnitus and hemiplegia may also be present.

Treatment

Calm Liver. Disperse Wind.

- LR 2 Xingjian Fire point disperses fire in the Liver.
- LR 3 Taichong Liver Source point. Balances Liver, moves Qi.
- GB 20 Fengchi expels Wind.
- BL 18 Ganshu Back Shu point for the Liver.
- LI 4 Hegu expels Wind. Used for face and neck.
- GV 20 Baihui used to calm the Liver and expel Wind.
- KI 3 Taixi tonifies Kidney Yin and Yang.
- KI 7 Fuliu tonifies both Kidney and Liver.
- BL 23 Shenshu Back Shu point for the kidneys.

Liver and Kidney Yin deficiency

This situation is often the precursor to Liver Yang rising. If the cooling Yin of the Liver is depleted the Yang becomes hyperactive and rises upwards, producing the symptoms of headache, dry eyes and tinnitus. The Heat also causes irritability and anger, emotions damaging to the Liver. This syndrome is a combination of both excess and deficiency, although the excess symptoms seem more obvious.

Liver Yang rising is a fairly common pattern and will be mentioned again in this book as it is closely associated with neurological damage. Stress, frustration, anger and resentment build up over a long period of time, obstructing the free flow of liver Qi. This produces heat, which dries up Yin. Yin thus cannot control Yang, which rises to the head. In contrast, the person could be relatively cool in the lower part of the body.

Symptoms will include: general frailty, dizziness, tinnitus, insomnia, headache, night sweats, low-back pain, stiff neck, back and knees and mental restlessness. Often also present will be lack of facial expression, poor memory and general physical clumsiness.

Treatment

Nourish Yin, dispel Wind, energize the meridians.
- CV 4 Guanyuan supports Kidney Yin
- BL 23 Shenshu Back Shu point for the Kidneys
- KI 3 Taixi nourishes Kidney Yin

- SP 6 Sanyinjiao nourishes Kidney Yin
- BL 18 Ganshu Back Shu point for the Liver
- LR 8 Ququan nourishes Liver Yin
- LR 3 Taichong Liver source point. Balances Liver, moves Qi.

Summary

Acupuncture treatment for MS seems to be endlessly complex but in reality follows the pattern of symptoms very closely, with Western medical acupuncture probably being most appropriate for the motor and sensory problems involving the limbs and the TCM theories more apposite when tackling the underlying disease process. It characterizes the best way of tackling most neurological conditions with acupuncture.

When deciding how best to organize treatment sessions, it must be borne in mind that MS patients can easily be overtreated and will become very fatigued after just a few points. Do not leave the needles in too long and limit the points used. Also remember the relapse/remission character of the disease and try to arrange for your patients to be able to refer themselves for more treatment immediately, if a relapse occurs.

Case study 8.1: level 1 case study

The patient was a 47-year-old woman, diagnosed with MS 4 years previously. She was still active and in part-time employment. She had a weak leg and forearm on the left side but she was generally mobile, normally using only a stick to help with her walking. She had a wheelchair to help when she was ill or particularly fatigued.

She presented for treatment in the wheelchair saying both her feet felt 'funny' and that she was afraid to walk as she felt as though she was 'walking in soft sand'. She had previously had successful acupuncture for a painful shoulder.

Impression

She had a local exacerbation of MS symptoms: Damp Heat in the meridians affecting the lower limbs. Apart from the changed sensation her legs were stiff and cold.

Treatment

Points used: Bilateral Bafeng and GB 34. This was kept simple in order to minimize fatigue. The needles were only left in for 10 minutes the first time.

She returned in 2 days and the treatment was repeated for 20 minutes as she had had no ill effects the first time. After the second treatment she said the strange sensation was going, the ground no longer felt soft but she was hesitant to leave the wheelchair.

Results

After three more treatments she attended for treatment using only the stick again and said her feet felt quite normal now. The range of knee and ankle movement and the skin temperature had returned to normal.

This woman returned for treatment about 6 months later with the same problem. It had come back after a holiday abroad where the weather had been particularly hot. It was resolved again after four treatments.

This was clearly not a cure, but the strong sensory stimulation provided by the Bafeng combination of points seemed to produce temporary relief of her symptoms.

Case study 8.2: level 3 case study

The patient

A 50-year-old female was referred to the community neurorehab team following a 6-month history of declining mobility, increase in muscle spasms and right leg pain causing falls at home. She had been diagnosed with relapsing-remitting MS several years previously, and stopped work 4 years after diagnosis. Prior to this deterioration, she lived alone and was independently self-caring. She took her dog for at least one walk daily, and was dependent on a friend only for shopping. She used an electric wheelchair and an adapted car and could walk up to 50 metres with two crutches.

Medications included baclofen 15 mg four times a day and tramadol as needed.

Assessment

Her main problems, due to the right leg pain and increase in right leg muscle spasms, were reported as:

- disturbed sleep
- daily falls
- unable to drive
- increased difficulty standing from armchair
- increased difficulty standing to cook meals.

Objective assessment revealed the following:

- right hip: 40° extension from neutral, severe pain at end of range active or passive movement
- tender on palpation all quadriceps muscles, with palpable taut bands of trigger points (TPs) in muscle bellies
- unable to lie prone due to pain
- right knee 20° extension, pain at end of range passive stretch
- right ankle: 15° dorsiflexion from plantigrade
- standing hips and knees flexed
- hips adducted
- right heel off ground
- mobility: only able to manage up to 5 metres due to pain; used upper limbs and elbow crutches to propel flexed legs forward
- function: slow, but independent with all transfers in the home.

Pain was made worse by standing for more than 5 minutes, or standing after sitting. Yoga helps; pain is worst in the evening, the patient has difficulty sleeping. Referrals were made to social services for meals on wheels, morning care, shopping and cleaning and to wheelchair services to review for an indoor wheelchair.

Impression

The patient's function was limited by pain caused by active TPs in the right quadriceps muscles due to underlying increase in lower-limb flexor muscle tone as the patient's MS progressed.

Treatment

Pain relief was the primary aim of treatment, with a view to review mobility indoors with crutches if pain and muscle spasms decreased.

Initially, treatment focused on deactivating the TP in the quadriceps muscles to provide pain relief for the right hip. Manual palpation of the TP caused severe pain so acupuncture was chosen as the treatment of choice for TP release, as manual release techniques would have been too painful.

See below for details of the first two treatments, focusing on local hip points for pain relief and deactivating quadriceps muscle TPs.

Treatment 1

5 minutes in left side lying.
Points: GB 30 Rt, GB 34 Rt, GB 39 bilateral + 4 TPs in quadriceps muscles.

Treatment 2

2 days later, 10 minutes in supine.
Points: GB 34 Rt, +7 TPs in quadriceps muscles.
Research has reported that treating patients with MS with acupuncture provoked spasms, clonus and even tonic-clonic muscle contractions of the extremity muscles [20]. Similarly, this patient experienced an increase in right leg flexor spasms during acupuncture, perhaps because a deep insertion was used, making the treatment very uncomfortable. This made it too difficult to insert needles on the anterior of the hip (such as at ST 31), and the needles were removed after 5 minutes of the first treatment.

There was some limited response but it was decided that a TCM approach utilizing the extra meridians might be more successful. The Conception Vessel meridian was used for pain on the anterior surface of the body, the Governor Vessel meridian to help the back and central nervous system, the Dai Mai to treat pain in the lower half of the body and the Chong Mai to help general circulation.

Treatment 3

3 days later; 15 minutes treatment in supine. LU 7 and KI 6 bilateral

Treatment 4

4 days later; repeated treatment +BL 62 (opening point for GV meridian)
The patient continued with treatment twice a week and eventually had eight treatments, during which the opening points for the extra meridians, GV, CV, Dai Mai and Chong Mai were slowly added. Thus by the last treatment the eight points used in diagonal were:

- LU 7 / KI 6
- BL 62 / SI 3
- GB 41 / TE 5
- SP 4 / PE 6, never left for longer than 20 minutes.

Deqi was achieved at all points and manual stimulation of the needles approximately every 5 minutes during treatment helped to maintain this.

Only a minimal increase in right leg flexor spasms was noted during acupuncture using distal points only.

Table 8.5 gives details of pre- and posttreatment measures for right hip pain. As can be seen from Table 8.1, acupuncture provided good temporary pain relief, lasting between 1 and 3 days. Some of the acupuncture-induced analgesia was maintained over the course of treatment. The client reported the worst pain was 40/100 on completion of the course of acupuncture, a 50% reduction from the worst pain experienced before acupuncture treatment commenced.

Table 8.5 Outcomes for each acupuncture treatment in case study 8.2

Treatment	VAS pretreatment	VAS posttreatment	Length of pain relief
1	80/100	40/100	1 day
2	60/100	25/100	2 days
3	60/100	40/100	2 days
4	70/100	20/100	3 days
5	50/100	40/100	2 days
6	45/100	30/100	2 days
7	40/100	30/100	2 days
8	40/100	30/100	2 days

VAS, visual analogue scale.

References

[1] Gilmore CP, Donaldson I, Bo L, et al. Regional variations in the extent and pattern of grey matter demyelination in multiple sclerosis: a comparison between the cerebral cortex, cerebellar cortex, deep grey matter nuclei and the spinal cord. J Neurol Neurosurg Psychiatry 2009;80(2):182–7.

[2] Hirst C, Swingler R, Compston DA, et al. Survival and cause of death in multiple sclerosis: a prospective population-based study. J Neurol Neurosurg Psychiatry 2008;79(9):1016–21.

[3] Callander M, Landtblom AM. A cluster of multiple sclerosis cases in Lysvik in the Swedish county of Värmland. Acta Neurol Scand 2004;110(1):14–22.

[4] Peterli B, Ristic S, Sepcic J, et al. Region with persistent high frequency of multiple sclerosis in Croatia and Slovenia. J Neurol Sci 2006;247(2):169–72.

[5] McKeage K. Interferon-beta-1b: in newly emerging multiple sclerosis. CNS Drugs 2008;22(9):787–92.

[6] Rojas JI, Romano M, Ciapponi A, et al. Interferon beta for primary progressive multiple sclerosis. Cochrane Database Syst Rev 2009; (1).

[7] NICE. Management of multiple sclerosis in primary and secondary care. National Collaborating Centre for Chronic Conditions, editor. Clinical Guideline 2003;8: 13-6-0009.

[8] van den Noort S, Holland NJ. Multiple Sclerosis in Clinical Practice. New York: Demos Medical Publishing; 1999.

[9] Donnellan CP, Shanley J. Comparison of the effect of two types of acupuncture on quality of life in secondary progressive multiple sclerosis: a preliminary single-blind randomized controlled trial. Clin Rehabil 2008;22(3): 195–205.

[10] Lee H, Park HJ, Park J, et al. Acupuncture application for neurological disorders. Neurol Res 2007;29(Suppl. 1).S49–54.

[11] Rabinstein AA, Shulman LM. Acupuncture in clinical neurology. Neurologist 2003;9(3):137–48.

[12] Hopwood V, White P. Poor reviews may not give a true reflection of the evidence. Physiotherapy 2001;87:549–51.

[13] Pucci E, Cartechini E, Taus C, et al. Why physicians need to look more closely at the use of complementary and alternative medicine by multiple sclerosis patients. Eur J Neurol 2004;11 (4):263–7.

[14] Kalavapalli R, Singareddy R. Role of acupuncture in the treatment of insomnia: A comprehensive review. Complement Ther Clin Pract 2007;13(3):184–93.

[15] Sjoling M, Rolleri M, Englund E. Auricular acupuncture versus sham acupuncture in the treatment of women who have insomnia. J Altern Complement Medicine (New York, NY) 2008;14(1): 39–46.

[16] Esmonde L, Long AF. Complementary therapy use by persons with multiple sclerosis: Benefits and research priorities. Complement Ther Clin Pract 2008;14(3):176–84.

[17] Jiao S. Scalp Acupuncture and Clinical Cases. Beijing: Foreign Languages Press; 1997.

[18] Blackwell R, MacPherson H. Multiple sclerosis. Staging and patient management. J Chin Med 1993;42:5–12.

[19] Maciocia G. The Practice of Chinese Medicine. Churchill Livingstone: Edinburgh; 1994.

[20] Steinberger A. Specific irritability of acupuncture points as an early symptom of multiple sclerosis. Am J Chin Med 1986;14(3–4):175–8.

Spinal cord injury and disease

9

KEY POINTS

- Spinal cord injury is both a serious and complex event treated intensively in physiotherapy departments, but with long-term support as the goal.
- Some of the residual problems will respond to acupuncture.
- Some of the side-effects produced by drug therapy will also respond to acupuncture.
- Treatment will be a mixture of traditional Chinese medicine and Western theory but since prognosis is so dependent on level of injury (or inflammation damage, as in transverse myelitis), often a Western approach is more helpful.

Part 1: Spinal cord injury (SCI)

This is clearly a devastating event which can have a major effect on the quality of the future existence of the patient. A complex neural network involved in transmitting, coordinating and modifying the sensory, motor and autonomic signals is abruptly disrupted.

Definition

SCI is defined in several ways; most simply, it is defined by the resulting loss of function. Paraplegia is the impairment or loss of motor, sensory or autonomic function of thoracic, lumbar or sacral segments of the spinal cord. Upper-limb function is spared but the trunk, pelvis and lower limbs will be affected.

Tetraplegia or quadriplegia will show similar damage, affecting the upper limbs as well. In high cervical lesions respiration will also be impaired.

Incidence and mortality

SCIs affect only a small percentage of the population, with a male-to-female ratio of 5:1. A total of 17.2 people per million of the population in Europe suffer a traumatic SCI and 8.2 per million experience a non-traumatic SCI (figures from 2001: [1]).

Risk factors

It is difficult to describe these causes as 'risk' exactly because this injury is so often the result of an accident: about 80% of SCIs are due to trauma. Gunshots and stabbings can cause this type of damage and falling from a height, whether accidentally or deliberately, is also a cause. However diseases where there is degeneration of the spinal structures such as cervical spondylosis also contribute to the statistics.

Diagnosis and prognosis

Diagnosis is dependent upon the completeness of the lesion and must take into account the infinite variations of this. Prognosis is irretrievably linked

Table 9.1 American Spinal Injuries Association (ASIA) impairment scale

A	Complete: no motor or sensory function is preserved in the sacral segments S4–S5
B	Incomplete: sensory but not motor function is preserved below the neurological level and extends through the sacral segments
C	Incomplete: motor function is preserved below the neurological level, and the majority of key muscles below this level have a muscle grade less than 3
D	Incomplete: motor function is preserved below the neurological level, and the majority of key muscles below this level have a muscle grade greater than or equal to 3
E	Normal: motor and sensory function is normal

with this. The most useful current classification is the American Spinal Injuries Association (ASIA) Impairment Scale (Table 9.1). This scale is reasonably predictive of diagnosis and makes for a logical subclassification of incomplete spinal column injuries into clinical syndromes:

- Central cord: upper limbs are more profoundly affected than the lower limbs. The condition is typically seen in older patients with cervical spondylosis. A hyperextension injury compresses the cord in a spinal canal that is already limited by osteophytes and other degenerative changes.
- Brown-Séquard: this is an incomplete lesion often affecting the cervical spinal. The hemisection damage to the cord is commonly caused by a stabbing injury, although it may result from infection or local inflammation. It is characterized by ipsilateral hemiplegia with contralateral pain and temperature sensation deficits. This is because of the crossing of the fibres of the spinothalamic tract. The associated morbidity and mortality will be related to the accompanying injuries. Morbidity is associated with the resulting paralysis whereas mortality may be the direct result of serious haemorrhage.
- Anterior cord syndrome: characterized by ventral cord damage affecting spinothalamic and corticospinal tracts. There is complete motor loss below the lesion and usually loss of pain and temperature sensation. Since the posterior tracts are preserved there will still be some proprioception and vibratory perception.

Motor recovery is generally poor unless evident within the first 24 hours.

- Conus medullaris and cauda equina syndromes are quite similar in that they offer a confusing mixture of signs and symptoms. The conus medullaris is the distal part of the spinal cord and injuries to this area often produce a mixture of upper motor neurone (UMN) and lower motor neurone (LMN) symptoms. Cauda equina lesions are predominantly LMN since they affect the peripheral nervous system [2].

Medical treatment

Early interventions

A recent study by Tederko et al. [3] came to the following conclusions:

> The primary zone of traumatic spinal damage enlarges due to local vascular disturbances, hypoxia, and the resulting inflammation. Secondly, inflammation in the region of secondary injury, apart from having a destructive impact, is the source of substances which may induce neural tissue repair, and finally the administration of methylprednisolone and surgical decompression of the spinal cord within several hours after SCI improves functional and neurological outcomes in patients with incomplete neurological deficits.

There are a number of things that must be checked and corrected, if possible, in the first 24–48 hours after injury. Haemorrhage from associated injuries must be dealt with quickly. Sympathetic paralysis below the level of the lesion can lead to neurogenic shock and hypotension. Thromboembolism can be prevented by elastic stockings and low-dose anticoagulants. Initial bladder management usually involves catheterization.

Pharmacology

Methylprednisolone is given at the time of the acute injury for up to 48 hours as one of the strategies for neuroprotection [4].

Surgery

Surgery, other than that required to stabilize the fracture site, is relatively rare. If pressure sores become serious, with infection, slow healing or infected bone, then surgery will be indicated.

SCI and physiotherapy

The following is a list of common medical problems which will delay or impede rehabilitation but is by no means exhaustive:

- Respiratory difficulty in the early stages is dealt with by assisted coughing to clear secretions and breathing exercises to prevent atelectasis or infection.
- Pressure sores: denervated skin is at risk from pressure damage within 30 minutes of injury. This means that pressure care is most important in this group of patients and a vigilant watch is kept for any areas of reddened skin. Where the patient retains the ability, pressure lifting is taught, with the patient lifting the buttocks clear from the wheelchair or chair every 30 minutes.
- Unilateral lower-extremity swelling with associated deep-vein thrombosis (DVT): prophylaxis, wearing pressure stockings and mobilizing as early as possible may help to prevent this.
- General mobility and independence will be enhanced by strengthening the unaffected muscles and encouraging standing and wheelchair use.
- Heterotopic ossification with possible fractures: calcification occasionally occurs in UMN-disordered muscles and may be confused with a DVT as the signs are often swelling and local heat. Most patients experience a degree of osteoporosis 2 years after injury, probably due to long periods of immobilization. Extra care must be taken during transfers and, if weight-bearing standing is undertaken after a long period, careful work progressing with the use of a tilt table is necessary.
- Spasticity: this is a common problem depending on the level of injury. Lower vertebral injuries, from the level of T12 downwards, give rise to LMN injuries and are generally classified as peripheral nerve damage presenting with flaccid paralysis or muscle weakness only. UMN injury, at the level of T12 or above, will involve damage to the cord itself and may present with a varying amount of spasticity in affected muscles.
- Autonomic dysreflexia: hypertension produced by a dysfunction in the sympathetic nervous system. This reaction may include palpitations, sweating, headache, piloerection and capillary dilation above the level of the lesion. Autonomic dysreflexia can occur with any noxious stimulus such as bladder or rectal distension. If it occurs

during treatment, the patient should be sat up, given appropriate medication and the underlying cause treated. This hypertension can be sufficient to induce cerebral haemorrhage so it should always be treated as an emergency. Very mild symptoms can indicate the need for toileting.

• Pain: where pain is present initially, for instance in fractured ribs, treatment including the application of transcutaneous electrical nerve stimulation may be used. Common syndromes include mechanical instability, muscle spasm, visceral pain and central dysaesthesia

syndrome – pain associated with the central nervous system and spinothalamic pathways.

• Contractures and malposition of the joints will be prevented by passive movements daily through full range.

Given the complexity of the possible changes, a clear knowledge of anatomy and associated nerve roots is vital. In order to know what can reasonably be expected by way of recovery, accurate location of the level of the spinal cord lesion is very important. Table 9.2 offers the range of possible goals and should be considered in conjunction with Table 2.2 in Chapter 2.

Table 9.2 Functional goals of rehabilitation in relation to the level of spinal cord lesion

Level	Key muscle control	Movement	Functional goals
C1–C3	Sternocleidomastoid Upper trapezius Levator	Neck control	Ventilator-dependent Electric wheelchair Verbally independent
C4	C3 plus diaphragm	Shoulder shrug	Electric wheelchair Verbally independent
C5	Biceps Deltoid Rotator cuff Supinator	Elbow flexion, supination Shoulder flexion, abduction	Manual wheelchair with capstans Electric wheelchair for long distance Independent brushing Teeth/hair/feeding with feeding strap
C6	Extensor carpi radialis longus Extensor carpi radialis brevis Pronator teres	Wrist extension, pronation	Tenodesis grip Manual wheelchair Independent feeding, grooming, dressing top half, simple cooking Same-height transfers
C7	Triceps Latissimus dorsi Flexor digitorum, flexor carpi radialis, extensor digitorum	Elbow extension Finger flexion/ extension	Manual wheelchair
C8	All upper limbs except lumbricals, interossei	Limited fine finger movements	Manual wheelchair Full dexterity
T1–T5	Varying intercostals and back muscles	No lower-limb movements	Full wheelchair independence Orthotic ambulation
T6–T12	Abdominals	Trunk control	Orthotic/calliper ambulation
L1–L2	Psoas major Iliacus	Hip flexion	Calliper ambulation
L3–L4	Quadriceps Tibialis anterior	Knee extension Ankle dorsiflexion	Ambulation with orthoses and crutches/sticks
L5	Peronei	Eversion	Ambulation with relevant orthoses
S1–S5	Glutei, gastrocnemius Bladder, bowel, sexual function	Hip extension Ankle plantarflexion	Normal gait

Management of psychological issues will be necessary and must take place with the help of qualified personnel. However the use of acupuncture may be valuable as long as the other staff know that it is being used. Maintaining a positive approach with realistic expectations is essential but hard to do.

Acupuncture in SCI

The use of acupuncture under these circumstances is by no means common and there has been little research. Acupuncture has been considered for pain control, a logical enough application, and also for bladder control, which might cause more comment.

The studies have been small but suggestive of a positive role for acupuncture [5]. A group of 22 patients with SCI who experienced moderate to severe pain of at least 6 months' duration were given a course of 15 acupuncture treatments over a 7-week period. In a more general review of complementary therapies for SCI, Nayak et al. suggest that, while acupuncture may have a place in pain control, massage has been shown to be even better and is apparently rarely used [6].

The combination of acupuncture technique and 'moving cupping' (see Chapter 12) could be very useful.

The same research group also looked into the effect of acupuncture on autonomic dysreflexia [7], and decided that, although none of their – admittedly small – sample of 15 patients went on to develop symptoms of autonomic dysreflexia, three of the total did display an acute elevation of blood pressure, making it desirable to monitor this type of patient carefully in future.

Achieving bladder control is an important issue for both the patients and their carers and there has been a preliminary study which offered a role for acupuncture. The potential mechanism, through afferent stimulation at the same segmental level using the points CV 3 and CV 4 and also reflex stimulation of the splanchnic nerves at sacral level using BL 32, seems logical in both anatomical and traditional Chinese medicine (TCM) terms. The trial has been criticized for general lack of rigour but they did observe in post hoc analysis that those patients receiving acupuncture within the first 3 weeks did better with achieving bladder balance [8].

Body acupuncture

Acupuncture points, mainly on Yang meridians, can be used, as in all neurological diseases, to tackle the superficial musculoskeletal symptoms. Both pain and movement problems can be addressed. The points can be selected according to symptoms and Table 9.3 gives some of the alternatives.

Many problems are directly caused by the medical interventions and points for these have also been listed. Electroacupuncture may be used at some of the points; the recommended frequency for body points is 2 Hz while that for scalp points is 100 Hz, although they may be alternated.

As with all the conditions in this book, there is a danger of the list of acupoints becoming endless, so only the most specific points are given. These are selected for completeness from both Western medicine approaches and those more traditionally Chinese. Those that relate directly to the following TCM syndromes are also mixed in.

Scalp acupuncture

The authors have been unable to find any convincing evidence for the use of scalp acupuncture in SCI. There is some anecdotal evidence, provided by practitioners of Yamamoto New Scalp Acupuncture (YNSA), of success with neurological conditions, but this technique of scalp acupuncture is slightly different to the Chinese version (see Chapter 12) and has a very limited evidence base. The main claim seems to suggest a change in neuroplasticity.

TCM approach

TCM regards injury to the spinal column as a direct injury to the Du meridian; thus points associated with that meridian, such as SI 3 Houxi and BL 62 Shenmai, can be used. The Huatuojiaji points are seen as valuable, being closely situated as they are, and this fits well with the neuroanatomy of the problem. The Huatuojiaji points are described as being able to 'activate the primordial energy' in the Du meridian [9]. Generally one would not needle the Du points but some authorities recommend this, choosing points above and below the level of damage and combining these with Huatuojiaji points.

The paralysed state is seen as a combination of obstruction to the meridian and the sudden stagnation

Table 9.3 Spinal cord injury, transverse myelitis, spinal stroke – useful points

Symptoms	Points	Rationale	Comments
Neurogenic bladder	Ren 3, Ren 4, UB 32	Indicated by nerve roots	Used by Cheng et al. 1998 (7)
Depression	Four Gates Ht 7 Ear Shenmen Sishencong Yintang	To lift the spirits and generally soothe and calm the psyche	Liver/Heart/Du influence
Cold and painful upper limbs	SJ 6	Local point	Treats poor circulation
Cold and painful lower limbs	Sp10, St 31	Circulation points	Treats poor circulation
Slow general circulation	Moxa to BL 17 Geshu	For general circulation	Ren 6, Qihai, can be used to support body Qi
Restless-legs syndrome	St 36, GB 34, Sp 10	Qi boost in lower limbs	UB 57 and UB 56
Complex regional pain syndrome	Local points on the opposite side, after ear acupuncture	Avoid overstimulation of a 'full condition'	Obtain a parasympathetic response
'Constricting' sensations in the trunk	SI 3 and UB 62 or GB 41 and SJ 5	Activation of Dai Mai, Du	Transverse myelitis
Fatigue	Any of the stimulating points Possible use of extra meridians	General acupuncture effects	Use in moderation, little surplus

of the Qi/Blood circulation, thus depriving the four limbs of nutrients and limiting normal movement. Needling the back Shu points and powerful points on the limbs themselves can be helpful. Passive and active movements are seen as part of the therapy.

Normal applications of acupuncture for pain, muscle hypertonicity, respiratory discomfort, insomnia and anxiety will include the usual points.

The most likely TCM syndromes involved will be Qi and/or Blood deficiency and Liver and Kidney Yin deficiency [10].

In practical terms this means that the symptoms of these syndromes, described elsewhere in this book, can be tackled with acupuncture and have a chance of influencing the well-being of the patient.

Case study 9.1: level 1 case study: partial spinal cord injury

A 53-year-old woman presented with difficulty sleeping. She had sustained a traumatic partial SCI 5 months previously at the level of L2. She presented with lower-limb weakness, no ankle movement and impaired lower-limb sensation; the left side was worse than the right.

Functional ability

The patient was able to walk short distances with two sticks and bilateral ankle foot orthoses. She was able to complete simple daily activities independently; she needed assistance with shopping.

Presenting symptoms

She had difficulty sleeping; she had problems falling asleep as well as waking frequently during the night. Her tongue had a purplish hue.

Treatment

Physiotherapy to improve mobility.

Seven acupuncture treatments were provided over 4 weeks.

Points: Bilateral ST 36, LR 3, LI4, SP6, SP9.

Manual acupuncture for 25 minutes; stimulated initially for Deqi then again at 5-minute intervals.

Outcome

The patient experienced a rapid improvement in sleep quality after two treatments; these improvements were sustained at the end of the course of treatment. She also reported feeling generally better and 'more like her old self' since before the accident.

Part 2: Transverse myelitis

Definition

This is a neurological syndrome caused by inflammation of the spinal cord at a specific level. The inflammation may have many causes and may occur in isolation or be associated with another illness.

Incidence and mortality

Transverse myelitis can occur at any age, in adults and children, male or female. Conservative estimates of incidence per year vary from 1 to 5 per million population [11].

Risk factors

There are many possible causes, including viral infections, abnormal immune reactions or insufficient blood flow through the blood vessels located in the spinal cord. Transverse myelitis may also occur as a complication of syphilis, measles, Lyme disease and some vaccinations, including those for chickenpox and rabies. It can also occasionally develop in association with human immunodeficiency virus (HIV).

Diagnosis

Differential diagnosis

As with many neurological conditions, diagnosis depends more on eliminating other possibilities than anything definite.

Tests

Magnetic resonance imaging (MRI) scans can be used to rule out lesions outside the spinal cord and can sometimes show an inflammatory lesion within the cord. Lumbar puncture may be performed to obtain fluid for studies including a white cell count, cultures to check for infections and tests to check for abnormal stimulation of the immune system. An MRI of the brain may be performed to screen for lesions suggestive of multiple sclerosis, even though it has been suggested that some sufferers from transverse myelitis may develop multiple sclerosis. If none of these tests is convincing the patient is presumed to have idiopathic transverse myelitis.

Medical treatment

Corticosteroids may be used in the early stages in an attempt to decrease the inflammation.

Prognosis

Recovery is often good and should commence within 1–3 months after onset. It may be partial or can be complete but the prognosis is relatively poor if there is no sign by 3 months [12]. In fact most patients will make a reasonable recovery but there may be a tendency to relapse if there is underlying serious illness.

Impact on the patient

Almost all patients will develop leg weakness of varying degrees of severity. The arms are involved in a minority of cases and this is dependent upon the level of spinal cord involvement. Sensation is diminished below the level of spinal cord involvement in most patients. Some experience tingling or numbness in the legs. Pain sensation and temperature sensation are diminished in most patients. Appreciation of vibration (as caused by a tuning fork) and joint position sense may also be decreased or spared. Bladder and bowel sphincter controls are disturbed in most patients. Many patients with transverse myelitis report a tight banding or girdle-like sensation around the trunk and that area may be very sensitive to touch.

Transverse myelitis and physiotherapy

As there is currently no effective cure for transverse myelitis, all that can be offered to patients is a support system in order to:

- treat any underlying cause, if known
- halt the progression of the damage to the spinal cord
- offer strategies and further support to cope with the physical and psychological issues that may result.

The common medical problems which will have an effect on rehabilitation include pressure sores, unilateral lower-extremity swelling with associated DVT, heterotopic ossification, possible fractures, spasticity, autonomic dysreflexia, orthostatic hypotension and pain.

Acupuncture in transverse myelitis

This will follow previous patterns, for stroke or for SCI, utilizing points for specific symptoms or those at appropriate spinal levels. Where pain is a major symptom, acupuncture should be utilized.

There is no supporting research for acupuncture in this condition but a very detailed case report was published recently where acupuncture was used to treat sleep disturbance and support a rehabilitation programme [13].

TCM approach

It is worth noting that the symptoms described are quite explicit and sound very like those associated with problems affecting the extraordinary meridians.

Needling GB 41 and TE 5 bilaterally would be helpful in opening the Dai Mai and Yang Wei Mai and encouraging the descent of Yang energy. The Yang Wei Mai is considered as a secondary vessel to the Urinary Bladder meridian and is described as a network winding around the body, keeping the muscles tight [14]. Alternatively the Du and Yang Chiao Mai meridians could be used, associated with the central nervous system as they are. Use SI 3 and BL 62 bilaterally to open this pairing.

As with all the conditions in this book, the addition of sundry Yang points to deal with local/superficial problems on the upper or lower limbs is always of benefit, particularly as sensation returns.

Part 3: Spinal cord stroke

Definition

A spinal cord stroke is a vascular event affecting the blood supply to the spinal cord. The spinal cord may be damaged due to blockage of the blood vessels leading to infarction of the cord, or due to haemorrhage within or around the cord causing damage. It more commonly affects the anterior spinal artery.

Aetiology

Spinal cord infarction is usually caused by arteriosclerosis of the major arteries of the spinal cord. Other causes include embolism, acute systemic hypotension, aortic pathology or associated with spinal or aortic surgery [15]. Spinal cord haemorrhage may be caused by coagulopathies, trauma or vascular malformations such as spinal artery aneurysms or dural arteriovenous malformation [16].

Incidence

Spinal strokes are rare, with an estimated incidence of 1–2% of all admissions for vascular pathology of the nervous system.

Mortality

Mortality figures range from 9% to 22% [15, 17].

Clinical presentation

Patients usually present with sudden onset of sharp spinal pain associated with weakness, sensory disturbance, loss of deep tendon reflexes and sphincter disturbance [18]. Presentation will be determined by spinal level involved. Most strokes affect the thoracic or thoracolumbar regions and will result in lower-limb weakness. Less commonly the cervical spinal cord is affected and this would result in weakness and sensory changes in all four limbs.

Treatment

Management will involve maximizing functional ability and minimizing the development of secondary complications. Physiotherapy and occupational therapy may be required to support the individual to regain as much functional ability as possible. Specific interventions to address continence issues may also be required, but these will be like those for SCI, described above. The pathology is vascular but the resulting disabilities are similar, depending on the severity of the presentation.

Prognosis

Recovery depends on the degree of spinal cord damage, as indicated by initial neurological examination. Presence of proprioceptive deficit, walking impairment or bladder dysfunction at outset is associated with poorer long-term outcome [18]. Some

authors suggest that female sex and advanced age are negative indicators for recovery [15, 17]. A long-term follow-up of 57 patients with spinal cord infarction showed that 41% of patients were fully ambulant, 30% were able to walk with walking aids and 20% were wheelchair-dependent [17]. Pain is often problematic in the longer term.

Spinal stroke and physiotherapy

This will be essentially supportive therapy, utilizing the capabilities of the patient and attempting to maximize those in order to support independence and mobility where possible.

Acupuncture in spinal stroke

This will follow previous patterns, for stroke or for SCI, utilizing points for specific symptoms or those at appropriate spinal levels. Where pain is a major symptom, acupuncture should always be tried.

There is no supporting research for acupuncture in this field.

References

[1] The University of Alabama National Spinal Cord Injury Statistical Center. Available online at:http://www.sci-info-pages.com/facts.html; 2002 [Accessed 24 November 2009].

[2] American Spinal Injuries Association. International Standards for Functional Neurological Classification of Spinal Cord Injury. Chicago: ASIA; 1992.

[3] Tederko P, Krasuski M, Kiwerski J, et al. Strategies for neuroprotection following spinal cord injury. Ortop Traumatol Rehabil 2009;11(2):103–10.

[4] Paddison F, Middleton F. Spinal cord injury. In: Stokes M, editor. Physical Management in Neurological Rehabilitation. Edinburgh: Elsevier Mosby; 2004. p. 125–52.

[5] Nayak S, Shiflett SC, Schoenberger NE, et al. Is acupuncture effective in treating

chronic pain after spinal column injury? Arch Phys Med Rehabil 2001;82(11):1578–86.

[6] Nayak S, Matheis RJ, Agostinelli S, et al. The use of complementary and alternative therapies for chronic pain following spinal cord injury: a pilot survey. J Spinal Cord Med 2001;24(1):54–62.

[7] Averill A, Cotter AC, Nayak S, et al. Blood pressure response to acupuncture in a population at risk for autonomic dysreflexia. Arch Phys Med Rehabil 2000;81 (11):1494–7.

[8] Cheng PT, Wong MK, Chang PL. A therapeutic trial of acupuncture in neurogenic bladder of spinal cord injured patients – a preliminary report. Spinal Cord 1998;36(37):476–80.

[9] Kong Y, Ren X, Lu S. High Paraplegia. The acupuncture treatment for paralysis. Beijing: Science Press; 1996. p. 191–2.

[10] Maciocia G. The Practice of Chinese Medicine. Churchill Livingstone: Edinburgh; 1994.

[11] Jeffery DR, Mandler RN, Davis LE. Transverse myelitis: retrospective analysis of 33 cases, with differentiation of cases associated with multiple sclerosis and parainfectious events. Arch Neurol 1993;50(5):532–5.

[12] Berman M, Feldman S, Alter M, et al. Acute transverse myelitis: incidence and etiologic considerations. Neurology 1981;8:966–71.

[13] Vaghela SA, Donnellan C. Acupuncture for back pain, knee pain and insomnia in transverse myelitis – a case report. Acupuncture Med 2008;26 (3):188–92.

[14] Hopwood V. The extra meridians – the deepest level. Acupuncture in Physiotherapy. Butterworth Heinemann: Edinburgh; 2004. p. 73–88.

[15] Salvador de la Barrera S, Barca-Buyo A, Montoto-Marques A, et al. Spinal cord infarction: prognosis and recovery in a series of 36 patients. Spinal Cord 2001;39 (10):520–5.

[16] Kim JS, Lee SH. Spontaneous spinal subarachnoid hemorrhage with spontaneous resolution. J Korean Neurosurg Soc 2009;45 (4):253–5.

[17] Nedeltchev K, Loher TJ, Stepper F, et al. Long-term outcome of acute spinal cord ischemia syndrome. Stroke 2004;35(2):560–5.

[18] Masson C, Pruvo JP, Meder JF, et al. Spinal cord infarction: clinical and magnetic resonance imaging findings and short term outcome. J Neurol Neurosurg Psychiatry 2004;75(10):1431–5.

Peripheral nervous system disorders

10

CHAPTER CONTENTS

KEY POINTS

- Peripheral neuropathies can occur almost anywhere in the body and for a multitude of reasons.
- Most are commonly associated with other neurological diseases; for instance, facial palsy often occurs with stroke, and pain in the trigeminal nerve is frequently found in multiple sclerosis patients.
- Some of the conditions described in this chapter, like Bell's palsy and restless-legs syndrome,

are also occasionally found on their own and in the case of Guillain–Barré syndrome are of sufficient seriousness to be considered as a separate disease.

- Acupuncture will be most effective if it is region- or meridian-specific.

Part 1: Guillain–Barré syndrome (GBS)

GBS is classified as a disease of the peripheral nervous system, those nerves controlling movement and senses, and is quite rare, with a prevalence of approximately 1 in 100 000 in European countries. It affects about 1500 people in the UK every year. It is slightly more common in men than women and can affect people of any age, including children. It is also sometimes referred to as acute inflammatory polyradicular neuritis.

The exact cause of GBS is unclear and there is no way to pinpoint who is most at risk from the condition. However, in most cases of GBS, the person affected will have had a viral or bacterial infection a few weeks before getting the condition. It is likely that the infection causes the immune system to attack the body's own nerves.

In GBS, the body's immune system attacks these nerves, causing them to become inflamed (swollen). Although axonal demyelination is an established pathophysiological process in GBS, the rapid improvement of clinical deficits with treatment is consistent with Na^+ channel blockade by antibodies or other circulating factors, such as cytokines [1]. Most people with GBS make a full recovery within a few weeks or months and do not have any further problems. Some people may take longer to recover and there is a possibility of permanent nerve damage.

Symptoms

Symptoms usually appear after a preceding infection. They increase in intensity over a period of time, varying from a few hours in serious cases to around 4 weeks in most patients. The symptoms also vary with regard to the pattern in which they appear. Their distribution is usually symmetrical and double-sided. This means that the symptoms appear on both the left and right side of the body, but they may also appear randomly, especially in the beginning. They may also appear and disappear quite randomly. Inflammation of the peripheral nerves leads to a tingly, numbing sensation in the arms and legs. This can eventually result in a short-term loss of feeling and movement (temporary paralysis).

Fever is not a symptom of GBS, but may be caused by the preceding infection that triggered the syndrome. GBS symptoms vary, depending on whether the syndrome has affected the sensory nerve fibres or the motor nerve fibres. When both motor and sensory nerves are affected, the patient experiences a mixture of symptoms. The patient may also experience disruption in the working of the autonomous nervous system.

Damage to sensory nerves

Symptoms generally begin in the patient's feet, hands or face, spread to the legs or arms, and increase in intensity as they move towards the centre of the body. They generally appear on both left and right sides of the body. However, GBS is unpredictable, and cases have been reported in which this 'glove and stocking' pattern is not followed. Instead, motor symptoms or disruptions in the autonomous system may be observed. GBS may also affect an arm or a leg alone, without spreading to the rest of the body.

Gradually muscle pain is experienced in the large muscles, such as the thighs, back and shoulders. Pain in the lower back, buttocks or thighs is common, and is often the earliest symptom. Stiffness and cramping pain or deep, aching muscle pain is common. The sensory symptoms then make themselves felt, as the sensory nerves are attacked. The patient experiences loss or reduction of the sense of touch, or abnormal sensations such as burning, tingling, pins and needles, 'ants under the skin', vibrations and numbness.

In some patients, the skin develops hyperalgesia, or tenderness to touch, made worse by bed covering, socks and tight-fitting shoes; in some cases, pain may limit walking. Patients with symptoms at first limited to the feet and ankles may observe similar symptoms in the fingertips; as the symptoms extend to the knees, they may also extend to the wrists. The symptoms usually remain peripheral, i.e. beyond the knee and the elbow. The patient loses the ability to tell the difference between hot and cold, and may feel cold or may sweat for no apparent reason. Minor injuries may occur without being noticed. The patient's sense of taste can be affected too.

Damage to motor nerves

The motor nerves control movement, and damage to them results in partially or completely blocked signals, causing reduced movement or coordination. The patient's muscles weaken and atrophy. Tendon reflexes are reduced or lost. Progressive weakening or paralysis may occur, typically beginning in the feet, hands or face. The paralysis characteristically involves more than one limb, most commonly both legs. The paralysis is progressive and usually ascending, spreading to the rest of the limb, and from there may spread to the legs, arms and the rest of the body.

It will be difficult to stand up or climb stairs, to walk or stand and the patient will often say that the legs feel heavy. The patient may have difficulty holding and manipulating small objects, and because the arms feel weak they can no longer lift heavy objects. The weakness is often accompanied by pain and muscle spasms. Constipation can sometimes be a problem, due to the reduced activity of the intestines, change of diet and weakened stomach muscles that resist efforts by the patient to empty the bowel.

Damage to the cranial nerves can affect the face, producing a form of facial palsy. The speech muscles and vocal cords may also be affected, causing unintelligible speech. If swallowing and breathing are involved then the disease becomes life-threatening. Admission to hospital may be necessary if the GBS develops very quickly. Patients showing signs of weakness are carefully observed for signs such as paralysis of the throat, which signals a potential respiratory failure. In this case a ventilator will be necessary and if the heart rhythm becomes unstable a heart monitor may also be used.

Diagnosis

There is no specific test for this disease. Diagnosis is made by the clinical features, characteristic changes in the spinal fluid (from a lumbar puncture (spinal tap)), and electrical studies of the peripheral nerves and muscles, a procedure known as electromyography. The final diagnosis reflects only the elimination of other possibilities. There does seem to be a link with human immunodeficiency virus (HIV) and acquired immunodeficiency syndrome (AIDS).

Physiotherapy treatment

Recovery generally begins within a month of the height of the illness and has the potential to be complete. Unfortunately approximately 30% of patients will retain a residual paralysis or paresis, most usually in the lower limbs. Statistically significant correlations have been found between the degree of residual motor deficit and the severity of the weakness in the acute phase, the duration of the plateau phase or the duration of artificial ventilation [2].

Complications such as contractures, particularly those around joints, will delay or prevent full recovery and physiotherapy often concentrates treatment on these. Gentle stretching is undertaken to prevent the patient remaining for long periods in a bent or contracted posture and positioning in bed or when seated needs to be carefully controlled to ensure a good position. Splints may be used and active-assisted exercises slowly introduced.

Another complication to recovery is fatigue, so any exercises need to be carefully graduated in order to strengthen without overtiring the muscles. Temporary use of mobility aids such as wheelchairs and orthoses may be desirable to prevent overstrain. Patients with GBS do seem to have a reduced quality of life and functioning with persistent levels of distress even after the recovery period [3].

Pain can also be a problem, mostly caused by the affected muscles. Correct positioning and comfortable support will assist with this but often analgesia is required, especially at night. Anxiety is undoubtedly a factor in such a sudden and serious illness and is associated with perceived slowness in recovery.

Acupuncture treatment

There is little or no useful research into the treatment of GBS by acupuncture, but it has been used in clinic. Chinese researchers claim that acupuncture used alongside medication improves the outcome during the rehabilitation phase [4]. A single case study was published some time ago by a couple of physical therapists and has some useful traditional Chinese medicine (TCM) ideas but carries little weight scientifically [5].

Taking the problems listed above into consideration, acupuncture could certainly be used for pain analgesia and might be preferable to drug control. All acupuncture treatments will tend to have a calming effect but additional points could be used with that effect in mind. Fatigue can be tackled with metabolic and immune points added to the prescription. With GBS it will be necessary to treat with care to avoid overtaxing the recovery system, rather as in multiple sclerosis.

TCM theories

The link is with the Wei syndrome since early stages are often characterized by fullness and febrile disease. Interestingly, antibiotics are sometimes thought to be a causative factor as they destroy bacteria but fail to expel the External Pathogenic factor, resulting in a residual or latent Damp Heat in the interior.

Empty patterns are likely to be the result, particularly Spleen Qi Xu or Spleen Yang Xu. The two given below are not specific for GBS but are likely to manifest in one form or another.

Deficient Spleen Qi

This set of symptoms may be due to all the dietary sins that normally affect the Spleen, but Spleen Qi Xu is a common diagnostic finding in Western patients and is a frequent complication of other syndromes. Since it can occur together with common syndromes such as Liver invading the Spleen, Spleen and Kidney Qi Xu, Stomach Heat and Qi Xu and Spleen Blood Xu, it is rare to see it in isolation and it can often be associated with GBS.

It may be diagnosed as chronic dysentery, gastric or duodenal ulcers, anaemia, hepatitis or just nervous dyspepsia.

Symptoms include:

- abdominal pain and distension, relieved by pressure
- poor appetite, lassitude, anaemia, blood in the stools, prolapse of the rectum or uterus
- uterine bleeding, chronic haemorrhage
- anorexia
- sometimes patients describe a bearing-down or sagging sensation in the abdomen
- chronic catarrh.

Tongue: pale, thin white coating
Pulse: empty

Treatment

Tonify Spleen Qi.

- SP 3 Taibai source point for the Spleen
- SP 2 Dadu tonification point
- SP 6 Sanyinjiao tonifies Sp and removes Damp
- LI 4 Hegu important Yang Ming point
- BL 20 Pishu Back Shu point for the Spleen
- BL 21 Weishu Back Shu point for the Stomach
- ST 36 Zusanli regulates Stomach and Spleen Qi
- LR 13 Zhangmen Front Mu point for the Spleen
- CV 12 Zhongwan to strengthen and regulate Qi.

Moxa can be used on all points.

Deficient Spleen Yang

This could be caused by general Spleen Qi deficiency consuming the Yin and these points will be helpful in re-establishing nutrition patterns in GBS. The syndrome is commonly associated with gastric or duodenal ulcers, gastritis, enteritis, hepatitis, nephritis or dysentery.

Symptoms can include cold limbs, abdominal pain and distension, relieved by heat or pressure. There is often undigested food in the loose stools. The patient may have diarrhoea, also anaemia, and poor appetite. Difficulty with urination, leucorrhoea and oedema are not uncommon.
Tongue: swollen, moist and pale.
Pulse: slow, weak.

Treatment

Tonify the Spleen, particularly the Yang energy.

- SP 3 Taibai source point for the Spleen
- SP 2 Dadu tonification point
- BL 20 Pishu Back Shu point for the Spleen
- ST 36 Zusanli regulates Stomach and Spleen Qi
- LR 13 Zhangmen Front Mu point for the Spleen
- CV 4 Guanyuan tonification of Yang.

Moxa should be used.

In addition, points could be used from the general collection for peripheral neuropathies (Table 10.1).

Table 10.1 Peripheral neuropathies – useful points

Symptoms	Points	Rationale	Comments
Stooping posture	GV 20 Moxa to GV 4 KI 3	GV meridian empty	Postural hypotension
Bradykinesia Slow and limited movement or difficulty initiating movement	ST 36 SP 6 KI 3	Qi and Blood deficiency, Kidney Yang deficiency	Used as both a tonic and boost
Uncoordinated movement	GV 20	Regulation of central nervous system	Add Sishencong
Depression	Four Gates HT 7 Ear Shenmen Sishencong Yintang	To lift the spirits and generally soothe and calm the psyche	Liver/Heart/Du influence
Cold and painful upper limbs	TE 6	Local point	Treats poor circulation
Cold and painful lower limbs	SP 10 ST 31	Circulation points	Treats poor circulation
Slow general circulation	Moxa to BL 17 Geshu	For general circulation	CV 6, Qihai, can be used to support body Qi
Restless-legs syndrome	ST 36 GB 34 SP 10	Qi boost in lower limbs	BL 57 and BL 56
Postherpetic neuralgia	LI 4 LI 11 SP 10 to remove Damp Heat	Ringing the Dragon	Add paired Huatuojiaji points at appropriate nerve root levels
Complex regional pain syndrome	Local points on the opposite side, after ear acupuncture	Avoid overstimulation of a 'full condition'	Obtain a parasympathetic response
Facial palsy	Local face points LI 4, major distal	ST 44 as distal if inflammation present	Bilateral needling can be helpful if not too many points involved
Drooling	HT 6 HT 7		For excess uncontrolled saliva
Dry mouth	CV 24		Drug side-effect
Fatigue	Any of the stimulating points Possible use of extra meridians	General acupuncture effects	Use in moderation, little surplus energy
Phantom limb	Acupuncture points on the opposite side, according to symptoms	Strong sensory input required	Use Baxie and Bafeng where appropriate
Non-specific neurological symptoms	SI 3 BL 62	GB 39 could be added	Influential points for GV meridian and central nervous system

Case study 10.1: level 1 case study: Guillain–Barré syndrome – pain in feet preventing walking

A 28-year-old man presented with severe pain and hypersensitivity in the soles of the feet. He was unable to put any weight through the feet due to pain. Pain also disturbed his sleep at night; pain medications had not helped with the foot pain. He was also feeling low in mood; he was very tired and irritable during the day. The patient was recovering from GBS which had developed 3 months previously.

Functional ability

There was upper- and lower-limb weakness. He was unable to stand or walk; he used an electric wheelchair for mobility. The patient needed the assistance of one person for all daily activities. He was previously in full-time employment.

Treatment

A course of five acupuncture treatments was provided over 4 weeks. Points used during the first two treatments included bilateral ST 36, KI 3, right LI 4, left LI 11 and Yintang. Bilateral LR 2, KI 3, KI 9, right LI 4, left LI 11 and GV 20 were used during treatments 3 and 4. Treatment 5 included the use of bilateral HT 7, ST 36, SP 6 and LR 3. Needles were stimulated initially for Deqi and then left in place for 30 minutes with no additional stimulation.

Outcome

The patient was sleepy at the end of each treatment. After two treatments he was feeling calmer and pain had reduced. After treatment 3 he was able to put some weight through the feet and walk a few steps in parallel bars. By treatment 5 he reported that he felt no pain in the soles of the feet as well as noting improved energy levels. At this stage he reported feeling calmer and happier and felt that acupuncture had played a significant part in reducing the pain.

Part 2: Diabetic neuropathy

Background

There can be many causes for peripheral neuropathy and GBS is only one of them. Perhaps more common is the type associated with the later stages of diabetes.

Research

Acupuncture has been used to control diabetic symptoms, most notably by Wang et al. [6], who treated the dyspeptic symptoms of gastroparesis by electroacupuncture at ST 36 Zusanli and LI 4 Hegu.

A small pilot study evaluated two clinical styles of acupuncture in the treatment of diabetic neuropathy. Japanese acupuncture, characterized by very shallow needle insertion, was compared to traditional Chinese acupuncture [7]. Interestingly, those given Japanese acupuncture reported decreased neuropathy-associated pain according to daily diary scores whereas those in the other group reported minimal effects. Both styles lowered pain as measured by the McGill Short Form Pain Score. The TCM style improved nerve sensation according to quantitative sensory testing while the Japanese style had a more equivocal effect. However, with such a small group – only 7 patients in all – no significant conclusions can be drawn. It remains possible that acupuncture could be useful in this situation.

Further work on peripheral neuropathy was undertaken by a German group [8]. This was a larger study, with 47 patients involved, all of whom were evaluated over 12 months. The results suggested that nerve conduction showed an objective improvement with treatment. Acupuncture analgesia has been compared with standard medication and proved as successful in alleviating the pain from this type of neuropathy [9].

Several ideas have been put forward, including the use of acu-magnets on acupuncture points, particularly for diabetes and insomnia [10].

Bearing in mind that regrowth of peripheral nerves is possible, if the conditions are favourable and destruction has not been complete, acupuncture to improve the local tissue condition and increase local circulation may be very helpful [11].

The following case study is not strictly illustrating diabetic neuropathy but demonstrates the general principles.

Case study 10.2: level 1 case study

This case report describes the treatment of knee pain in a 43-year-old man with alcoholic peripheral neuropathy with axonal damage. He had bilateral dorsiflexor muscle weakness and wore bilateral ankle foot orthoses. He had poor balance but walked independently with one stick. He had been diagnosed with epilepsy 4 years previously.

Main complaint

The patient presented with dull aching pain in both knees which was worse in cold and damp weather. He rated the pain as 7/10 on a numerical rating scale for pain. He was always worse in the winter but reported only mild symptoms in the summer. He also reported feeling irritable when the knee pain was worse. X-rays of the knee were normal. In addition he reported anxiety, restless sleep, generalized fatigue and a poor memory.

Treatment

Assessment suggested Bi syndrome of his knees involving the Pathogens of Damp and Cold. Treatment aimed to clear obstruction of channels around the knee and involved needling of bilateral SP 10, SP 9, ST 34 and ST 36. In additional bilateral LR 3 and LI 4 were needled to aid smooth flow of Qi and Blood and for generalized pain-relieving and calming effects. Needles were stimulated for Deqi initially. No further stimulation was given. The patient received three treatments of 30 minutes over 1 week. After this he was unable to attend for further treatment.

Outcome

Pain reduced to 4/10 and the patient reported that it bothered him much less during the day. He also reported feeling more relaxed and was sleeping very deeply each night after treatment. It was unfortunate that this man was unable to attend for additional treatments.

Part 3: Bell's palsy

Bell's palsy is defined as a weakness in one side of the face, causing the facial muscles on that side to droop. There may also be an accompanying feeling of numbness in the area. The patient may have difficulty closing the eye fully and closing the mouth to retain saliva. Occasionally, in addition to the paralysis there is a loss of taste, increased sensitivity to sound and pain or discomfort in or around the ear.

Causes

The specific cause is not really known. This problem can occur after stroke or a transient ischaemic attack simply because of the muscle weakness involved in those conditions but true Bell's palsy is thought to be caused more by an inflammatory episode in the facial nerve. The most common situations which may lead to this inflammation are systemic viral infections, local infections, trauma, surgery, diabetes, tumour, immunological disorders or drugs [12]. It is also thought that a persistent cold draught on the side of the face can cause this type of inflammation.

Differential diagnosis

This relies upon the presence of typical symptoms and signs, blood chemical investigations, cerebrospinal fluid investigations, X-ray of the skull and mastoid, cerebral magnetic resonance imaging or nerve conduction studies. Bell's palsy may be diagnosed after exclusion of all secondary causes, but causes of secondary facial nerve palsy and Bell's palsy may coexist [12, 13].

Medical treatment

As Bell's palsy is often associated with a viral infection, antivirals such as aciclovir may be prescribed. Corticosteroids may also be given to reduce the inflammation.

Physiotherapy treatment

Care must be taken of the eye surface when the eyelid is disabled; there may be either excessive tear production or a dry eye. An eye patch is often used.

Otherwise gentle stretching, massage and active exercises when possible are all techniques used by physiotherapists. Electrical stimulation is an intervention used to encourage the return of activity to the muscles and the artificial contractions help to maintain circulation and tissue condition.

Acupuncture treatment

Simple application of needles to local points is the best form of treatment. The most commonly used points are those on the Stomach, Small Intestine and Gall Bladder meridians. Appropriate distal points should be used and low-frequency electro-acupuncture (2–4 Hz) can be applied to the facial points, producing a treatment effect very like that obtained by electrical stimulation in physiotherapy.

Case study 10.3: level 1 case study – acute facial palsy

The patient was a 27-year-old female who had a middle- and outer-ear infection that was also diagnosed as shingles which affected balance and caused nausea. Her ear became red and swollen. She was given painkillers and antibiotics by her GP. Six days later she noticed that her mouth did not feel right when she was cleaning her teeth. She could not spit properly. Her parents also noticed she looked odd. She realized something was wrong with her facial muscles when she went to wipe her eye and touched her eyeball. Two days later she was unable to close her eye and the left side of her face had slumped. Her smile was asymmetrical. She went to her GP who diagnosed shingles/herpesvirus and gave her antiviral medications. She was also referred to an ear, nose and throat (ENT) specialist who prescribed prednisolone. She was advised that the problem could take 6 months to go – or might not go at all.

Presenting symptoms

- Unable to close left eye (demonstrated one-quarter closing – rolling the eye up into the eyelid). Unable to blink (flicker only). Unable to raise eyebrows.
- Only able to drink through a straw.

- Unable to maintain a mouth seal – air escapes.
- Diagnosed with grade 5 Bell's palsy by an ENT consultant.

Objective assessment

Photographs were taken (no facial electromyogram was available) to record progress.

Treatment

Acupuncture was used as the first line of treatment. Before starting acupuncture, we had to wait until her GP indicated that the infection was no longer in its contagious phase. Verbal and written consent was gained.

Acupuncture point selection – affected side only

TE 21, SI 19, GB 2, LI 20, ST 2, ST 6, ST 7, EX-HN 4, LI 4 (bilateral)

TCM texts suggested that only the affected side should be needled to direct flow to this area.

Outcomes

At the frst session needling started at the ear, then over the face and finally in the forehead (EX-HN 4, Yu Tao). For insertion of the 'fish spine' the patient needed to look straight ahead but she kept having to be asked to keep the eye open – it was after asking several times that it was realized that this meant that she was shutting her eye! This was truly astonishing – and a very promising sign. The face and ear felt warm during treatment (35 minutes of needling).

LI 4 was stimulated manually but, for fear of bruising, the facial needles were left alone. Further photographs were taken after and these showed some early signs of improvement.

The next day the same points were used for 50 minutes. Two days after this the same needles were used for 45 minutes. Photos were taken afterwards that showed more symmetry in smiling; the eyebrow moved on the eyebrow raise. The puckering of her lips (kiss) was more centralized and she was closing eyes to 1–2 mm off sealed.

She was seen again on the Sunday, a week after starting the acupuncture, and had another 45 minutes of needling. The Friday before she had seen her ENT consultant who was very impressed and said that the grade 5 palsy was now reduced to grade 1. Within a further week the paralysis had completely disappeared. The acupuncture points were not changed because the results were achieved very rapidly. The patient was thrilled with the outcome.

Part 4: Restless-legs syndrome (RLS)

This syndrome is described as a common sensorimotor disorder of unknown aetiology. It is sometimes associated with multiple sclerosis. It ranges in severity from merely causing annoyance in the patient to actively affecting sleep and quality of life. Lifestyle changes such as decreased use of caffeine, alcohol and tobacco together with regular sleep and exercise are frequently recommended and these provide some relief. In about half of the patients there seems to be some family tendency.

Symptoms

RLS is characterized by unpleasant sensations in the legs and an uncontrollable urge to move when at rest in an effort to relieve these feelings. The distinctive aspect of this condition is that the condition is much worse when the patient is lying down or trying to relax.

RLS sensations are often described by people as burning, creeping, tugging, or like insects crawling inside the legs. These sensations are often called paraesthesias (abnormal sensations) or dysaesthesias (unpleasant abnormal sensations) and the sensations range in severity from uncomfortable to irritating or truly painful.

If it is a severe case it is thought to warrant medical treatment. Restless-legs symptoms are dramatically relieved with levodopa and dopamine agonists, which are first-line treatment for this disorder. In addition, opioids have been shown to provide a marked symptomatic relief. This unique responsiveness of RLS to both dopaminergic agents and opioids places it at the crossroad of the two systems implicated in the placebo response. Indeed, in recent large-scale studies a substantial placebo response was observed [14].

RLS and acupuncture

With the clear response to dopamine agonists produced by acupuncture it is logical to suppose that acupuncture may be of value in this condition and indeed there is a current Cochrane review, although only two trials, with a total of 170 patients, met the inclusion criteria [15]. Borderline positive findings are recorded but, as with most reviews, it is agreed that further work is needed. Even if this is classified as a 'placebo' response by the researchers, the clinical use of acupuncture would still seem to be warranted.

The points used were ST 36, GB 34, SP 10, BL 57 and BL 56, with the addition of scalp acupuncture using motor treatment zones.

Part 5: Postherpetic neuralgia

This is a complication of herpes zoster or shingles, and seems to occur most often in middle-aged to elderly patients. It is characterized by persistent pain following the course of the intercostal nerve at the level which was originally infected by the virus. It can be shooting or burning in nature and can sometimes lead to allodynia, a supersensitivity to non-noxious stimuli in the area. This can make normal clothing very uncomfortable. This pain can be very debilitating, often leading to fatigue, insomnia, anxiety and depression.

Treatment is started when the rash first appears and may continue for many months, or even years, once this condition becomes chronic.

Acupuncture research

There has been little research of note in this condition although, clinically, acupuncture has a good reputation. Two well-written case studies offer some information [16, 17]. A small group of patients of mixed acute and chronic conditions demonstrated that acupuncture had diminished the pain [18].

Acupuncture treatment

In common with all other viruses in TCM, the herpes zoster virus is considered as an invasion of Damp Heat. It often occurs together with some form of Liver stagnation. The most important action to take is to expel the Heat in the Blood using LI 4 Hegu, LI 11 Quchi and SP 10 Xuehai. ST 36 Zusanli and PE 6 Neiguan could also be added.

'Ringing the Dragon' is a technique often recommended for dealing with the large area of painful skin. This involves the superficial, oblique insertion of many small needles around the inflamed or painful area. Huatuojiaji points can be added in pairs above and below the affected nerve root. The best results are obtained when treatment is given in the acute phase of the disease but it is always worth trying in a chronic situation and even when the course of the virus has not been confined to an intercostal nerve.

Case study 10.4: level 2 case study

The patient was a school teacher, aged 58. He had retired early due to postherpetic neuralgia from which he had suffered for 4 years. This was atypical in that the area most affected seemed to be concentrated on his right eye. He was often forced to cover the eye with an eye patch as he found light painful and he took over-the-counter painkillers constantly to control a 'burning, stabbing' pain in that area. This was often spread over the right side of his face.

Impression

This was an old herpes zoster infection affecting the seventh cranial or facial nerve. A very slight mottling of the skin could be seen but there was no other visible sign. The whole nerve appeared to have been damaged, judging by the pain distribution. This was considered as a local disturbance of nerve tissue and treated geographically. However points were also considered for their TCM actions and some added for the elimination of Pathogenic Heat.

Acupuncture treatment

An attempt was made to 'Ring the Dragon' by using needles to circle the right eye socket, extending the contained area back towards and around the ear. This was very approximate and guided by the patient's description of his symptoms. This circle closed anteriorly at Yintang (Extra) and included

GB 14 Yangbai, ST 2 Sibai, GB 2 Tinghui, GB 8 Shuaigu, GB 20 Fengchi and a pair of Huatuojiaji points at the C4 level. Two distal points were used to expel residual Heat, LI 4 Hegu and GB 43 Xiaxi. This resulted in more than 10 needles but after the first treatment gaps were left in the circle and the points continued to be effective.

Outcome

After the first treatment the patient said he had slept much better than he had done for years. He was a physiotherapy outpatient so he returned weekly for treatment. Within six treatments he no longer covered his eye and was back to wearing his glasses in order to enjoy his restored visual comfort. His pain had mostly gone, returning only briefly if he was fatigued. He was cheerful and relaxed and quite aggrieved that he had not been offered acupuncture earlier as he might have remained at work longer. He had a relapse 3 months later after a stressful family crisis but after one further treatment he telephoned to say all was well and did not return.

Part 6: Phantom limb pain

This is the pain felt by the patient in a non-existent limb after amputation, whether accidental or surgical. In fact the limb does not need to be physically lost since this also occurs in conditions in which the brain is dissociated from the body such as in peripheral nerve injury and after spinal cord injury when an area loses sensation and usually movement too. It can be very distressing to the patient and, while it clearly originates in the spinal column, it is usually described in terms of the perceived locality as in 'my hand is burning' or 'my foot feels as though it's being crushed'.

Mechanism

The usual cause lies with damage to the nerve endings and may involve subsequent regrowth leading to painful discharge of neurons in the stump and faulty connections with the spinal segment. There is evidence for altered nervous activity within the brain as a result of this loss or change in sensory input.

Treatment

The condition is generally described as chronic and intractable and there are few medical remedies. Surgery involving the destruction of nerve tissue is sometimes used but is rarely of permanent value. Some new treatments are available, particularly that of using a 'mirror box' where the mirrored limb is reversed to look like the amputated one, giving the impression that the loss has been somehow reversed for the duration of the treatment. This is thought to be effective since changes to the way the peripheral areas of the body are represented on the cortex may lead to changes in pain sensation. The neuroplastic changes and the pain itself seem to be increased if a chronic painful situation has preceded them [19]. Stimulation of the sensorimotor cortex does seem to be able to reduce the pain [20].

Acupuncture in phantom limb pain

There is little supporting research evidence for the use of acupuncture in this situation but it is nonetheless well known to be effective in clinic. Some case study work has been published, but not enough [21, 22].

Points are selected on the existing limb to correspond to the sites of pain in the missing limb. One would expect that mostly Yang meridians would be used with emphasis on the powerful analgesic points, such as L 4 Hegu, SI 3 Houxi, ST 44 Neiting and BL 62 Shenmai. There is a case for using a really strong sensory stimulus such as the Baxie points on the hand or Bafeng on the foot as long as the skin remains viable.

References

[1] Vucic S, Kiernan MC, Cornblath DR. Guillain–Barré syndrome: an update. J Clin Neurosci 2009;16 (6):733–41.

[2] deJager AE, Minderhoud JM. Residual signs in severe Guillain–Barré syndrome: analysis of 57 patients. J Neurol Sci 1991;104 (2):151–6.

[3] Rudolph T, Larsen JP, Farbu E. The long-term functional status in patients with Guillain–Barré syndrome. Euro J Neurol 2008;15 (12):1332–7.

[4] Zou H. Clinical observation on 38 cases with Guillain–Barré syndrome treated with acupuncture combined with medicine. International Journal of Clinical Acupuncture 2001;12 (2):171.

[5] Elgert G, Olmstead L. The treatment of chronic inflammatory demyelinating polyradiculopathy with acupuncture. Am J Acupuncture 1999;27:15–22.

[6] Wang C, Kao C, Chen W, et al. A single-blinded, randomized pilot study evaluating effects of electroacupuncture in diabetic patients with symptoms suggestive of gastroparesis. J Altern Complement Med 2008;14 (7):833–9.

[7] Ahn AC, Bennani T, Freeman R, et al. Two styles of acupuncture for treating painful diabetic neuropathy – a pilot randomised control trial. Acupunct Med 2007;25(1–2):11–7.

[8] Schroder S, Liepert J, Remppis A, et al. Acupuncture treatment improves nerve conduction in peripheral neuropathy. Eur J Neurol 2007;14(3): 276–281.

[9] Abuaisha BB, Costanzi JB, Boulton AJM. Acupuncture for the treatment of chronic painful peripheral diabetic neuropathy: a long-term study. Diabetes Res Clin Pract 1998;39(2):115–21.

[10] Colbert AP, Cleave J, Brown KA, et al. Magnets applied to acupuncture points as therapy a literature review. Acupunct Med 2008;26(3):160.

[11] Green J, McClennon J. Acupuncture: an effective treatment for painful diabetic neuropathy. Diabetic Foot 2006;9 (4):182.

[12] Finsterer J. Management of peripheral facial nerve palsy. Eur Arch Otorhinolaryngol 2008;265 (7):743–52.

[13] He L, Zhou MK, Zhou D, et al. Acupuncture for Bell's palsy (update). Cochrane Database Syst Rev 2007;4: CD002914.

[14] Fulda S, Wetter TC. Where dopamine meets opioids: a meta-analysis of the placebo effect in restless legs syndrome treatment studies. Brain 2008;131(Pt 4):902–17.

[15] Cui Y, Wang Y, Liu Z. Acupuncture for restless legs syndrome. Cochrane Database Syst Rev 2008;(4): CD006457.

[16] Key S. A single case study of an 82 year old woman with depression and post-herpetic neuralgia. J Acupunct Assoc Chartered Physiotherapists 2002;2002(2):47.

[17] Valaskatgis P, Macklin EA, Schachter SC, et al. Possible effects of acupuncture on atrial fibrillation and post-herpetic neuralgia – a case report. Acupuncture Med 2008;26 (1):51–6.

[18] Coghlan CJ. Herpes zoster treated by acupuncture. Cent Afr J Med 1992;38(12):466–7.

[19] Flor H. Maladaptive plasticity, memory for pain and phantom limb pain: review and suggestions for new therapies. Expert Rev Neurother 2008;8(5): 809–818.

[20] Mackert BM, Sappork T, Grusser S, et al. The eloquence of silent cortex: analysis of afferent input to deafferented cortex in arm amputees. NeuroReport 2003;14(3):409–12.

[21] Bradbrook D. Acupuncture treatment of phantom limb pain and phantom limb sensation in amputees. Acupunct Med 2004;22 (2):93–7.

[22] Monga TN, Jaksic T. Acupuncture in phantom limb pain. Arch Phys Med Rehabil 1981;62 (5):229–31.

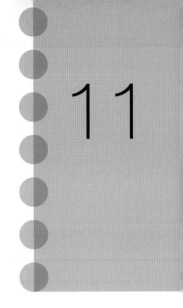

Motor neurone disease

CHAPTER CONTENTS

- Motor neurone disease (MND) is less commonly treated by physiotherapists.
- The aim is to manage the course of the disease as well as possible.
- Respiratory problems are common.
- Some of the symptoms will respond to acupuncture.
- Treatment will be a mixture of traditional Chinese medicine (TCM) and Western theory.
- In TCM terms MND is associated with both Feng and Wei syndromes.

Introduction

Definition

Motor neurone disease (MND) is characterized by the progressive deterioration of the anterior horn cells of the spinal cord and the corticospinal tracts, causing lower motor neurone lesions and upper motor neurone lesions respectively. Certain motor nuclei of the brainstem may also be affected, leading to bulbar paralysis. Degeneration of the motor neurones leads to weakness and wasting of muscles, a loss of mobility in the limbs and difficulties with speech, swallowing and breathing.

Incidence

The incidence is about 2 per 100 000, with a familial form found in about 1% of all cases [1]. MND tends to be a disease of later middle life; the mean age of onset is 58 years, with a slightly higher percentage of males affected.

Mortality

The mean duration of survival after diagnosis is 3–4 years, although this can vary greatly according to the type of MND and the part of the nervous system most seriously affected.

Amyotrophic lateral sclerosis (ALS)

This is the most common form of MND, accounting for about 66% of all patients [2], with both upper and lower motor neurones affected. It is characterized by weakness and wasting in the limbs, often first indicated by clumsiness in walking or handling things. Most commonly the upper limbs and hands are affected first with evident wasting of the thenar eminence. Average life expectancy with this form can be between 2 and 5 years from onset of symptoms.

Progressive bulbar palsy (PBP)

PBP involves both upper and lower motor neurones and affects about a quarter of the patients diagnosed. This form of MND often causes difficulties with speech or swallowing. If the lower motor neurones are affected, the tongue tends to atrophy with visible fasciculation and reduced mobility. This results in a rather nasal type of speech. If the upper motor neurones are affected the tongue is spastic and tends to cause dysarthria, difficulty with the mechanics of speech, i.e. stuttering.

Wild mood swings may also occur with little apparent cause. The limbs are less affected but as the disease progresses the patient may experience weakness in the arms and legs [3]. Life expectancy is between 6 months and 3 years from the onset of symptoms.

Progressive muscular atrophy (PMA)

PMA affects only a small group of people, with damage mainly occurring in the lower motor neurones. It tends to start earlier, predominantly affecting men below the age of 50 years. It first presents with wasting in the arms, manifesting as weakness and clumsiness of the hands. There may be progression to the lower limbs but bulbar involvement is rare until late in the disease. The rate of progression is much slower, with patients living 5–10 years after diagnosis.

There are other much less common variants: Kennedy's disease, Guam variant MND and primary lateral sclerosis.

Although ALS, PBP and PMA are the three main forms of MND there is an enormous variation in symptoms between patients. Control of bladder or bowels is rarely affected. Mental deterioration and dementia are found in less than 5% of patients [3]. There is increasing evidence of frontal lobe involvement which may lead to emotional lability. Anxiety and depression are quite commonly found, unsurprisingly, in such a serious disease.

Risk factors

There are no apparent risk factors although, as mentioned above, there can be, rarely, a familial link.

Diagnosis

Differential diagnosis

MND presents some problems with diagnosis for several reasons: primarily because it is comparatively rare, but also because the early symptoms do not appear serious to the patient. These can include clumsiness, mild weakness or slightly slurred speech, all of which could have an innocent cause. It may be some time before a doctor is consulted.

The classification and terminology used to describe the different MND syndromes are not always clear or consistent, with ALS being frequently used in US information sources as the general title.

Tests

There is rarely a clear pattern or a single indicative symptom and no definitive test. MND does not usually affect the bladder or bowel. It can be confirmed by electromyography later in the progress of the disease when the motor action potentials are of increased amplitude and duration but fewer in number than normal. Other investigations may be necessary to exclude syringomyelia or cervical spondylosis, both of which may present with weakness in the upper limbs.

Medical treatment

Pharmacology

The National Institute for Clinical Excellence has recommended the use of riluzole (Rilutek) to treat ALS. It is thought to prolong life for a couple of months and may delay the need for a tracheostomy, but it does not really help with many of the symptoms. The drug reduces the natural production of the neural transmitter glutamate, which carries signals to the motor neurones. It is believed that too much glutamate can damage these and inhibit nerve signalling.

Other medicine may help with symptoms. Muscle relaxants such as baclofen, tizanidine and the benzodiazepines may reduce spasticity. Glycopyrrolate and atropine may reduce the flow of saliva. Quinine or phenytoin may decrease cramps. Anticonvulsants and non-steroidal anti-inflammatory drugs may help relieve pain, and other drugs can be prescribed to treat depression. Tranquillizers often help with sleeping problems.

Some patients with PPS develop sleep apnoea (a potentially life-threatening condition characterized by interruptions of breathing during sleep), which can be treated with decongestant therapy or assisted breathing at night. Panic attacks over fears of choking to death can be treated with benzodiazepines. Botulinum toxin may be used to treat jaw spasms or drooling. Amitriptyline and other anticholinergic drugs can help control excess drooling. Some patients may eventually require stronger medicines such as morphine to cope with musculoskeletal abnormalities or pain, and opiates are used to provide comfort care in terminal stages of the disease.

Surgery

Surgery can occasionally be used to remove any blockage to the airway but is not generally applied to this disease.

Prognosis

As stated previously, the prognosis is a poor one for sufferers of this disease, with a small variation according to the focus of the disease. Symptom control is undertaken by the multidisciplinary health team and the main goal is greater comfort for the patient.

Impact on the patient

The manifest problems can be subdivided into the following categories.

Pain

This is a common problem, with up to 73% of patients reporting pain of some kind [4]. The causes are mainly muscular, muscle cramps, spasticity or spasms as a result of weakening muscles. These produce abnormal stresses on the joints and often result in changed posture, leading to further stresses and pain. If the patient is unable to change position easily then areas of pressure will also lead to pain. Chronic back pain produced by poor posture is very common.

Breathing problems

Dyspnoea or the dysfunction of breathing muscles can occur in nearly half these patients. While this is due mainly to the weakening of muscles around the neck, shoulder girdle and in the thorax, anxiety can certainly make it much worse.

Impaired swallowing

This is due to the impairment of the motor nuclei in the medulla combined with spasticity and poor coordination. Slow, careful feeding is essential to prevent choking episodes. Speech and language therapists can make a great contribution with careful assessment and positioning of the patient in order to prevent inhalation of food.

Dysarthria or difficulty speaking

Often considerable patience and care are required to understand the speech of patients with this condition, particularly in the later stages. Assessment by a speech and language therapist will help to make the most of remaining abilities. There is a wide range of aids now available including computers with especially sensitive controls for those with minimal movement in the upper limbs.

Constipation

Constipation is largely due to the lack of easy movement. Physical inactivity combined with a diet often lacking in roughage, because of choking problems, will make evacuation of the bowels difficult and less frequent. Weakness in the abdominal walls will also affect the ability to raise intra-abdominal pressure sufficiently to open the bowels.

Insomnia

This is a common problem, reported in 48% of patients admitted to a hospice [5]. There are of course many reasons why this might be so. Firstly, any breathlessness will tend to get worse when it is time to sleep, especially if there is associated anxiety. Again, this is often linked to weak musculature. It may also be associated with depression and may respond to antidepressants or sedatives.

Fatigue

A form of general fatigue occurs in most patients and can in itself be seriously disabling. Any physical activity needs to be undertaken with care but 'a little and often' is very useful. Corticosteroids are sometimes prescribed for fatigue but if they are used for long periods that may produce unwanted side-effects of their own.

Other less common problems may include sore eyes resulting from the weakness of the eye muscles. Urinary retention may occur, due more to the weakness of the abdominal walls rather than to problems with the kidney or bladder. Catheterization is sometimes necessary. Pressure sores may result if movement is severely limited and regular turning and the use of pressure-relieving cushions and mattresses are vital.

MND and physiotherapy

Physiotherapists are part of a multidisciplinary team dealing with the problems of MND and the main thrust of physical management is the control of symptoms.

The pain can be dealt with in several ways. As discussed previously, a lot of it is due to the weakening of muscle, the imbalance caused by this and the subsequent inappropriate increase in muscle tone, leading to cramps and spasticity. Correct positioning, education of handlers in moving and handling and encouragement of physiological movement with adequate rest periods underpin the treatment programme. Gentle stretching to maintain soft-tissue length can sometimes alleviate pain. Acupuncture may also now be routinely considered as part of the pain relief [6]. Transcutaneous electrical nerve stimulation (TENS), hot packs or even warm baths can all be useful.

Respiratory problems are difficult to treat and many modalities are used. Fundamental failure of chest expansion is dealt with by maximizing ventilation and gas exchange and assisting with the removal of secretions. Physical methods will include non-invasive ventilation, drug therapy, advice and education for the family as well as the patient.

Acupuncture in MND

There is not much evidence supporting the use of acupuncture in MND, or ALS. This is surprising considering the manifestations of the disease but probably reflects the overall rarity of the condition. It is possible that much of the recorded acupuncture research on patients receiving palliative care does include a fair number of MND sufferers. Specific problems, such as anxiety, depression, insomnia and shortness of breath, are fairly common in this unfortunate group [7]. The calming and anxiolytic effect of acupuncture will contribute significantly in this situation.

A recent Cochrane review included five acupuncture studies and decided that there was low evidence that acupuncture and acupressure were useful [8]. Acupuncture certainly is used [9], but precise details of the interventions are often lacking.

Body acupuncture

Local points are used in dealing with the pain to facilitate freer joint movement; a concentration on the major Yang meridians will be helpful, with the addition of the powerful distal points. The limbs are thought to be regulated through the Governor Vessel so acupuncture can be used to strengthen and augment the flow of Qi which may be blocked by pathogenic invasion. Table 11.1 offers a selection of useful points.

Scalp acupuncture

Some authorities use scalp acupuncture but MND is not generally cited as an indication. However Jiao suggests that two variations of bulbar paralysis will respond [10]. What he terms as 'true bulbar paralysis' with symptoms of dyslalia, dysphagia and the disappearance of the pharyngeal reflex can be treated by stimulating the balance areas bilaterally. What he terms 'false bulbar paralysis', with additional symptoms of dysphagia, choking and excess salivation, requires the addition of the lower two-fifths of the motor area on each side (see Chapter 12). Good results are claimed, but there is no very convincing research evidence as yet.

TCM approach

The picture in traditional Chinese medicine (TCM) literature for MND is unclear. The disease itself is not commonly described in TCM and certainly not in terms that Western medicine would be comfortable with. The links to the Wei syndrome are tenuous but seem to be the best match. Wei syndrome

refers to weakness and motor impairment of the limbs, possibly accompanied by numbness and muscular atrophy. The fact that this seems to be localized in either the upper or lower portions of the body serves to confuse the picture somewhat, although there are well-established methods for balancing Qi in the two halves of the body, often by using the extraordinary meridians: in this case the Dai Mai might be helpful.

The most likely syndromes will be Lung and Spleen Qi Xu, Qi and Blood deficiency or Liver and/or Kidney Blood deficiency.

Nicholas Haines provides a good example of a case history in the book *Acupuncture in Practice* [11]. In a useful flow diagram (Figure 11.1) he indicates how a succession of pathogenic influences may produce the right circumstance for the symptoms of MND. It is not suggested that these are the root cause of the disease but the TCM points to treat them will be useful as part of the wider management of the patient.

Deficient Lung and Spleen Qi

Symptoms

Deficient Lung and Spleen Qi affects the voice. The voice is low, there is no desire to talk. In addition there is weak respiration, weak cough, shortness of breath, spontaneous sweating, weakness and general lassitude and low resistance to cold.
Tongue: pale; thin white coating
Pulse: weak

Treatment

Tonify Lung and Spleen Qi.

- LU 7 Lieque used for throat infection and cough.
- (Could be used with LI 4 Hegu in allergic asthma.)
- LI 4 Hegu used to strengthen Wei Qi.
- ST 36 Zusanli regulates Stomach and Spleen Qi.
- BL 13 Feishu Back Shu point for the Lungs.
- BL 20 Pishu Back Shu point for the Spleen.
- CV 17 Shanzhong regulates Qi in the Upper Jiao.
- LR 13 Front Mu point for the Spleen.

Explanation

A combination of both Lung Yin and Qi deficiency is often seen in clinical practice. Recurrent coughing tends to weaken the Spleen. Failure to clear the secretions may also cause Spleen problems. It is rare to see Spleen Qi Xu in isolation.

Table 11.1 Motor neurone disease – useful points

Symptoms	Points	Rationale	Comments
Postural changes 'Dropped-head' syndrome	GV 22 Xinhui BL 6 Chengguang GB17 Zhengyang GB10 Fubai	Extrapyramidal effect	Hard to influence weak neck muscles
Stooping posture	GV 20 Baihui Moxa to GV 4 Mingmen KI 3 Taixi	GV meridian empty	Postural hypotension
Spinal acupuncture Combine GV points and Huatuojiaji points	Use on alternate days	Stimulate Qi in the GV meridian, link with central nervous system	Method of Dr Wang Leting
Uncoordinated movement	GV 20 Baihui GV 14 Dazhui	Regulation of central nervous system	Add Sishencong
Depression, anxiety and breathing problems	Four Gates HT 7 Shenmen Ear Shenmen Sishencong Yintang	To lift the spirits and generally soothe and calm the psyche	Liver/Heart/GV influence
Cold and painful upper limbs	TE 6 Waiguan	Local point	Treats poor circulation
Cold and painful lower limbs	SP10 Xuehai ST 31 Biguan	Circulation points	Treats poor circulation
Upper/lower balance	TE 5 Waiguan GB 41 Zulinqi	Opening Dai Mai	Extra meridian
Stiff tongue, rapid exhaustion when speaking	HT 5 Tongli	Associated with speech	Stimulate Spirit
Involuntary tremor	LR 3 Taichong SI 3 Houxi GV 16 Fengfu	Weakness	GV 16 expels Wind
Drooling	HT 6 Yinxi HT 7 Shenmen		For excess or uncontrolled saliva
Fatigue	Any of the stimulating points Possible use of extra meridians	General acupuncture effects	Use in moderation; little surplus energy available

Qi and Blood deficiency

Common symptoms include chronic tremor of a limb or limbs, sallow complexion, reluctant speech and lack of facial expression. Also found are stiff neck, cold painful limbs, general poverty of movement, unsteady gait with difficulty in taking the first step, dizziness and blurred vision.

Treatment

Tonify Qi, nourish Blood, energize the meridians and dispel Pathogens.

- ST 36 Zusanli tonifies Qi and Blood.
- SP 6 Sanyinjiao tonifies Qi and Blood.
- LR 8 Ququan nourishes Liver Blood.

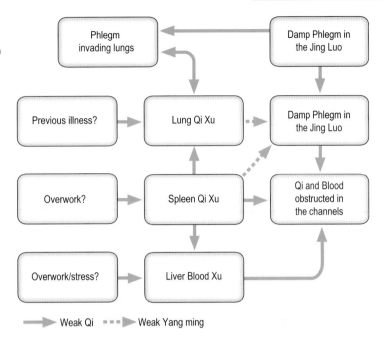

Figure 11.1 • An example of generation of motor neurone disease in traditional Chinese medicine terms. (After Haines [11].)

- CV 4 Guanyuan nourishes Blood generally.
- SP 10 Xuehai improves Blood circulation in the lower limb.

Explanation

A poor or absent circulation of Qi and Blood is seen in TCM as the cause of both pain and also poor movement ability. The blockage may in fact be caused by early manifestations of Phlegm Heat. Local points on the most affected limbs will also be useful.

Summary

In TCM terms MND provides an unpleasant list of symptoms. Most interventions are aimed at making life more bearable for the sufferer without being able to offer hope of a cure. It is true that occasionally a patient with the PMA form does survive for a good number of years but this form is unfortunately rare. It is, however, reasonable to suppose that the known physiological effects of acupuncture may help with symptom control.

It is always best to combine acupuncture with the type of physical treatment described in the physiotherapy section of this chapter. Much of the muscle pain will respond to acupuncture and one of the well-documented side-effects of acupuncture

is the improvement in mood. Anything that can help with panic attacks and depression will be helpful.

Case study 11.1: level 1 case

The patient was aged 44, and had been diagnosed with MND 2 years previously. He was coping in sheltered accommodation and living alone. He was receiving community physiotherapy visits.

Presentation

The patient was experiencing trunk and lower-limb stiffness and difficulty in walking. He found it hard to initiate movement and his legs felt stiff and painful. He was experiencing great difficulty with breathing and speech. His upper limbs were almost useless.

On examination it was found that he had poor circulation in the lower limbs, which were blue and cold to the touch.

TCM impression

Qi and Blood deficiency.

Treatment

Points used bilaterally were:

- SP 10 for lower-limb circulation
- SP 6 and ST 36 boost to system
- ST 44 and GB 43 for leg pain.

Outcome

Within two treatments his legs were warmer to touch. The patient stated that walking was 'looser and less painful'.

His mood was generally better, despite his problems, and after six treatments he was encouraged to seek 'maintenance' acupuncture privately as it was recognized that the NHS would not provide enough community physiotherapy visits to cover this. He continued to live semi-independently for a further year.

Case study 11.2: level 2 case

The patient, aged 65, had had MND for 4 years and was now in the terminal phase.

He was urgently referred with respiratory distress, following a 'cold', which resulted in a severe chest infection. He had audible secretions and extensive pulmonary congestion bilaterally. Breathing was rapid and shallow. He was using oxygen at 2 l/min via a nasal mask. He was anxious and gasping and unable to expectorate.

The most important issue for him was that he wished to make his will and needed to be fully in control of his faculties to do so. The medical team had offered medical treatment which might have aided his respiratory difficulties but might also have made him too drowsy to complete this task. Acupuncture for respiratory distress was suggested and agreed on.

The aim of treatment was to clear phlegm, improve lung function and reduce anxiety.

Treatment 1

The patient was using apical muscles of respiration excessively. He had audible secretions: he was too weak to expectorate. He was restless and distressed.

Acupuncture was given to ST 40, LU 5, LI 4 bilaterally and CV 17 for 20 minutes.

Clinical reasoning

- ST 40 to clear Phlegm
- LU 5 to transform and drain dampness, and reduce shortness of breath
- CV 17 to open chest, and also to reduce shortness of breath.

Outcome

Next day the patient was much more settled. Shortness of breath at rest and secretions were reduced. The patient was now feeling able to complete the task of writing his will with the solicitor.

Treatment 2

ST 40, LU 5, LI 4 bilaterally for 20 minutes.

Outcome

The patient was very settled. No medication was given for respiratory symptoms.

Treatment 3

Acupressure to LU 9 bilaterally using Seabands.

Clinical reasoning

The patient was now in the dying phase. Needling was not now appropriate but Seaband treatment was agreed with the family to maintain a settled breathing pattern.

The patient and family were delighted with acupuncture being used effectively in the terminal management phase. The patient died with minimal distress 3 days later.

This case history shows a different dimension for the use of acupuncture in MND. Respiratory symptoms are commonplace and acupuncture can be a viable and preferable alternative to medication for some patients, as demonstrated here.

Case study 11.3: level 3 case

The patient was female, aged 45 and married, with three children aged from 7 to 13. She had been diagnosed with MND and spinal muscular atrophy 3 years previously; she was currently presenting with muscle weakness. She was psychologically distressed, reluctant to acknowledge the diagnosis and cutting herself off from all family and friends apart from her husband and children. She refused to see any doctors or leave her study or bedroom. She spent most of the day in an inappropriate wooden rocking chair (the rocking mechanism enabled her to rise to stand with her husband for short periods to relieve sacral pressure).

At initial assessment she could just stand with the assistance of one person. She could no longer speak, and communicated via text messages or a lightwriter.

History

She was previously a fit healthy businesswoman running her own business, living a rural lifestyle, eating organic food and interested in 'healthy living'. She was open to complementary therapies but against pharmacology. She had a previous medical history of osteoarthritis of the spine and a possible prolapsed spinal disc; the level was not known by her husband.

Physical assessment

She appeared to be very tall, even when seated. She seemed cachectic or wasted and uncommunicative; she was looking down at the floor, although she was able to extend her neck fully and had good head control when awake. She was wary of health professionals. She was sleeping upright in the rocking chair for periods during the day, refusing neck support, collar or neck pillows. Consequently her head dropped forward and she tended to waken with neck pain. She refused all medication because she viewed it as 'poisoning the body'.

Presenting symptoms

- pain 1: frequent spasms in muscles (predominantly limbs)
- pain 2: neck pain
- pain 3: right shoulder pain
- pain 4: back pain.

All pains were difficult to score or evaluate due to her psychological state. Most questions were answered with a nod or eyes directed upwards nonchalantly.

Other symptoms were as follows:

- breathless
- impaired swallow, cachectic, tolerating soft diet only
- insomnia, but refusing sleeping tablets
- psychologically and spiritually distressed
- constipated
- reducing muscle power and loss of grip.

She was referred specifically for acupuncture, having had previous experience of it given by a friend.

Treatment 1

Simple acupuncture for pain relief and muscle spasm was offered and given. It was a minimal initial treatment to ascertain her acupuncture tolerance.

She refused to lie on a bed so the treatment had to be given in her rocking chair. Access to certain appropriate points was therefore restricted. Consent was agreed and her husband was also present to support her and aid with communication difficulties.

Points chosen

Due to accessibility as well as for clinical reasoning, and to build trust with patient, the following points were chosen: auricular Shenmen and TH5 Waiguan bilaterally for 25 minutes.

Clinical reasoning

Shenmen is the 'wonder point' of the ear, and is readily accessible. It enhances relaxation, relieves pain and is pertinent to relax muscle spasm, pains and anxiety. Supplementary *Vaccaria* seed plasters were used to enhance treatment between sessions.

TE 5 was used for general pain relief and also to clear lower Jiao (constipation) although TE 6 might have been a better choice for this symptom alone.

Outcome

The acupuncture was effective for a short time only. Her pains were still aggravated by the poor posture forced on her by the hard wooden rocking chair. (She persistently refused a more appropriate chair, or cushions or a fleece to pad chair, reasoning that if she did not have the ability to rock she could not continue to stand.) She refused all manual handling advice and aids offered.

Treatment 2

It was becoming apparent that the patient was very angry, possibly depressed and obstructive to most guidance offered. She was fatigued with a poor sleep pattern.

The acupuncture extended to address her psychological status as well as her painful areas

- right shoulder visual analogue scale (VAS) 7
- left buttock VAS 9
- low back VAS 9, eased by massage but nothing else.

Points chosen

ST 38, ST 36, SP 6, GB 34, LI 4, BL 11, auricular Shenmen bilaterally for 25 minutes.

Clinical reasoning

- ST 38 is a reflex point for shoulder pain.
- ST 36 and SP 6 are a supportive combination for depression/anxiety.
- GB 34 for muscle spasm is an influential point for muscles and tendons.
- LI 4 is a major distal pain control point.
- BL11 is an influential point for bone (The patient was known to have had osteoarthritis of the spine and disc collapse 2 years previously).

Additional recommendations were made, including placing sheepskin in the chair. The patient was referred to occupational therapy for hoist assessment and comfort issues. She was supplied with a resting collar for periods of sleep in her chair. Passive limb movements were shown to her husband.

Outcome

She was still reluctant to try a collar or pressure relief or protection for her spine. She had a better response to the second treatment:

- right shoulder VAS 5
- low back (base of spine) VAS 7
- thoracic spine (due to pressure on wooden chair) VAS 7.

Treatment 3

- BL 23 bilaterally (through spokes in chair!)
- LI 15, TE 14, LI 11, LI 4 right side only for 25 minutes.

Clinical reasoning

- BL 23 segmental treatment for low-back pain
- LI 15, TE 14 eyes of shoulder, with LI 11 and LI 4 for shoulder pain (the patient was becoming progressively weaker and all movements were becoming more difficult, aggravating the pain).

Outcome

There was slight improvement, although it was difficult to evaluate due to ongoing issues with the chair.

Treatment 4

- pain in right shoulder and base of spine, both VAS 5
- BL 62, SI 3, GB 34
- auricular Shenmen and auricular shoulder point right ear for 25 minutes
- auricular plasters to support treatment applied.

Clinical reasoning

- BL 62 and SI 3 together for back pain
- GB 34 muscle spasms, auricular treatment for general and shoulder pain

Further advice with regard to positioning and manual handling was given.

Outcome

There was minimal improvement in pain levels. Her back pain scored VAS 4 and her shoulder pain VAS 5. Her spasms were less frequent but her muscles were becoming weaker.

At this point the value of offering further acupuncture was discussed, considering the confounding issues of reluctance to accept appropriate advice regarding the chair, comfort measures, pressure relief, passive movements, neck supports and manual handling advice. She had psychological and spiritual distress, but refused any of the psychological support offered. To some extent she used her pain as a way of gaining attention.

This case history demonstrates the complexities of MND, especially in a younger person. The symptoms were reduced with acupuncture but the multiple confounding issues were limiting factors. However she did accept and appreciate this treatment modality. It was effective within the limits she imposed.

Other options which could have been considered were Seabands HT 7 for insomnia and anxiety and TENS but it was felt that they would probably have been dismissed without a fair trial.

Sadly the patient died 3 months later due to respiratory failure.

References

[1] Borasio GD, Miller RG. Clinical characteristics and management of ALS. Semin Neurol 2001;21 (2):155–66.

[2] Stokes M. Physical Management in Neurological Rehabilitation. 2nd ed. Edinburgh: Elsevier Mosby; 2006.

[3] Tandan R. Clinical features and differential diagnosis of classical motor neurone disease. In: Williams AC, editor. Motor Neurone Disease. London: Chapman & Hall; 1994. p. 3–27.

[4] Oliver D. The quality of care and symptom control – the effects on the terminal phase of ALS/MND. J Neurol Sci 1996;139: (Suppl):134–6.

[5] O'Brien T, Kelly M, Saunders C. Motor neurone disease: a hospice perspective. BMJ 1992;304 (6825):471–3.

[6] Wasner M, Klier H, Borasio GD. The use of alternative medicine by patients with amyotrophic lateral sclerosis. J Neurol Sci 2001;191 (1–2):151–4.

[7] Molassiotis A, Sylt P, Diggins H. The management of cancer-related fatigue after chemotherapy with acupuncture and acupressure: A randomised controlled trial. Complement Ther Med 2007;15 (4):228–37.

[8] Bausewein C, Booth S, Gysels M, et al. Non-pharmacological interventions for breathlessness in advanced stages of malignant and non-malignant diseases. Cochrane Database Syst Rev 2008;(2).

[9] Vardeny O, Bromberg MB. The use of herbal supplements and alternative therapies by patients with amyotrophic lateral sclerosis (ALS). J Herb Pharmacother 2005;5(3):23–31.

[10] Jiao S. Scalp Acupuncture and Clinical Cases. Beijing: Foreign Languages Press; 1997.

[11] Haines N. Treating the untreatable. In: MacPherson H, Kaptchuk T, editors. Acupuncture in Practice. Churchill Livingstone: Edinburgh; 1997. p. 83–92.

Section 3

Marrying East and West

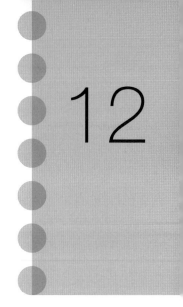

Pulling it together

KEY POINTS

- This chapter deals with the arrival of the patient: how are we to apply all these ideas and theories? We suggest ways of organizing our thoughts, according to the response we are hoping to encourage.
- For instance, if the presentation seems to have a Western medical feel to it then it will be best to consider it in that way, checking off the systems that are demonstrating damage and attempting to place the needles in sites that will elicit a change in physiology.
- Western medical acupuncture, as described in Chapter 2 by White [1], will support the choices, whether aiming for a local, spinal or supraspinal effect.
- The first part of Chapter 12 deals with the direct application of Western ideas.
- When the picture is complex with many different symptoms competing for the chief problem, or the picture changes from hour to hour, day to day, it may be that the philosophies of Chinese medicine have as much to offer, specializing as they do in interactivity, complicated interactions and results that may progress through further syndromes before resolving.
- The second part of Chapter 12 offers a loose structure to support the traditional Chinese medicine treatment model.

The Western therapist

The Western approach is summed up perfectly by the following quotation:

Acupuncture is a valuable method of complementary medicine with broad application in neurology. It is based on the experiences of traditional Chinese medicine as well as on experimentally proven biological (biochemical and neurophysiological) effects. Acupuncture-induced analgesia is mediated by inhibition of pain transmission at a spinal level and activation of central pain-modulating centers by release of opioids and other peptides that can be prevented by opioid antagonists (naloxone). Modern neuroimaging methods (functional MRI) confirmed the activation of subcortical and cortical centers, while transcranial Doppler sonography and SPECT showed an increase of cerebral blood flow and cerebral oxygen supply in normal subjects. Clinical experience and controlled studies confirmed the efficacy of acupuncture in various pain syndromes (tension headache, migraine, trigeminal neuralgia, posttraumatic pain, lumbar syndrome, ischialgia, etc.) and suggest favorable effects in the rehabilitation of peripheral facial nerve palsy and after stroke. Appropriate techniques, hygiene safeguards and knowledge of contraindications will minimize the risks of rare side effects of acupuncture which represents a valuable adjunction to the treatment repertoire in modern neurology. There is sufficient evidence of acupuncture to expand its use into conventional medicine and to encourage further studies of its pathophysiology and clinical value [2].

Although broadly encouraging, this raises a number of questions, the first being safety. Are we certain that acupuncture is safe? We do have results from a couple of very important safety trials, mentioned elsewhere in this book [3, 4], which support clinical practice and we also have additional anatomical work where skeletal anomalies have been examined and confirmed for prevalence. The two most important are the possibility of a sternal foramen at the level of CV 17 Shanzhong, and the thinning and occasional hole in the subspinal area of the scapula [5]. Once aware of the existence of these problems, and recognizing that the general bulk of muscle tissue can be greatly diminished in neurological disease, needling can be adjusted to avoid inflicting damage to the patient in any way.

Other safety issues are concerned with the physiological actions of acupuncture, such as increases in blood flow and velocity, sudden changes in blood pressure, unrealistic expectations produced by pain relief or euphoric responses to needling. Reviews of safety have concluded that, while acupuncture is not free of adverse events, they are rare, and it remains a relatively safe procedure [6].

It is also worth remembering that some of the recorded side-effects of acupuncture can be positive, the chief among them being described in a study of acupuncture as used by Swedish physiotherapists as 'a pleasant feeling of fatigue' [7].

Western supporting techniques

Ear acupuncture

This is a technique claimed by both Western and Eastern camps and probably belongs equally well in both. It is probably the best-known microsystem in acupuncture. It was first recognized as a reflex system by Paul Nogier in the 1950s. There are two distinct classifications of points, those according to Nogier, adapted by Bahr, and those according to traditional Chinese medicine (TCM).

The ancient Chinese recognized that some channels passed around or through the ear and described all the Yang meridians as having some connection but had not fully appreciated the reflexes involved. Nogier on the other hand spent many years studying the ear and slowly built up his concept of the 'man in the ear', in which he described a human fetus in an upside-down position with the head in the region of the earlobe and the limbs towards the top of the ear (Figure 12.1).

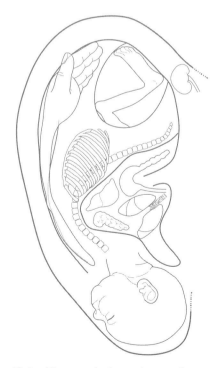

Figure 12.1 • 'The man in the ear' according to Nogier. (From Hopwood V. Acupuncture in Physiotherapy. Oxford: Butterworth-Heinemann, 2004, p. 142.)

Nogier's ideas were imported into China in the mid-1950s and barefoot doctors were trained in auricular therapy techniques, using the map of points as illustrated, and enabled to treat a large range of problems.

Nogier postulated that if there is a change in the body system due to pathology then a corresponding change can be shown in the ear, on the appropriate region. In the case of pain the areas where pain is felt in the body have been shown to have a high correlation with tenderness in the points on the ear that correspond with the sites. Oleson et al. provided the statistical evidence for these defined regions with a 74% accuracy rate in defining the musculoskeletal pains of 40 patients [8]. This applies to many kinds of pathology, not just pain [9]. The area occupied on the ear surface is proportional to that in the cortex, so the upper limb, particularly the hand and face, seems well represented.

The standardization of nomenclature for ear acupuncture points has been slow: the two main schools, that of Nogier and the TCM point locations, have now been joined by the work of Frank and Soliman [10, 11] who built on the original Nogier extended work which described three basic phases – mesodermal, ectodermal and endodermal. The theory underlying this division is that the ear is composed of three different kinds of tissue in the developing embryo and each of these types is involved in differing somatotropic responses relating to the ear. Further, the different phases are associated with acute, intermediate and chronic pain conditions. An acupuncture atlas [12] just gives all the points with little or no explanation, leading to much confusion among students.

Auricular therapy is defined as a physical reflex therapy which detects somatic level disturbances on the auricle. There are precise zones of representation of organs, though these are not thought of as fixed points as they tend to have fluctuating boundaries, depending as they do on the metabolism of the organ. The right ear is said to represent the left hemisphere of the brain whereas the left ear represents the right hemisphere. Thus treatment will be on the same side as the problem.

The ear is associated with the parasympathetic nervous system, effectively modulating the sympathetic responses. The innervation of the central part of the ear links directly into the vagal nerve (the 10th cranial nerve). This means that rather than the 'fight or flight' response it tends to reduce the heart rate, lower blood pressure and facilitate

digestion and excretion, thus returning the body processes to their normal rate. In short, in times of danger, the sympathetic system prepares the body for violent activity; the parasympathetic system reverses these changes when the danger is over.

Nogier discovered that there was a change in the amplitude of the human pulse as monitored at the wrist when tactile stimulation of the ear occurred. This was evidence of a sympathetic reflex affecting peripheral blood vessel activity. He referred to this as the auricular cardiac reflex. The changes detected are in waveform or amplitude, not in pulse rate. It is an involuntary arterial reflex and also known as the vascular autonomic signal, and is found as a vascular cutaneous reflex in response to other stimuli. This response to any form of tactile stimulus may explain the soothing effect of rubbing the ears, in both small children and dogs!

Acupuncture technique in the ear is slightly different to any other body surface. Short, fine needles are preferable and these are inserted carefully without piercing the cartilage of the ear. The reason for this care is that the cartilage has a poor blood supply so if it becomes infected it is difficult to eliminate the infection. This has led to recommendation of alcohol swabs to clean the surface before needle insertion.

Originally auriculotherapy was recommended for the treatment of nicotine or alcohol addiction and subdermal needles like tiny tacks were left in situ from one treatment to the next and covered by a small piece of plaster. This is discouraged nowadays because the risk of infection is too great.

The Chinese ear charts differ quite radically from those produced by Nogier, leading to considerable confusion among acupuncturists (Figure 12.2). There are many points on the TCM ear, located by way of a grid system and requiring a fine location skill. Chinese texts recommend the use of the points according to TCM principles, i.e. the Kidney point to treat bones, but since this appears to be a true reflex system this use is not supported scientifically.

More important is the nerve supply to each part of the structure. The ear has an abundant innervation, being supplied by the sensory fibres of the trigeminal, facial and vagus nerves. The endings of these nerves are closely interwoven and can influence many distant body areas. Bourdiol gives an explanation based on embryology, emphasizing the fact that these nerves travel only a short distance to the reticular formation of the brainstem [13].

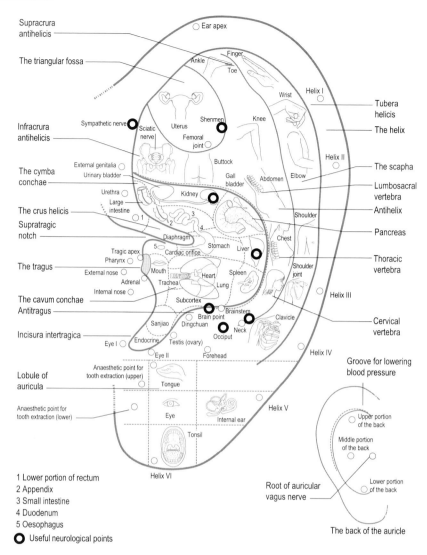

Figure 12.2 • Chinese map of ear points (from Hopwood V. Acupuncture in Physiotherapy. Oxford: Butterworth-Heinemann, 2004, p. 14.)

There are several ways of classifying the points. Oleson and Kroening [14] suggested nomenclature that depends on whether the points are located on raised, depressed or hidden areas in the ear. Otherwise the Chinese or Nogier maps are commonly used.

The mechanism appears to be the same as in the rest of the body. Ear acupuncture has been shown to affect the endorphin concentration and to be reversible by naloxone [15]. The study by Simmons and Oleson investigated changes in dental pain threshold after electroacupuncture stimulation to the ear, showing that true electroacupuncture produced a significant rise in the pain threshold while the placebo, using inappropriate ear points, did not.

All areas of the ear surface are utilized, with some points being located on raised areas, some in the depressions and some in hidden areas under folds of tissue and still others on the posterior surface of the ear.

When the two maps, that of Nogier and the TCM map, are compared it can be seen that some regions are similar but there are many single points that do not seem to tally. In physiotherapy practice the most commonly used auricular point is Shenmen, common to both, a sedative point located in the navicular fossa. As might be deduced from the name, this has similar applications to Heart 7 Shenmen, being used to calm anxious patients, often before further acupuncture is undertaken. The musculoskeletal zones are also frequently used, perhaps because they are easily located.

These points are used in conjunction with body acupuncture in many protocols for musculoskeletal acupuncture. They offer an alternative when points are inaccessible, either because of medical problems or plaster, or simply because of the difficulty of positioning or undressing the patient.

Points derived from the Chinese system of ear acupuncture are regularly used in drug addiction withdrawal programmes. The National Acupuncture Detoxification Association protocol uses five points – Shenmen, Liver, Lung, Sympathetic and Kidney – and is supported by some research [16]. This combination of points can produce profound relaxation in distressed patients so it has an application beyond that of drug withdrawal. It may owe more to the fact that the pinna is richly innervated and offers a good site to stimulate the central nervous system in a general way, but it has been utilized successfully in palliative care patients with serious anxiety states.

Technique

The indications of pathology are similar to those elsewhere in the body. Among these are changes in the appearance of the skin, redness or small skin lesions, changes in tenderness or sensitivity of the skin and changes in the electrical resistance of the skin. The usual way of detecting these tender points is to use manual pressure via the blunt end of an acupuncture needle or a blunt spring-loaded instrument. Care must be taken to maintain an even pressure and the location of tender spots indicates both the area of the body in trouble and the point in the ear to insert the needle.

Electrical point finders are often recommended for use in the ear. Where the points are so close together distinguishing between one and the next might be a critical factor in treatment. While theoretically a good idea, these are difficult to use in practice because it is easy to produce a false impedance reading if the pressure on the skin is too great or if the patient is sweating. It is also possible to burn a low-resistance pathway through the dermis if the current is too high, also producing a false point.

Treatment is usually most effective with the least number of needles. The tiny needles are usually left in for 10–20 minutes, normal treatment time and, as explained previously, it is not recommended that they be left between treatments. Slight bleeding may occur after removal of the needles; an alcohol swab can be used to clear this.

If a longer effect is required patients can be asked to stimulate the point themselves. Sterilized mustard seeds or small ionic beads (Magraine) may be left securely stuck to the ear with small plaster patches. This makes it possible for the patient to apply acupressure in between treatments, whenever the presenting problem recurs.

If body acupuncture is to be combined with the use of ear points, the points on the ear must be located first as the delicate organ cutaneous reflex can be altered by body needling and the ear points will be harder to locate.

Research

The original work supporting this theory was performed by Oleson et al. [8]. In a blinded trial it was found that body pathology in patients could be detected with 74% accuracy by testing for tenderness in the ear and measuring changes in the electrical resistance of the skin. The result was highly statistically significant and anecdotal evidence from the same trial indicated that old pathology that the patients themselves had forgotten about was also detected.

A more recent study has taken this apparent correlation further. Given that the pathology of a particular organ appears to give rise to changes in the electrical impedance of the skin on the ear over the corresponding point, the researchers tested the validity of this reflex with patients undergoing surgery [17]. Forty-five patients, admitted for surgery for cholecystectomy, appendectomy, partial gastrectomy or dilatation and curettage after miscarriage, were tested. The initial value of skin resistance was estimated at the auricular organ projection area on five occasions: (1) before premedication; (2) after medication; (3) under general anaesthesia; (4) after skin incision; and (5) after surgery. Two healthy organ projection areas were measured on each patient each time as a control. The examiners performed all measurements without knowledge of the corresponding points.

Of more relevance to neurological disease, a recent systematic review has now indicated that auricular acupuncture appears to be effective for treating insomnia [18]. Ear acupuncture is a useful addition to the needling skills of a physiotherapist. It seems to have a reasonable evidence base and lends itself to use on nervous or debilitated patients. Since it can also be utilized in patients where access to the normal body points is not possible for some reason, for instance in cases of pain after major surgery, during childbirth or extensive application of plaster fixation, it can be versatile. It also provides a means of treating a patient where mobilization is difficult and normal transition from chair to bed presents problems with increased muscle tone.

Trigger point acupuncture

Trigger point acupuncture is a phrase loosely used in acupuncture circles. It needs to be made clear whether one is referring to the use of Ah Shi points in TCM terms (where there is a single painful spot needled in the usual manner) or whether one is using Western-type trigger point acupuncture, which is often referred to as 'dry needling'. This term is often misunderstood but it is only used to distinguish it from other forms of medical use of needles where fluids may be administered or extracted.

Trigger points are points within the muscles, tendons, ligaments and joint capsule that demonstrate hypersensitivity and pain. These points may be latent, not actually referring pain, or active, referring pain in clearly recognizable patterns.

Myofascial pain, commonly treated by trigger point needling, appears to be modulated by local or segmental effects, perhaps not always requiring a fully intact nervous system. It is worth noting that the myofascial pain points described as trigger points often correlate with traditional acupuncture points [19]. The best textbook, detailing both patterns and treatment techniques, is that by Peter Baldry [20] describing a minimally invasive form of needling which can be very effective and often preferable to the deeper kind when treating neurogenic conditions.

Trigger points are recognized by physiotherapists and appear to form when there is disruption at the motor endplate causing increased adrenocorticotrophic hormone release with sarcomere contraction and compression of blood vessels and a resulting sort of 'energy crisis'. The clinical characteristics of these points include local tenderness, a palpable taut band and a local twitch response in the

contracted band on palpation with a concentration of acetylcholine. Pain is referred distally and there is restricted movement and muscle weakness. There is also often autonomic dysfunction with possible trophoedema.

There are two ways of dealing with this. Since they have not been scientifically compared and both seem to have a clinical effect they are described below.

Superficial needling [20]

The trigger point is first palpated. Either the patient may exhibit a disproportional response, the so-called 'jump and shout' response, and/or the operator may be able to palpate a taut band in the muscle. Using a short needle, the point is introduced subdermally and the needle allowed to fall against the skin. No manipulation is given and the Deqi sensation is not elicited. This needle is retained for only 30 seconds, removed and then the point is palpated again. If the sensation remains unchanged, the needle can be reinserted (provided it has not been in contact with anything else in the meantime) and left for a further 30 seconds before final removal. This often appears to deactivate the tender trigger point after the first application [21].

Deep trigger point needling [22]

This involves deep needling into the palpated taut band and a visible muscle twitch is often produced. Quite a long needle is used and, to facilitate easy insertion and prevent contact with the shaft of the needle, a tubular guide is used. Needle grasp conforms to muscular spasm and the accuracy of the insertion. The patient experiences a strong sensation rather like a muscle cramp which can be very painful but does guarantee the eventual success of the intervention. The needle is vigorously manipulated. This manipulation is aimed at disrupting the dysfunctional endplates in order to provoke a healing response. The needle is left for 10–20 minutes and then removed once relaxation has occurred. This may be obtained more quickly with manual stimulation, particularly with 'pecking' movements, although it may cause the spasm to intensify initially. Although placing the needle at the motor zone or musculotendinous junction is most effective for releasing spasm, in neuropathy extrajunctional acetylcholine receptors or 'hot spots' are formed throughout the entire length of the muscle.

Thus a needle inserted almost anywhere into a shortened muscle can relieve spasm [23].

Both types of treatment depend on knowledge of the muscle innervations, nerve roots and the distribution of referred pain from trigger points. Neither really involves Deqi and they are not dependent on knowledge of the meridians and their actions.

Recently published work [24] has offered links between the distal acupuncture points and changes in the painful loci within the trigger point regions. These loci are probably located in the endplate zone and endplate 'noise' in trapezius muscles in patients with chronic pain has been shown to decrease after acupuncture is applied to Waiguan and Quchi. The story is not yet fully explored and use of the major distal points remains important whichever school of acupuncture is followed.

Electroacupuncture

Electroacupuncture involves the electrical stimulation of acupuncture points by passing a current through acupuncture needles. It was developed into its modern form in China in the 1950s, when it was used for surgical anaesthesia. Since then it has been used for acupuncture analgesia and many other clinical presentations. It allows the provision of a stronger, more continuous level of stimulation and can be less time-consuming for the practitioner. In some conditions it may produce more rapid and prolonged treatment effects. This form of acupuncture is widely used in research studies since the level of stimulation provided may be carefully standardized [25].

Application of electroacupuncture

The effects of electroacupuncture are influenced by the frequency of stimulation used and the intensity selected. The application of low frequencies of 2–8 Hz will stimulate small-diameter afferent fibres and provide analgesic effects by the release of β-endorphin, enkephalin and orphanin, whilst high frequency, of 80–100 Hz, stimulates large afferent fibres, causing the release of dynorphin [26]. Other neurotransmitters are released and probably include noradrenaline (norepinephrine), dopamine and serotonin [25]. Intensity of stimulation may be varied.

Strong stimulation is often used for pain relief, particularly in situations of chronic nociceptive pain which has failed to respond to milder stimulation. Strong stimulation will increase sympathetic tone, whereas milder stimulation may enhance parasympathetic activity. Electroacupuncture has been used for many situations other than pain, including spasticity, tissue repair and bladder dysfunction.

Electroacupuncture in neurological conditions

Electroacupuncture has been used widely for neurological conditions in China and has also been used in many of the research trials on acupuncture for stroke. Studies relevant to neurological conditions have been considered in Chapter 4. In practical terms electroacupuncture seems to be useful for sensory and motor problems. Evidence shows that lack of afferent information from areas of impaired sensation or movement results in reorganization of cortical maps. Interventions to increase somatosensory stimulation are being used increasingly to influence sensory and motor function, with promising results in some studies [27]. Electroacupuncture could provoke a strong stimulus in this regard, providing afferent information from skin and muscle contraction.

Contraindications and safety specific to neurological conditions

In addition to the usual contraindications and precautions there are particular considerations when using electroacupuncture in neurological conditions. Electroacupuncture may be used in well-controlled epilepsy with caution, although the option of choice would be manual acupuncture. Strong or sustained muscle contraction should be avoided in this condition as well as stimulation applied over the scalp [25].

Caution should also be exercised when considering electroacupuncture stimulation in those with spinal cord injury at T6 and above. Noxious stimulation below the level of the spinal lesion may precipitate autonomic dysreflexia in some individuals. Therefore mild stimulation or perhaps manual acupuncture would be preferred options. Monitoring the patient's blood pressure before and after treatment would provide valuable information if the practitioner was concerned about this possibility. Reports by the patient of pounding headache, nausea, anxiety and blurred vision require immediate action since this condition may progress rapidly and lead to seizures, intracranial haemorrhage or death.

Intensity of stimulation needs to be considered carefully when treating patients with spinal spasticity, for example in multiple sclerosis or spinal cord injury. Stimulation may provoke disinhibited spinal reflexes, resulting in spasms in the legs, most commonly flexor spasms [28]. Needling should consider the possibility of limb movement during treatment and the practitioner may need to stay immediately by the patient to stabilize the limb and prevent movement if spasms occur.

Transcutaneous electrical nerve stimulation (TENS)

TENS is the application of an electrical current to the body through surface electrodes. There are similarities between electroacupuncture and TENS and the electrodes are frequently applied to acupuncture points. However their physiological effects are different, since TENS can only effectively stimulate nerve endings near the body surface. In general electroacupuncture has stronger and more long-lasting effects than TENS. Even so, TENS may have useful applications in neurological conditions for relief of pain, spasms and spasticity as well as improvement in motor and sensory function [29–31]. TENS is a useful option to provide sensory stimulation over a longer period of time and can be used by the patient as part of a home maintenance programme. Further research is required to clarify the most beneficial applications.

Scalp acupuncture

The insertion of needles into points on the Governor Vessel channel as it runs over the scalp is as old as acupuncture itself. However scalp acupuncture as a distinct system is a relatively new technique which emerged in China and Japan in the early 1970s. It is variously reported as being invented by Jiao Shunfa in 1971, Fang Yunpeng in 1970 and Toshikatsu Yamamoto in 1970. Jiao outlined a system based on the premise that needling points on the surface overlying an organ could produce beneficial effects on the underlying organs in the same way as needling mu points could benefit the associated organ. He extended this thinking to disorders of the brain and incorporated modern awareness of the functional divisions of the cerebral cortex to devise a system of stimulating the scalp to influence the brain [32].

Jiao's system seems to have some logic to it – needling over the sensory homunculus to influence sensation and over the motor homunculus to influence movement. The system is reported to be particularly useful for neurological conditions such as stroke and Parkinson's disease, with benefits noted for motor, sensory and speech problems, chronic muscle spasm, balance problems and tremor (see Figures 7.1 and 7.2 in Chapter 7).

Yamamoto's system, called Yamamoto New Scalp Acupuncture, involves the needling of various points on the scalp according to zones which are reported to influence different parts of the body. It is based on a combination of Chinese medicine, Five Phases principles and Yamamoto's microsystem theory. The important 'brain' points are located either side of the midline just inside the frontal hairline [33]. Yamamomoto's system is reported to be useful for musculoskeletal and neurological conditions but has not been subjected to rigorous research protocols.

Practical application of Jiao's system

The hair needs to be parted and skin sterilized with a solution of 2.5% iodine and 75% alcohol. The use of needles up to 7 cm in length is described, with insertion just under the skin of the scalp into the space between the epicranial aponeurosis and the periosteum. However Western practitioners usually use three or four short needles inserted obliquely along the line (see Figure 6.2 in Chapter 6). Needles may be stimulated manually. However, electroacupuncture is commonly applied, usually to each end of the line being stimulated. A frequency of 100–200 Hz is usually used, although some report using lower frequencies. Treatment lasts 20–40 minutes. Some people find scalp acupuncture to be a strong stimulation. However many experience a general warmth, tingling, pins and needles or buzzing sensation and find it relaxing. Sometimes general warmth is also felt in the body part being targeted [34].

Contraindications to scalp acupuncture

Scalp acupuncture should not be applied in the immediate acute phase after stroke until cerebral bleeding has stopped. Otherwise contraindications and precautions are the same as for manual and electroacupuncture. One short paper detailed the development of angina in two cases involving scalp acupuncture with electrostimulation provided to the highest tolerance [35]. Less intense stimulation is recommended.

Research

Anecdotal reports from China indicate miraculous results for scalp acupuncture in neurological conditions. Indeed, there are many trials from China reporting benefits from scalp acupuncture in a range of conditions such as stroke and cerebral palsy. However, virtually no rigorous research has been conducted in the West. Some trials have combined body acupuncture with scalp acupuncture but failed to indicate significant benefits for the acupuncture group compared to control group [36]. Rapson et al. [37] reported a substantial reduction in neuropathic pain in spinal cord injury following electroacupuncture at 1 Hz for 30 minutes to a number of Governor Vessel points on the scalp. This was a retrospective review of cases and represented usual clinical practice.

Clinical reasoning

It is impossible to escape the medical diagnosis and all the associated information available in the Western system. This is all useful to the acupuncture practitioner, supporting the choices we make and allowing us to estimate progress accurately. Refer back to Table 5.1 in Chapter 5 to remind yourself of the options. To return to our definition of clinical reasoning:

> a cognitive process of critical analysis and reflection that supports decision making. The purpose of this process is the well-being of the patients. The treatments are tailored to meet their individual needs, skills and priorities.

As medical acupuncture practitioners we may be more familiar with the scientific reasoning process and should not be afraid to apply it. Understanding the mechanisms and differing techniques, it will be possible to formulate a treatment plan for our neurology patients that will bear close scrutiny.

To make our reasoning process truly comprehensive we should draw in the TCM ideas and clinical practice and make sure we do not ignore some aspects that may add something important to the mixture.

The Eastern way

> Chinese medicine provides a particularly attractive model for holistic health care. It sees health and well-being as a state of balance between a person and every

aspect of that person's context. This indicates primarily a respectful and caring relationship with the natural environment and a lifestyle appropriate to the exigencies of natural forces and climates. It can also be extrapolated to include relationships between the body's constitution and the way we work and play, where we live, what we eat, how we modulate our relationships with others and so on. The interdependence of mind and body goes without saying in such a comprehensive view of health. Illness is not usually an arbitrary and unlucky event but an expression of a lack of balance, and as such it is up to the individual to take care of their lifestyle to keep their health [38].

General application of TCM ideas and techniques

Probably the most useful thoughts to begin with will be those concerning Pathogens. Which Pathogen do the symptoms most remind you of? Given that we are dealing with the neurology syndromes, which is the most predominant subpattern? Is it more to do with Wind or Feng, or does the situation make you think more of Wei or withering, with a clear decrease in muscle activity? Or finally, is it more that nothing seems to be working very well, there is a 'stuckness' of Qi or Blood and the Bi syndrome seems dominant?

The two types of stagnation may be manifest in the superficial layers of the body, and both will respond to acupuncture treatment. There is a TCM saying: 'The Blood nourishes the Qi and the Qi leads the Blood'. Qi is more Yang than Blood, which tends to be Yin. If the predominant symptom is pain it is relatively easy to distinguish between them; the main points are given in Table 12.1.

The acupuncture points generally recommended for moving stagnation of the blood are listed in Table 12.2.

All stagnation is considered as a Shi (Full, or Excess) condition but since it may occur only locally this could be happening within a context of overall Xu or deficiency. It may, of course, simply be due to local trauma. A visible haematoma would be a good example of this. When drugs produce a similar visible effect, for instance warfarin or heparin, the effect in TCM terms is similar. The Excess may vary in type. It may be full or empty in nature.

A Full or Shi situation is characterized by pain that is worse on waking in the morning or after a period of inactivity.

Table 12.1 Qi or Blood stagnation?

Qi stagnation	Blood stagnation
Dull pain	Sharp, strong
Less severe	Severe pain
Mobile	Fixed
Palpable changes less likely	Clearly palpable by therapist, dry, scaly skin. Possible varicosities
Patient vague about location	Patient indicates painful point(s) clearly
Affected by stress or emotion	Unaffected
Improves with gentle massage	No immediate improvement with light massage but deep, invigorating massage may help in treatment
Responds to acupuncture	Responds to acupuncture
Distal acupuncture points are the most important	Fixed local points are more effective; these may include Ah Shi and Extra points
Overall regulation of body energy required	Does not affect internal functions

Table 12.2 Blood stagnation points

Upper body	LI 11, LI 4, LU 7, LU 5
Lower body	ST 36, ST 41, SP 10, SP 6

An Empty or Xu condition is worse after activity. There is little energy and what there is, is soon used up. This pain comes on in the evening or after activity.

There is a need to identify the type of stagnation in order to be able to treat it successfully. However it will be clear that this is a problem associated with most diseases of the elderly and many of a neurological origin. Consequently it will be quite difficult to treat since, due to a general decrease in the abundance and energy of Qi, there will be a tendency to relapse.

From a physiotherapeutic point of view the use of light massage to stimulate the superficial circulation makes good sense. Using the TCM adjunctive technique of cupping is also relevant. Improving the oxygen exchange in the tissues by increasing subcutaneous perfusion will clearly improve the health of the tissues and increase their resistance to minor injury or infection.

Moving cupping

In particular, the technique known as 'moving cupping' or Tui Guan Fa is an excellent way to mobilize connective tissue and offers an easy way to provide a type of massage which will assist in moving Blood stagnation. The most effective way to provide this is by the use of glass cups with a flexible rubber bulb to provide the vacuum that allows them to stick to patients' skin. With a light application of suitable massage oil, the massage delivered when the cup is slid along the muscle surface is both effective and comfortable.

This type of cupping can be applied where there is sufficient muscle for the connective tissues to be mobilized in this way. This may be over the scapula, on the back (Figure 12.3), on the thighs or, even, if the cup is small enough, over the facial muscles in the case of facial paralysis. It should not be used if the patient is physically frail or weak and never over open or infected skin.

Bell's palsy with all the classic symptoms can also be treated by 'flash' cupping, where the small cups remain in contact for less than 30 seconds. Plastic vacuum cups may be used for this. The short duration is enough to stimulate the Qi and Blood but not enough to drain [39].

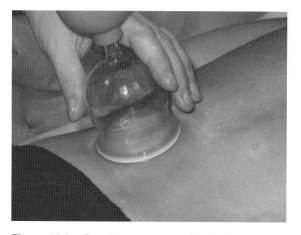

Figure 12.3 • Cupping massage on the back.

Gua Sha

Gua Sha is another Chinese technique for dealing with stagnation of the circulation. It is quite similar to an old-fashioned physiotherapeutic technique known as connective tissue massage [40].

It is also similar to cupping in that it aims to produce a deliberate increase in superficial circulation, bringing blood visibly to the surface in a red heat rash (Figure 12.4).

This is done in order to bring the Pathogenic Heat and Wind to the surface. 'Gua' means to scrape or scratch and 'Sha' translates as cholera, heat, skin rash [41]. Gu Sha is thought to mobilize the Wei Qi in the tissues.

Gua Sha is performed with a smooth-surfaced instrument, traditionally a porcelain Chinese soup spoon (Figure 12.5).

Before treating the desired area, a thin application of oil or talcum powder will ensure smooth contact. Long gentle strokes are applied until there is a visible change in the tissues, like light bruising.

This technique will increase superficial circulation in the same way as cupping but it is clear that by dispelling one form of stagnation, another, more

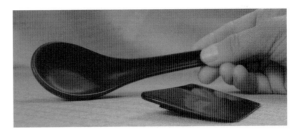

Figure 12.5 • Gua Sha equipment.

superficial one, is being produced so further general movement of the tissues will be necessary. Gu Sha can be used for muscular pain in the arms and legs where cupping can be difficult either because of small areas of muscle or the possibility of uncontrolled movements.

Making sense of it

Figure 12.6 offers an overview of the links between the major syndromes involved in the treatment of neurological conditions.

It can be seen that the balance and interplay between the Spleen, Kidney and Liver are of particular importance. This is a complex diagram because no organ works in isolation and Chinese theory teaches us that, where there is Xu or a deficiency, there will be Shi or an excess elsewhere in the system. It is not possible to put the main neurological conditions dealt with in this book exactly on the map. The syndromes have all been mentioned in the different chapters. It would be misleading to suggest that the Heart, Pericardium and Lungs play no part in this picture but, nonetheless, in the light of experience it has become apparent that the Spleen underpins the ability of the body to recover, Kidney is closely concerned with the damage to the central nervous system and the Liver has an important part to play both in preventing and treating stagnation and, in tandem with the Spleen and Stomach, in maintaining muscle function.

A neurology syndrome

It makes sense to consider this whole complex as a new syndrome, a neurology syndrome, where respect is paid to the underpinning Chinese theories but our new understanding of neurophysiology is also acknowledged.

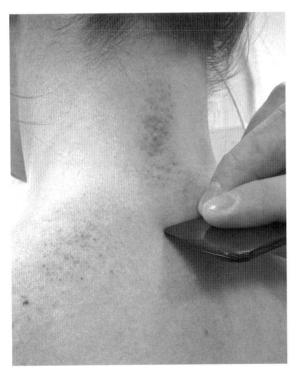

Figure 12.4 • Gua Sha effects on skin.

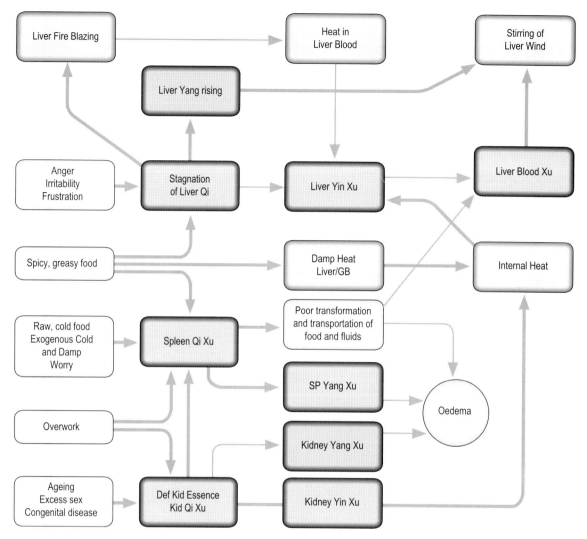

Figure 12.6 • Neurology syndrome (spleen, liver and kidney syndromes and relationships). The main syndromes are shaded and the contributing factors are in clear boxes. The dangerous Heat syndromes are in lighter shaded boxes.

The more one examines the literature and the evidence base in both Western and Eastern publications, the clearer it becomes that there is little difference in how most neurological diseases are considered. Even when the supporting theories owe perhaps more to the prevailing cultural influences, frequently the same points are chosen.

And finally, as this manuscript goes to print, new Cochrane review protocols have been made public [42]. These include:

- acupuncture for acute management and rehabilitation of traumatic brain injury
- acupuncture for attention-deficit hyperactivity disorder in children and adolescents

- acupuncture for autistic spectrum disorder
- acupuncture for Guillain–Barré syndrome
- acupuncture for myopia in children and adolescents
- acupuncture for postherpetic neuralgia.

Recently published systematic reviews not yet appraised by the Cochrane research database include:

- a systematic review of the effects of acupuncture in treating insomnia
- acupuncture for lowering blood pressure: systematic review and meta-analysis
- acupuncture for obesity: a systematic review and meta-analysis

- auricular acupuncture for insomnia: a systematic review
- effectiveness of acupuncture for Parkinson's disease: a systematic review
- efficacy and safety of acupuncture for idiopathic Parkinson's disease: a systematic review.

Some of these have been cited in this book and it is encouraging to see them being investigated more fully. While we await their eventual outcomes with much interest, we feel that the science has evidently been sufficient to prompt their endeavours and, even before the results are published, our patients can only gain if we include acupuncture in their treatments. Acupuncture has been proved to be safe; now would be a very good time to add further clinical evidence of its value in neurological conditions.

References

[1] White A. Western medical acupuncture: a definition. Acupunct Med 2009;27(1):33–5.

[2] Jellinger KA. Principles and application of acupuncture in neurology. Wiener Medizinische Wochenschrift (1946) 2000;150 (13–14):278–85.

[3] MacPherson H, Thomas K, Walters S, et al. The York acupuncture safety study: prospective survey of 34 000 treatments by traditional acupuncturists. BMJ 2001;323:486–7.

[4] White A, Hayhoe S, Hart A, et al. Adverse events following acupuncture:prospective survey of 32 000 consultations with doctors and physiotherapists. BMJ 2001;323:485–6.

[5] Peuker E, Cummings M. Anatomy for the acupuncturist – facts and fiction. 2. The chest, abdomen, and back. Acupuncture Med 2003;21 (3):72–9.

[6] Birch S, Hesselink JK, Jonkman FA, et al. Clinical research on acupuncture. Part 1. What have reviews of the efficacy and safety of acupuncture told us so far. Journal Of Alternative And Complementary Medicine (New York, NY) 2004;10(3):468–80.

[7] Odsberg A, Schill U, Haker E. Acupuncture treatment: side effects and complications reported by Swedish physiotherapists. Complement Ther Med 2001;9:17–20.

[8] Oleson TD, Kroening RJ, Bresler DE. An experimental evaluation of auricular diagnosis: the somatotopic mapping of musculoskeletal pain at ear acupuncture points. Pain 1980;8:217–29.

[9] Nogier PMF, Nogier R. The Man in the Ear. Sainte-Ruffine: Maisonneuve; 1985.

[10] Frank BL, Soliman NE. Atlas of Auricular Therapy and Auricular Medicine. Richardson, TX: Integrated Medicine Seminars; 2000.

[11] Frank B, Soliman N. Zero point: A critical assessment through advanced auricular therapy. Journal of the Acupuncture Association of Chartered Physiotherapists 2001;61–5.

[12] Hecker H-U, Steveling A, Peuker E, et al. Color Atlas of Acupuncture. Stuttgart: Thieme; 2000.

[13] Bourdiol RJ. Elements of Auriculotherapy. Moulin-le-Metz, France: Maisonneuve Editions; 1982.

[14] Oleson T, Kroening R. A new nomenclature for identifying Chinese and Nogier acupuncture points. Am J Acupuncture 1983;12:325–44.

[15] Simmons M, Oleson T. Auricular electrical stimulation and dental pain threshold. Anesth Prog 1993;40:14–9.

[16] Smith MO, Khan I. An acupuncture programme for the treatment of drug addicted persons. Bull Narc 1988; XL:35–41.

[17] Szopinski JZ, Lukasiewicz S, Lochner GP, et al. Influence of general anesthesia and surgical intervention on the parameters of auricular organ projection areas. Medical Acupuncture 2003;14 (2):40–2.

[18] Chen HY, Shi Y, Ng CS, et al. Auricular acupuncture treatment for insomnia: a systematic review. Journal of Alternative and Complementary Medicine (New York, NY) 2007;13(6):669–76.

[19] Dorsher PT, Fleckenstein J. Trigger points and classical acupuncture points: part 3: relationships of myofascial referred pain patterns to acupuncture meridians. Deutsche Zeitschrift fur Akupunktur 2009;52(1):9–14.

[20] Baldry PE. Acupuncture, Trigger Points and Musculoskeletal Pain. 3rd ed Edinburgh: Churchill Livingstone; 2004.

[21] Edwards J, Knowles N. Superficial dry needling and active stretching in the treatment of myofascial pain. A randomised controlled trial. Acupuncture in Medicine 2003;21(3):80–6.

[22] Gunn C. Treating Myofascial Pain. Seattle: University of Washington; 1989.

[23] Gunn CC. Treatment and Needle Technique. Treating myofascial pain. Seattle, USA: University of Washington Medical School; 1989. p. 37–44.

[24] Chou LW, Hsieh YL, Kao MJ, et al. Remote influences of acupuncture on the pain intensity and the amplitude changes of endplate noise in the myofascial trigger point of the upper trapezius muscle. Arch Phys Med Rehabil 2009;90(6):905–12.

[25] Mayor DF. Electroacupuncture: a practical manual and resource. Edinburgh: Churchill Livingstone; 2007.

[26] White A, Cummings M, Filshie J. An introduction to western

medical acupuncture. Edinburgh: Churchill Livingstone; 2008.

[27] Conforto AB, Cohen LG, dos Santos RL, et al. Effects of somatosensory stimulation on motor function in chronic cortico-subcortical strokes. J Neurol 2007;254(3):333–9.

[28] Donnellan CP, Shanley J. Comparison of the effect of two types of acupuncture on quality of life in secondary progressive multiple sclerosis: a preliminary single-blind randomized controlled trial. Clin Rehabil 2008;22 (3):195–205.

[29] Miller L, Mattison P, Paul L, et al. The effects of transcutaneous electrical nerve stimulation (TENS) on spasticity in multiple sclerosis. Multiple Sclerosis 2007;13(4):527–33.

[30] Ng SSM, Hui-Chan CWY. Transcutaneous electrical nerve stimulation combined with task-related training improves lower limb functions in subjects with chronic stroke. Stroke 2007;38 (11):2953–9.

[31] Yan T, Hui-Chan CW. Transcutaneous electrical stimulation on acupuncture points improves muscle function in subjects after acute stroke: a randomized controlled trial. J Rehabil Med 2009;41(5): 312–316.

[32] Jiao S. Scalp Acupuncture and Clinical Cases. Beijing: Foreign Languages Press; 1997.

[33] Feely RA. Yamamoto new scalp acupuncture: principles and practice. New York: Thieme; 2006.

[34] Yau PS. Scalp-Needling Therapy. Beijing: Medicine & Health Publishing; 1990.

[35] Li CD, Jiang ZY. Angina pectoris induced by electric scalp acupuncture: report on two cases. International Journal of Clinical Acupuncture 1998;9(1):53–4.

[36] Hopwood V, Lewith G, Prescott P, et al. Evaluating the efficacy of acupuncture in defined aspects of stroke recovery: a randomised, placebo controlled single blind study. J Neurol 2008;255(6):858–66.

[37] Rapson LM, Wells N, Pepper J, et al. Acupuncture as a promising treatment for below-level central neuropathic pain: a retrospective study. J Spinal Cord Med 2003;26 (1):21–6.

[38] Lyttelton J. Of molecules, meridians and medicine: the feminist influence – putting the yin back into health care. Am J Acupunct 1992;20(3):237–43.

[39] Chirali IZ. Empty (flash) cupping. Traditional Chinese Medicine; Cupping Therapy. Edinburgh: Churchill Livingstone; 2007. p. 87.

[40] Brattberg G. Connective tissue massage in the treatment of fibromyalgia. Eur J Pain 1999;3 (3):235–44.

[41] Nielsen A. Gua Sha, a traditional technique for modern practice. Edinburgh: Churchill Livingstone; 1995.

[42] NHS Evid CAM Newsletter, Available online at: http://www.library.nhs.uk/CAM/NHSLibrary; 2009.

Appendix: Outcome measures in neurological rehabilitation

This appendix provides a brief description of outcome measures which may be encountered in the research literature or which may be useful in clinical practice when recording acupuncture effect.

Beck Depression Inventory (BDI)

BDI is a 21-item self-rated screening tool for depression. It evaluates symptoms of depression covering emotions, behaviours and somatic symptoms. The BDI is valid and sensitive but has low specificity, i.e. high scores cannot be interpreted as diagnostic of depression. It is an extremely valuable depression-screening tool.

Fatigue Impact Scale (FIS)

FIS is a self-rated symptom-specific measure of health-related quality of life. It assesses the impact of fatigue on three domains of daily functioning: cognitive, physical and psychosocial. It is used within a wide range of conditions where fatigue is a significant problem. The scale has been modified specifically for use in the multiple sclerosis population, and this is called the Modified Fatigue Impact Scale (MFIS). The FIS and MFIS are valid, reliable and regularly used in clinical practice and research.

Fugl–Meyer Assessment (FMA)

FMA is a 155-item stroke-specific observer-rated scale assessing five domains of motor function, balance, sensation, joint range and joint pain. It may take 45–60 minutes to administer the entire scale.

Individual domains may be assessed separately. The FMA is reliable, valid and widely used in research and in clinical practice.

General Health Questionnaire-12 (GHQ-12)

GHQ-12 is a shortened version of the well-validated GHQ-60. It is a 12-item self-rated scale, designed to detect psychological distress in community or medical settings. It may be scored to detect cases on a binary scale (0, 0, 1, 1, i.e. total score of 0–12). Alternatively it may be scored on a Likert scale (0–3, i.e. total score of 0–36) to provide information on the degree of disorder. It demonstrates good reliability, validity and responsiveness.

Hamilton Rating Scale for Depression (HAM-D)

HAM-D is a 21-item multiple choice questionnaire administered by the clinician to assess the severity of depression in those already diagnosed with the disorder. It includes questions on mood, insomnia, agitation, anxiety and weight loss. It demonstrates adequate validity, and good reliability and responsiveness. It is widely used in research.

Hoffman Reflex (H-Reflex)

H-reflex is a spinal reflex that can be elicited by electrical stimulation over a mixed peripheral nerve. Stimulation causes impulses to travel up the primary sensory fibres from the muscle spindle (Ia afferents), into the dorsal horn of the spinal cord and synapse on the alpha motorneurones. The impulse then continues out of the ventral horn of the spinal cord to activate the muscle fibres. The H-reflex amplitude or latency may be assessed. The H-reflex provides information about the excitability of the spinal motor neurone pool. Shorter H-reflex latency and greater amplitude indicate greater excitability in the spinal cord as might be seen in people with spasticity. The H-reflex is moderately reliable.

Insomnia Severity Index (ISI)

ISI is a brief seven-item self-rated symptom-specific scale for assessment of sleep disturbance and its impact on daytime functioning. It is a valid and reliable measure for assessing perceived insomnia severity.

Measure Yourself Medical Outcome Profile-2 (MYMOP-2)

MYMOP-2 is a brief individualized questionnaire assessing symptoms, activity and well-being. Patients are required to identify and rate their most problematic symptoms, their activity restriction and well-being. The questionnaire is applicable to a wide range of conditions and was originally designed for use by primary care practitioners. It has been validated for acupuncture patients and trialled in Parkinson's disease. The measure is reliable and responsive.

Motor Assessment Scale (MAS)

MAS is an eight-item observer-rated scale of ability to perform functional motor tasks such as rolling, sitting up in bed, balance in sitting, moving from sitting to standing, walking, upper-limb function and hand function. The scale is valid and reliable. The final (ninth) item observing muscle tone is not reliable and is usually not scored.

Motricity Index (MI)

MI is a brief six-item observer-rated measure of motor ability. It is based on the Medical Research Council scale of muscle strength and is applied to

the upper and lower limbs. It is most commonly used in stroke rehabilitation. It is valid, reliable and easy to score.

Multidimensional Fatigue Inventory (MFI)

MFI is a 20-item self-rated symptom-specific questionnaire which assesses five dimensions of fatigue, including general fatigue, physical fatigue, reduced activity, reduced motivation and mental fatigue. It is a valid and reliable measure and useful in a variety of neurological conditions.

Multiple Sclerosis Impact Scale-29 (MSIS-29)

MSIS-29 is a disease-specific 29-item self-rated questionnaire assessing the impact of multiple sclerosis on the individual. It comprises two distinct subscales which assess physical and psychological functioning. It is valid, reliable and responsive.

Numerical rating scale (NRS)

NRS is an 11-point numerical rating scale from 0 to 10 which may be rated by the patient or carer. It may be used to assess symptoms such as pain intensity or fatigue or to assess activities such as ease of getting dressed or confidence when walking. The NRS may be selected instead of a visual analogue scale (VAS). Studies suggest that patients who have difficulties with abstract thought may have difficulty with a continuous measure such as a VAS and may find an NRS easier to comprehend. The NRS is valid and reliable.

Parkinson's Disease Questionnaire-39 (PDQ-39)

PDQ-39 is a disease-specific 39-item self-rated questionnaire assessing health-related quality of life. It comprises eight scales relating to mobility, activities of daily living, emotional well-being, stigma, social support, cognition, communication and bodily discomfort. The scale is valid and reliable. A short form of this scale has been developed, with just eight items: the PDQ-8. It is considerably quicker to administer and produces results that are almost identical to the longer scale, although with less detail.

Pittsburgh Sleep Quality Inventory (PSQI)

PSQI is a nine-item self-rated symptom-specific measure for assessing sleep quality and sleep disturbance over the previous month. It is a valid and reliable measure of subjective sleep quality.

Scale of Pain Intensity (SPIN)

SPIN is a six-point vertically oriented pictorial patient-rated pain scale using six circles with different inner circles in red of proportionately smaller size. This scale is useful for people with cognitive or communication difficulties who struggle with conventional visual analogue or numerical rating scales for pain. It has been validated for people with communication and cognitive deficits.

Visual analogue scale (VAS)

VAS is a patient-rated measure of severity of symptoms. It is widely used for pain but may also be used to rate other symptoms such as sleep, fatigue, anxiety or breathlessness. It is usually represented as a 10-cm horizontal line, anchored by word descriptors at either end. It may also be represented by a vertical line and studies have indicated similar reliability of these different formats. Patients place a mark on the line at a point representing the severity of their symptoms. VAS is valid, reliable and responsive.

Index